Psychosis:
Global Perspectives

Psychosis
Global Perspectives

Edited by

Craig Morgan
Professor of Social Epidemiology and Co-Director, ESRC
Centre for Society and Mental Health, Institute of Psychiatry,
Psychology, and Neuroscience, King's College London, UK

Alex Cohen
Senior Lecturer, Centre for Global Mental Health,
London School of Hygiene and Tropical Medicine, UK

and

Tessa Roberts
Post-Doctoral Research Fellow, ESRC Centre for Society
and Mental Health, Institute of Psychiatry, Psychology, and
Neuroscience, King's College London, UK

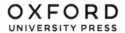

OXFORD
UNIVERSITY PRESS

OXFORD
UNIVERSITY PRESS

Great Clarendon Street, Oxford, OX2 6DP,
United Kingdom

Oxford University Press is a department of the University of Oxford.
It furthers the University's objective of excellence in research, scholarship,
and education by publishing worldwide. Oxford is a registered trade mark of
Oxford University Press in the UK and in certain other countries

Published in the United States of America by Oxford University Press
198 Madison Avenue, New York, NY 10016, United States of America

British Library Cataloguing in Publication Data
Data available

Library of Congress Control Number: 2022945866

ISBN 978–0–19–873558–8

DOI: 10.1093/med/9780198735588.001.0001

Printed in the UK by
Ashford Colour Press Ltd, Gosport, Hampshire

Oxford University Press makes no representation, express or implied, that the
drug dosages in this book are correct. Readers must therefore always check
the product information and clinical procedures with the most up-to-date
published product information and data sheets provided by the manufacturers
and the most recent codes of conduct and safety regulations. The authors and
the publishers do not accept responsibility or legal liability for any errors in the
text or for the misuse or misapplication of material in this work. Except where
otherwise stated, drug dosages and recommendations are for the non-pregnant
adult who is not breast-feeding

Links to third party websites are provided by Oxford in good faith and
for information only. Oxford disclaims any responsibility for the materials
contained in any third party website referenced in this work.

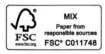

Foreword

Ezra Susser

This engaging book provides a landmark for the progress of sociocultural research on psychotic disorders up to the present time. It synthesizes what we know now, and what remains to be learned. It underscores, in particular, how much more knowledge could be gained by diversifying the locales where this research is done. We surely need a better understanding of the ways in which the causes and manifestations of psychotic disorders vary across sociocultural settings (Martínez-Alés & Susser, 2022; Susser & Martínez-Alés, 2018). This is, in fact, a precondition for achieving global equity, a primary goal of global health and mental health. Although the book focuses primarily on sociocultural research, an equally if not more compelling case could be made for more inclusiveness in other dimensions of research on psychotic disorders, a prominent example being genomic research (Gulsuner et al., 2020).

The book also serves as a landmark for how far we have to go. We are still awaiting the proliferation of studies required to capture anything close to the true variation in psychoses across the diverse populations of the globe. The vast majority of psychosis research is being done in a small minority of high-income countries. These few countries have living conditions and cultures that are similar to one another, but markedly different from most of the world. This limited focus of research is self-reinforcing. As results accumulate ever more rapidly from a few countries, and research methods continually advance, investigators want to apply new methods to pursue questions raised by previous studies, which might only be feasible within those countries. Meanwhile, the gap in the foundation of knowledge across countries becomes ever wider.

Thanks to the cumulative work of many investigators like the ones writing the chapters in this book, the capacity to do such research in most other countries is now either present or could be readily developed. Yet there remains a common (mis)perception that it is sufficient to conduct research in a few countries and generalize the results to all others. Why is that?

We first need to recognize that this blind spot is not specific to psychosis research (Gaudillière et al., 2020). The concentration of health research in a few countries is pervasive (The Lancet Global Health, 2021). Although it may be more salient in psychosis research, it is evident to some degree in all health research. We must therefore look outside of the field of psychosis research to find the underlying reasons for it. My own view, similar to the book authors, is that the blindspot reflects structural inequities between countries. Military and financial strength, manifest in lender/debtor relationships among other ways, maintains the dominance of a few countries over most others. Many though certainly not all of these power relationships are a legacy of the colonial era that had its heyday from about 1850 to 1950. Colonized populations were subjugated and the power held over them was justified on the grounds that they were not the equals of those who ruled them. After the colonies won their independence, largely the same power relationships persisted, though without direct subjugation and under different camouflage (Richardson, 2019). For this reason, a growing social movement that seeks to promote diversity and equity in research is sometimes folded under the banner of 'decolonizing' global health (Büyüm et al., 2020). The term implies that the legacy of colonialism is the primary contributor to the blindspot. This legacy is present not only in direct and plainly visible actions, but also in more subtle ways that may not even be seen by the actors, such as in the hegemony of concepts and credibility. I am not entirely comfortable with branding the goal as 'decolonization', because not all power relationships derive from the colonial era, and the term itself implies reversing policies of former colonizing countries more than empowerment of the formerly colonized (Turcotte-Tremblay et al., 2020). Nonetheless, I find much to agree with in that emerging movement.

Second, we need to recognize that while underlying power dynamics foster a narrow perspective in psychosis and other health research, this perspective is by no means immutable. The transformation of HIV/AIDS research since the beginning of this century provides an example. This was largely due to a coincidence of two forces. The United States and other rich countries came to perceive the growing pandemic as a threat to global security. At the same time, social activists across the globe mounted a remarkably successful campaign, demanding that treatments restricted to rich countries be extended to all countries. Although research on HIV/AIDS was not fully 'decolonized', significant gains were achieved towards that end.

It is of course discouraging to witness the inequity that has emerged during the current COVID-19 pandemic (Mascayano et al., 2021). It is generally recognized by scientists that the pandemic could only be brought to an end by vaccination of the global population. Until that happens, it is likely that the SARS-CoV2 virus will continue to mutate to produce new variants that pose a threat to vaccinated rich countries as well as to other countries. Despite that, we are witnessing the emergence of one of the most stunning inequities in health since the Second World War. Rich countries are hoarding vaccines for their own populations, and enriching the pharmaceutical companies that have been allowed to patent them after being publicly funded, while entire regions of the world are being left without sufficient access to vaccines and remain vulnerable to devastating effects of the pandemic (Padma, 2021). But this setback is also not immutable. Rich countries face increasing pressure to share vaccines, waive pharmaceutical patents, and facilitate the manufacture of vaccines in all regions. At some point, they surely will. By then a great deal of damage will have been done to health and living conditions and whatever trust there was in the beneficence of rich countries will have been undermined. Yet in the long run, the profound damage wrought by this glaring inequity may serve as a crucial historical lesson that health for all is beneficial to the few as well as the many.

Pressure for change can be brought to bear from many angles. This book exemplifies one of them. It is an excellent work of scholarship. At the same time, by revealing how a greater diversity of settings in psychosis research would benefit all countries, it plays a role in advocacy. Thus, we need not be complacent about power relationships that impede advances in the health of everyone. The more evident we can make the benefits of diversifying research on psychosis, the stronger the grounds we have to challenge the limited scope of psychosis research, and to promote investment in health equity for this field as well as others.

References

Büyüm, A. M., et al. (2020). Decolonising global health: if not now, when? *BMJ Global Health*, 5, e003394.

Gaudillière, J. P., et al. (eds) (2020). *Global health and the new world order: Historical and anthropological approaches to a changing regime of governance* [Internet]. Manchester (UK): Manchester University Press. Retrieved from https://www.ncbi.nlm.nih.gov/books/NBK564276/

Gulsuner, S., et al. (2020). Genetics of schizophrenia in the South African Xhosa. *Science*, 367(6477), 569–573.

The Lancet Global Health (2021). Global health 2021: who tells the story? *Lancet Glob Health*, 9(2), e99.

Martínez-Alés, G. & Susser, E. S. (2022). A useful construct to improve the lives of people with schizophrenia. *Schizophr Res*, 242, 91–93.

Mascayano, F., Bruni, A., & Susser, E. (2021). Global and local inequalities in COVID-19 vaccine distribution for people with severe mental disorders in Latin America. *JAMA Psychiatry*, 78(9), 945–946.

Padma, T. V. (2021). Covid vaccines won't reach poorest countries before 2023. *Nature*, 595, 342–343.

Richardson, E. T. (2019). On the coloniality of global health. *Med Anthropol Theory*, 6(4), 101–118.

Susser, E. & Martínez-Alés, G. (2018). Putting psychosis into sociocultural context: an international study in 17 locations. *JAMA Psychiatry*, 75(1), 9–10.

Turcotte-Tremblay, A.-M., et al. (2020). Global health is more than just 'public health somewhere else'. *BMJ Glob Health*, 5, e002545.

Contents

List of abbreviations

ANEP	Asian Network of Early Psychosis	EIP	Early Intervention in Psychosis
ARMS	At-risk mental state	EIS	Early intervention service
BELL	Butabika East London Link	FEP	First-episode psychosis
BREC	Butabika Recovery College	GDP	Gross domestic product
CAARMS	Comprehensive assessment of at risk mental states	GINGER	Global Initiative for Neuropsychiatric Genetics Education in Research
CAP	Complementary and alternative mental healthcare providers	GPC	Genomics of Psychiatry Consortium
CAR	Cortisol awakening response	GSHS	Global School-based Student Health Survey
CBR	Community-based rehabilitation	GWAS	Genome-wide association study
CBT	Cognitive-behavioural therapy	HDI	Human Development Index
CEE	Central and Eastern Europe	HIC	High-income countries
CMD	Common mental disorder	HKMMS	Hong Kong Mental Morbidity Survey
CMHC	Community mental health centres	IIBDGC	International Inflammatory Bowel Disease Genetics Consortium
CMHS	China mental health survey		
CNV	Copy number variations	IPSS	International Pilot Study of Schizophrenia
COSIMPO	COllaborative Shared care to IMprove Psychosis Outcome	ISoS	International Study of Schizophrenia
CRPD	Convention on the Rights of Persons with Disabilities	JCEP	Jockey Club Early Psychosis
CSP	Cooperative Studies Program	LD	Linkage disequilibrium
CTO	Community treatment orders	LMIC	Low- and middle-income countries
CZEMS	CZEch Mental health Study		
DALY	Disability-adjusted life years	MHC	Multi-Histocompatibility Complex
DFID	Department for International Development	MLS	Madras Longitudinal Study
DOSMeD	Determinants of Outcome of Severe Mental Disorders	MVP	Million Veteran Program
		NAPD	Non-affective psychotic disorder
DSM	Diagnostic and Statistical Manual of Mental Disorders	NARP	Non-affective remitting psychosis
DUP	Duration of untreated psychosis	NMDA	N-methyl-D-aspartate
EBQ	Economic burden questionnaire	PACE	Personal Assessment and Crisis Evaluation

PANSS	Positive and Negative Syndrome Scale	SHARP	Shanghai-At-Risk-for-Psychosis
PE	Psychotic experiences	SMI	Severe mental illness
PEIP	Psychosis Early Intervention Programme	SNP	Single Nucleotide Polymorphism
PEPP	Prevention and Early Intervention Program for Psychosis	SOFAS	Social Functioning Assessment Scale
PGC	Psychiatric Genomics Consortium	SOHO	Schizophrenia Outpatient Health Outcomes
PHC	Primary health centre	SSFI	SCARF social functioning index
PHCP	Primary healthcare providers	SWAP	Support for Wellness Achievement Programme
PIPE	Psychological Intervention Programmes in Early Psychosis	TFH	Traditional and faith healers
PPHS	Psychiatric and personal history schedule	THP	Traditional health practitioners
PRS	Polygenic risk scores	UHR	Ultra-high-risk
PSE	Present state examination	UPSIDES	Using Peer Support in Developing Empowering Mental Health Services
PSW	Peer Support Work		
QC	Quality control	VHA	Veterans Health Administration
RCT	Randomized controlled trial		
SAD	Separation and divorce	WHO	World Health Organization
SEPEA	Social Epidemiology of Psychoses in East Anglia	WNUSP	World Network of Users and Survivors of Psychiatry

List of contributors

Atalay Alem, PhD, Addis Ababa University, Ethiopia

Stephanie Beards, PhD, Centre for Evidence and Implementation, London, UK

Jonathan K. Burns, PhD, University of Exeter, UK

Geraldo Busatto, PhD, Universidade de Sao Paulo, Sao Paulo, Brazil

Sherry Chan, MBBS, FRCPsych, Mphil, MD (HKU), FHKCPsych, FHKAM (Psych), The University of Hong Kong, Hong Kong

Wing Chung Chang, MBChB (CUHK), MD (HK), FRCPsych(UK), FHKCPsych, FHKAM(Psychiatry), The University of Hong Kong, Hong Kong

Eric Chen, MA(Oxon), MBChB(Edin), MD(Edin), FRCPsych, FHKAM (Psychiatry), The University of Hong Kong, Hong Kong

Bonginkosi Chiliza, PhD, University of KwaZulu-Natal, South Africa

Alex Cohen, PhD, London School of Hygiene and Tropical Medicine, London, UK

Erminia Colucci, PhD, MPhil, CPsychol, BPsySc(Hons), PGCAP, PGDip, DipEd SFHEA, Middlesex University London ,UK

Paola Dazzan, MBBS, MRCPsych, M.Sc,PhD, King's College London, UK

Cristina Marta Del-Ben, MD, University of São Paulo, São Paulo, Brazil

Oluyomi Esan, MBBS, MSc, PhD, DSc, FRCPsych, University of Ibadan, Nigeria

Charlotte Gayer-Anderson, PhD, King's College London, London, UK

Oye Gureje, MBBS, MSc, PhD, DSc, FRCPsych, University of Ibadan, Nigeria

Charlotte Hanlon, PhD,Addis Ababa University, Ethiopia

Cyril Höschl, DrSc., FRCPsych, Charles University, Prague, Czech Republic

Christy Hui, BSocSci (Psychology), PhD (Psychiatry), The University of Hong Kong, Hong Kong

Gerard Hutchinson, PhD, University of the West Indies, St Augustine campus, Mount Hope, Trinidad

Conrad Iyegbe, BSc Biochemistry, PhD, Icahn School of Medicine at Mount Sinai, New York, USA

Srividya N. Iyer, BA MA, PhD, Douglas Research Centre & Prevention and Early Intervention Program for Psychosis (PEPP-Montreal), Canada

Sujit John, MA, Schizophrenia Research Foundation, Chennai, Tamil Nadu, India

James Kirkbride, BA, MSc, PhD, FHEA, University College London, London, UK

Dzmitry Krupchank, MD, MSc, PhD, Medical Officer at World Health Organization, Geneva, Switzerland

Edwin Lee, MBChB (CUHK), MSc (CUHK), MRCPsych, FHKCPsych, FHKAM (Psychiatry), the University of Hong Kong, Hong Kong

Ashok Malla, MBBS, FRCPC, MRCPsych, McGill University, Montreal, Quebec, Canada

Paulo Rossi Menezes, MSc, PhD, University of São Paulo, São Paulo, Brazil

Greeshma Mohan, PhD student, Schizophrenia Research Foundation, Chennai, Tamil Nadu, India

Merve Mollaahmetoglu, BA, MSc, PhD, University of Sheffield, Sheffield, UK

Craig Morgan, BA, MSc, PhD, King's College London, UK

Neely Anne Laurenzo Myers, BA, PhD, Southern Methodist University, Dallas, Texas, USA

Lu Niu, PhD, The Chinese University of Hong Kong, Hong Kong

Akin Ojagbemi, MBBS, PhD. MSc, University of Ibadan, Nigeria,

Ramachandran Padmavati, MBBS, DPM, MD., Schizophrenia Research Foundation, Chennai, Tamil Nadu, India

Jan Pfeiffer, PhD, Charles University, Prague, Czech Republic

Oksana Plevachuk, PhD, Danylo Halytsky Lviv National Medical University, Ukraine

Vijaya Raghavan, MD, Schizophrenia Research Foundation, Chennai, Tamil Nadu, India

Ursula M. Read, BA, PG Diploma, MSc, MRes, PhD, Warwick Medical School University of Warwick, UK

Ulrich Reininghaus, PhD, MSc, Dipl.-Psych., Central Institute of Mental Health (CIMH), Mannheim, Germany

Tessa Roberts, BA, MSc, PhD, King's College London, UK

Giulia Segre, MSc, King's College London, London, UK

Rosana Shuhama, PhD, University of São Paulo, São Paulo, Brazil

Ezra S. Susser, MD, DrPH, Columbia University, New York, USA

Orest Suvalo, MD, Institute of Mental Health Ukrainian Catholic University, Ukraine

Rangaswamy Thara, MBBS, PhD, FRCPsych, Schizophrenia Research Foundation, Chennai, Tamil Nadu, India

Sarah Tosato, MD, PhD, University of Verona, Verona, Italy

Els van der Ven, PhD, PGDip, Vrije Universiteit, Amsterdam, Netherlands

Petr Winkler, PhD, National Institute of Mental Health, Klecany, Czech Republic

Shuiyuan Xiao, PhD, Central South University, Changsha, China

Part I

Psychosis by Topic

1

Psychosis across place: The madding crowd—urban living and psychosis

Ozden Merve Mollaahmetoglu and
James B. Kirkbride

Introduction

Human populations are increasingly becoming urban dwellers, with over half the world's population living in cities, a figure projected to rise to two-thirds by 2050, with over 90% of this rise taking place in the Global South, particularly in Asia and Africa (United Nations Department of Economic and Social Affairs, 2019). In research conducted to date, mostly in the context of settings in the Global North, including Europe, North America, and Australia, there is evidence of a strong association between exposure to urban life and the incidence of psychotic disorders. A key question for public mental health is whether such associations are evident in different global contexts. If they are, this may result in a rise in the incidence of psychotic disorders around the world over the next two to three decades, particularly in the Global South which may have the fewest resources to provide treatment and intervention for people with psychosis. If rural–urban differences in the incidence of psychotic disorders are not universal, as some recent evidence may suggest (DeVylder et al., 2018), this may provide vital clues about the aetiology of psychotic disorders in different contexts. Despite the strong associations in the Global North between being born, brought up, and living in cities and the incidence of psychotic disorders (March et al., 2008), we still do not know whether this is a consequence of susceptibility to disorder or a consequence of living in urban environments, or interplay between the two.

In this chapter, we present an overview of evidence on variation by place in the incidence of psychotic disorders. Our scope ranges from local—i.e. variation between small area neighbourhoods—to global, and our lens attempts to be both descriptive and critical. In the first two sections, we review the historical and contemporary evidence for variation in incidence rates, and the search for the drivers of these patterns. In the third section, we consider some of the major limitations of the current epidemiological evidence and the extent to which this evidence supports a causal association between place and psychosis. In the penultimate section of this chapter, we consider emerging evidence from neuroscience, which provides adjunct findings from experimental paradigms testing the role of urban living on psychosis-related phenomena. Finally, we balance the available evidence in the context of public mental health, and consider whether we are yet able to suggest putative prevention strategies within the city to reduce the future incidence of psychotic disorders.

Historical perspectives: emerging evidence of variation by place

The finding that psychotic disorders such as schizophrenia tend to cluster in inner cities is not new. In their pioneering work almost eight decades ago, Faris and Dunham (1939) conducted an ecological study of nearly 35,000 first admissions to hospitals in Chicago between 1922 and 1934 with a diagnosis of schizophrenia, manic-depressive psychoses, or alcohol and drug-induced psychoses. By linking each person admitted for one of these disorders to the census tract in which they lived, they were able to map crude (unadjusted) hospitalization rates onto Chicago's neighbourhoods. Their results revealed a strikingly close relationship between the distribution of schizophrenia and substance use disorders, and the ecological structure of the city (Faris & Dunham, 1939). For instance, schizophrenia rates ranged from 111 per 100,000 population in more affluent parts of the city, to 1995 per 100,000 population in downtown, inner-city areas. Incidentally, such rates would be considered extremely high by today's standards, where schizophrenia rates are more typically in the region of 15 per 100,000 (McGrath et al., 2004; Kirkbride et al., 2012). This highlights possible issues with the validity of case definitions (incidence versus prevalence cases, diagnostic validity) in this sample. Nevertheless, their data revealed a strong centripetal gradient which suggested that inner-city areas exhibited higher rates of schizophrenia in neighbourhoods characterized by homelessness, social isolation, high population turnover, poverty, and alcoholism. Moreover, schizophrenia rates were higher for people of white ethnicity living in areas predominantly occupied by Black ethnic groups, as well as for foreign-born individuals living in areas with fewer foreign-born residents. This phenomenon has become known as the 'ethnic density effect' (Cochrane & Bal, 1988), and has been found to moderate risk of psychosis in a number of ethnic groups (Boydell et al., 2001; Faris & Dunham, 1939; Kirkbride et al., 2014; Veling, 2006;

Dykxhoorn et al., 2020). Faris and Dunham (1939) concluded that extreme social disorganization in inner-city areas was most likely causally related to higher
rates of schizophrenia, a view that has subsequently been challenged (see next).

Faris and Dunham's work set in motion further epidemiological studies with
varying methodologies, all of which examined the relationship between psychotic disorders and urbanicity across Europe and North America, including notable work in Bristol and Nottingham (UK), Mannheim (Germany), and Boston
(USA) (Giggs, 1973, 1986; Giggs & Cooper, 1987; Hare, 1956; Maylaih et al.,
1989; Mintz & Schwartz, 1964). Hare (1956) set out to test the observations of
Faris and Dunham in the first methodologically comparable study conducted
in England, using data collected in the city of Bristol. In a critical advance over
Faris and Dunham's (1939) study, Hare (1956) was able to exclude age–sex differences in the composition of neighbourhoods as an explanation for higher
rates in more urban parts of Bristol. As in Faris and Dunham's work, neighbourhoods with the highest schizophrenia rates were clustered in the city centre,
and were positively correlated with indices of social and economic status (Hare,
1956). This relationship appeared stronger for markers of social isolation than
economic prosperity, leading Hare (1956) to conclude that social isolation may
be more relevant to schizophrenia aetiology than economic factors.

Nevertheless, during the latter half of the twentieth century, worse economic
conditions were found to predict schizophrenia incidence in several cities,
including Nottingham (Giggs, 1973; Giggs, 1986; Giggs & Cooper, 1987) and
Mannheim (Maylaih et al., 1989), although not in Boston (Mintz & Schwartz
1964). Here, no association was found between median monthly rent and
the incidence of schizophrenia or 'manic-depressive' psychoses. Mintz and
Schwarz also investigated the role of ethnic density, as they considered Faris
and Dunham's original investigation to have failed to take into account generally higher psychosis rates in foreign-born individuals and, moreover, had
treated all foreign-born individuals as a single group. To overcome these issues,
Mintz and Schwartz (1964) measured psychosis incidence in one particular migrant group—first and second-generation Italians—living in 27 communities
in Boston. Their findings revealed that this group had lower hospital admission
rates for schizophrenia and 'manic-depressive' psychosis when they lived in
neighbourhoods with higher concentrations of other Italian immigrants, consistent with an ethnic density effect.

As research in this area progressed, researchers began to question whether
the strong socioeconomic gradients which psychotic disorders exhibited were
a cause or consequence of schizophrenia and related disorders. This gave rise
to social causation and social drift (selection) hypotheses. Social causation
posits that socioeconomic factors are aetiologically relevant to schizophrenia,

whereas the social drift hypothesis proposes that deterioration in mental state results in lower socioeconomic position. Early support for the latter hypothesis came from Goldberg and Morrison (1963), who found that the socioeconomic environment in which individuals with schizophrenia grew up was very similar to the general population, whereas the individuals affected themselves held lower-skilled jobs, indicative of downward drift. By contrast, Hollingshead and Redlich (1954) reported that the vast majority of individuals with schizophrenia originated from the same social class as their families, leading them to disregard social drift as an explanation.

In high-income countries, therefore, there is now a large literature suggesting that rates of schizophrenia and other non-affective psychoses are not uniform, but vary across urban and rural areas (with higher rates observed in the former) as well as within cities across neighbourhoods (Heinz et al., 2013; Kirkbride et al., 2012; March et al., 2008; Vassos et al., 2012). Recent findings further suggest that urbanicity may confer increased risk of psychosis independently of (Newbury et al., 2022; Solmi et al., 2020; Paksarian et al., 2018), or in interaction with, genetic risk (Grech et al., 2017; van Os et al., 2004) in high-income countries, and area-level variation in rates of psychotic disorders can primarily be explained by exposures such as social deprivation and fragmentation, as well as an interaction between individual-level (e.g. ethnicity) and area-level (e.g. ethnic density) exposures (Heinz et al., 2013). This raises the question of whether rates of psychosis are equally heterogeneous in terms of place in low- and middle-income countries (LMICs) and, if so, what the factors are that account for this heterogeneity.

Turning, first, to findings on variation in rates of psychotic disorders across countries, the World Health Organization (WHO) Ten-Country Study (Jablensky et al., 1992) included 12 centres in 10 countries, covering both urban and rural settings, and—using the terminology employed at the time—developed and developing nations. It was a ground-breaking study, using stringent epidemiological criteria, but the incidence data generated was only deemed of sufficient quality in 8 of the 12 centres. The authors reported no clear pattern of higher or lower incidence of schizophrenia in the participating centres from LMICs (Chandigarh, India; and—at the time—Moscow, Russia) compared with those from high-income countries, although it should be noted that the study was not originally designed to investigate incidence and as such it may have been underpowered. Across all study sites, incidence rates of narrowly-defined schizophrenia ranged from 7 (Aarhus, Denmark) to 14 (Nottingham, UK) per 100,000 population at-risk, while a broader definition, including all non-affective psychotic disorders, was associated with slightly more variation, from 16 to 42 per 100,000 population at-risk, in Honolulu (USA)/Aarhus

(Denmark) and rural Chandigarh (India), respectively. Focusing on narrowly-defined schizophrenia, findings from the WHO-10 country study have been interpreted as evidence of homogeneity in the incidence of schizophrenia across cultures and geographical areas (Jablensky et al., 1992). This interpretation has been strongly challenged, however (McGrath et al., 2004).

Recently, another large cross-national study, the European Network of National Schizophrenia Networks Studying Gene-Environment Interactions (EU-GEI) study, employed a similar methodology across 17 settings in 6 countries (England, France, Netherlands, Spain, Brazil, Italy) (Jongsma et al., 2018). This study reported more than an eightfold variation in the incidence of all psychotic disorders between settings, with the highest rates in the most urban Northern European sites (Paris, London, Amsterdam) and the lowest in Southern European cities (Madrid, Barcelona, Palermo, Bologna) and Brazil (Ribeirao Preto) as well as more rural sites throughout Northern and Southern Europe. This variation was not attributable to differences between these populations by age, sex, or ethnic composition (Jongsma et al., 2018) or population density, but there was evidence that higher rates were associated with lower levels of home ownership (Jongsma et al., 2018), as well as higher levels of cannabis use amongst controls (Di Forti et al., 2019). These patterns suggest social determinants which give rise to more adverse neighbourhood environments, through greater exposure to deprivation, social fragmentation, or substance use may affect the population rates of psychosis.

One setting in the EU-GEI study—Ribeirao Preto in Brazil—was located in a LMIC. Despite being an urban setting, rates of psychotic disorder were lower here than in similarly-sized urban settings in Northern Europe (London, Amsterdam, Paris). Lower rates of psychotic disorders have also been reported in Sao Paolo, Brazil (Menezes et al., 2007). While the authors noted that incidence may have been slightly underestimated (Menezes et al., 2007), emerging evidence suggests global patterns of psychosis risk may differ from the Northern European observations of higher rates in more urban settings (DeVylder et al., 2018; Kirkbride et al., 2018). For example, using World Health Survey data, DeVylder et al (2018) reported no overall urban-rural differences in the prevalence of psychotic experiences in 42 LMIC countries, though this association varied depending on context, with five positive associations (higher prevalence in urban settings), five negative associations (lower prevalence in urban settings) and the remainder of countries (N = 32) showing null results. Other studies in LMIC countries have reported higher levels of psychotic experiences in more urban settings. For example, Binbay et al. (2012) reported some evidence that urban upbringing was associated with increased odds of low-impact psychotic symptoms and psychotic disorder in a large household survey conducted in

Izmir, Turkey (Binbay et al., 2012). In line with this, current urban living was found to be associated with a higher prevalence of psychotic experiences in Timor Leste (Soosay et al., 2012) and non-affective psychosis in Nigeria (Gureje et al., 2010) and Ethiopia (Kebede et al., 2004). Overall, however, evidence on variation in the occurrence of psychosis across urban and rural areas in LMIC remains mixed, and more longitudinal incidence studies are required.

The incidence of psychotic disorders also appears heterogeneous between low- and middle income countries. For example, a recent systematic review on the incidence of non-affective psychotic disorders in LMIC settings found substantial variation in rates across 23 studies which met inclusion criteria, ranging from just 10.0 per 100,000 in Sao Paolo (Brazil) to 42.0 in rural Chandigarh (India) (Bastien et al., 2023). Whether this variation is due to methodological differences in study design and case ascertainment or can be attributed to systematic differences in exposure to social or environmental risk factors requires further investigation, but work on this issue is emerging.

Very recently, for example, the INTREPID-II study conducted in three sites in Trinidad, Nigeria and India has revealed new, important findings about the incidence of psychotic disorders in the Global South (Morgan et al., 2023). The study identified variation in age-sex standardised rates, ranging from just 14.4 per 100,000 in Ibadan, Nigeria, and 20.7 per 100,000 in Kancheepuram, India, to 59.1 per 100,000 in Trinidad. These findings contrast with earlier evidence of higher rates in rural India (Jablensky et al., 1992) and comparatively lower rates in Trinidad (Bhugra et al., 1996). Several reasons may account for these differences, including differences in the specific contexts and populations in which these studies were conducted, differing methodologies, and/or changes in the underlying pattern of risk factors over time in the same settings. The authors of the INTREPID-II findings noted, for example, that in the intervening period between their study and that of Bhugra et al., (1996), Trinidad has witnessed dramatic increases in violence, deprivation and substance use, all of which could contribute to the higher rates recently observed.

In the community-based WHO World Mental Health Surveys of 31,261 respondents, McGrath et al. (2015) found significant variation in the prevalence of psychotic experiences across 18 countries. Specifically, this study reported a higher prevalence of psychotic experiences in upper-middle and high-income countries compared with low- and lower-middle-income countries. However, the prevalence estimates of psychotic experiences varied markedly within each of these income levels (e.g. low- and lower-middle-income countries, range 1.2–7.5%; upper-middle-income countries, 1.0–14.9%; high-income countries, 2.8–10.8%) (McGrath et al., 2015). This mirrors findings from another systematic review and meta-analysis by Supanya et al. (2016), which found marked heterogeneity in prevalence estimates and a pooled lifetime prevalence of 4%, 8%, and 6% for low-, middle-, and high-income countries (Supanya et al., 2016), and a review of incidence studies that similarly reported marked heterogeneity in rates without any clear association with country-level GPD (see the section 'Incidence studies in other places' in Morgan et al., 2016). Notably, the WHO cross-national World Health Survey conducted in 52 countries found a slightly higher prevalence of psychotic experiences in low- and lower-middle-income countries (12.9%) than in upper-middle and high-income countries (8.8%) (Nuevo et al., 2012).

Consistent with findings in high-income countries, area-level social deprivation seems to account for some variation in psychosis risk by place. For example, in the WHO Ten-Country Study, the rural areas of Chandigarh (India), for which incidence of schizophrenia was reported to be higher, were also the most socioeconomically deprived areas compared with all other participating centres (Jablensky et al., 1992). Similarly, in an ecological study from South Africa, Burns and Esterhuizen (2008) found higher rates of psychosis in geographical regions characterized by higher poverty and income inequality, independent of urbanicity (Burns & Esterhuizen, 2008). While speculative, this tentatively suggests that, even if the pattern of urban–rural differences in the occurrence of psychosis may be reversed in some LMICs compared with what has been found in high-income countries, the area-level factors that account for this variation (such as social deprivation) may be similar across LMICs and high-income countries. This highlights the need for more robust research that allows for more detailed investigation of the heterogeneity in incidence of psychosis in terms of place and its determinants in LMICs.

In general, early epidemiological studies found less evidence that affective psychoses varied with respect to place; thus, in Faris and Dunham's (1939) analysis of Chicago data, they observed random variation in rates, not predicted by any given socioenvironmental factors, although this was challenged in re-analysis of their data by Mintz and Schwartz (1964). A relatively smaller amount of spatial variation in affective psychoses has been found in several subsequent studies (Kirkbride et al., 2007; Kirkbride et al., 2012, 2014; Mortensen et al., 2003; Pedersen & Mortensen, 2006; Scully et al., 2004; Wainwright & Surtees, 2004), although given that their incidence is rare (in the order of magnitude of 12.4 new cases per 100,000 people per year; Kirkbride et al., 2012) some studies may have lacked sufficient sample sizes to detect effects. Recent larger studies conducted in Europe suggest some variation in incidence of affective psychoses may be apparent close to the time of onset (Jongsma et al., 2018; Richardson et al., 2018), but a large, nationwide population cohort in

Denmark found no association between urban birth and subsequent risk of these disorders (Mortensen et al., 2003).

Contemporary research: the hunt for social determinants

Contemporary studies of the incidence of psychotic disorders have investigated the roles of chance, bias, confounding, and reverse causation in explaining elevated rates in more urban areas. For example, studies have measured exposure to urban living at various points over the life course, including at birth, during upbringing and in adulthood. Those which have measured urbanicity close to the time of presentation for disorder have generally found an association between city living and psychosis. For example, using Swedish population-based registers, researchers found an almost 70% increase in the risk of non-affective psychotic disorders among individuals living in the most densely populated parts of Sweden at the time of hospitalization compared with those living in the least urban regions (Sundquist et al., 2004). This association remained evident after adjusting for age, sex, marital status, education level, and immigration status. In England, researchers found increased crude and age-sex adjusted incidence rates of affective and non-affective psychotic disorders in Southeast London compared with Nottingham and Bristol (Kirkbride et al., 2006). Further, and importantly, this excess was not explained by the larger proportion of ethnic minority groups in London, groups in which there is also evidence of increased incidence (Fearon et al., 2006; Kirkbride et al., 2012). Reviewing the available epidemiological data from England between 1950 and 2009, a systematic review found strong and consistent evidence for geographical variation in non-affective psychoses, particularly schizophrenia (Kirkbride et al., 2012), with higher rates concentrated in urban settings. Similarly, incidence rates of schizophrenia, but not affective psychoses, have also been found to be raised in urban populations in Ireland (Kelly et al., 2010), while in France, the incidence rates of both affective and non-affective psychoses were elevated in urban versus rural settings (Szöke et al., 2014). In Italy, non-affective psychosis rates were not associated with urbanicity (Lasalvia et al., 2014). However, a twofold variation by socioeconomic deprivation was observed. Moreover, there is evidence that some rural communities, e.g. in Finland, have particularly high rates of schizophrenia. However, this could be driven by strong genetic isolation, and may be a cohort or period effect, since in Finland urbanicity appears to be an emerging risk factor for schizophrenia in this country (Haukka et al., 2001; Perälä et al., 2008). Together, these findings suggest that urbanicity may be only one component of variation in risk of psychosis, and that other ways in which we structure our societies (via factors such as deprivation, inequality, or social ties and social capital) may also affect the manifestation of psychotic disorders.

One important limitation of these studies is that urbanicity is usually measured close to psychosis onset. This makes it impossible to determine the extent to which more deprived, isolated, or fragmented urban environments *cause* psychosis, or alternatively, simply harbour people who develop psychosis, having drifted socially and economically into such environments. In an attempt to isolate these effects, a number of Danish and Swedish studies have been able to use longitudinal population-based register data to examine the association between urban birth and upbringing and subsequent risk of psychosis (Lewis et al., 1992; Mortensen et al., 1999; Pedersen & Mortensen, 2001, 2006). For example, Lewis et al. (1992) used Swedish conscript data to first show that men brought up in urban areas as children were at elevated risk of schizophrenia, providing initial evidence against the *social drift* hypothesis. Crucially, this association persisted after adjustment for other aspects of city living thought to influence risk, including cannabis use, parental divorce, and family history of psychotic disorders (Lewis et al., 1992). Mortensen and colleagues have contributed further seminal advances to this research using Danish population cohorts, demonstrating that higher degrees of urbanization—both at *birth* and *during upbringing*—increase risk of schizophrenia in adulthood, independent of many confounders (Mortensen et al., 1999; Pedersen & Mortensen, 2001, 2006). They further found that cumulative exposure to urbanicity during childhood and adolescence was associated with a dose-response relationship with risk of schizophrenia (Pedersen & Mortensen, 2001).

While these studies have been influential in demonstrating that exposure to urban environments at birth and during upbringing are associated with increased risk of schizophrenia later on, we need to look elsewhere for clues as to the precise aspects of city living which may drive these associations. Hypothetical underlying mechanisms include greater exposure to adversities during prenatal development (infections, vitamin D deficiency, and obstetric complications) (Cannon, 2002; McGrath, 1999; Sham et al., 1992) and socioenvironmental stressors in urban environments (inequality, deprivation, social fragmentation (Allardyce et al., 2005; Curtis et al., 2006; Kirkbride, Morgan, et al., 2007; Kirkbride et al., 2014). The former hypothesis has, however, not generally been matched by corresponding empirical support (Eaton et al, 2000; McDonald et al., 2001; see Kelly et al., 2010 for a review). Moreover, the critical window of exposure to these factors is thought to be *in utero* and early life, whereas urban upbringing may have a stronger association with later risk of psychosis than urban birth (Lewis et al., 1992; Mortensen et al., 1999; Pedersen & Mortensen, 2001). Social and economic aspects of urban environments have received greater attention in the psychosis epidemiology literature. Socioeconomic deprivation has been consistently linked to increased risk of onset of psychotic disorders (Croudace et al., 2000; Kirkbride et al., 2014; Sariaslan et al., 2015; Wicks et al., 2005), although some studies suggest a non-linear association may be present, with excess risk confined to the most deprived communities (Croudace et al., 2000; Kirkbride et al., 2017). Moreover, absolute levels of deprivation may only be one aspect of economic disadvantage which increases risk; one recent study in inner-city East London found that rates of non-affective psychoses were also higher in neighbourhoods with greater levels of economic inequality—differences between rich and poor—independent of absolute deprivation (Kirkbride et al., 2014). This suggests that in addition to absolute poverty, relative poverty across socioeconomic gradients may be associated with psychotic disorders.

Corresponding research in the Global South is sparse. Similar findings on inequality have been observed in South Africa (Burns & Esterhuizen, 2008), where increased municipal income inequality was associated with increased incidence of first-episode psychosis; however, this study only measured treated incidence rather than true incidence, which is likely to be greater (Burns & Esterhuizen, 2008). Research in this region, as well as other LMIC settings, has additional challenges. In South Africa, for example, patients were excluded from the study by Burns and Esterhuizen (2008) if they had a psychosis diagnosis secondary to a general medical condition, e.g. HIV. Given the high prevalence of such conditions in people with psychosis in South Africa, this may affect the generalizability of such results to those whose psychosis has an organic cause (Mashaphu & Mkize, 2007). Globally, there is evidence that national incidence rates of schizophrenia are associated with income inequality as measured by the Gini coefficient, even after adjustment for other known risk factors such as urbanization, migration, unemployment rate, GDP per capita, and population density (Burns et al., 2014). Countries with the highest Gini coefficients—indicating higher levels of inequality—such as Costa Rica, Trinidad, and Tobago, Jamaica, and Singapore were also reported to have higher rates of schizophrenia.

If exposure to material deprivation and social inequality creates conditions of stress, then perceived social support may help mitigate its effects. At the neighbourhood level, several studies have attempted to operationalize levels of social support. For example, areas indexed by high levels of social fragmentation—a putative proxy for a lack of available social support—have been shown to have higher rates of psychotic disorders in both the USA and Europe (Allardyce et al., 2005; Drukker et al., 2006; Silver et al., 2002). Furthermore, in one study adjustment for social fragmentation and deprivation attenuated urban–rural differences in psychosis incidence, suggesting that these factors may partially explain the urbanicity effect (Allardyce et al., 2005). Social capital—levels of civic participation, trust, reciprocity, and cohesion in society—has also been proposed as a putative predictor of risk of psychosis (McKenzie et al., 2002; Drukker et al., 2006; Kirkbride et al., 2007; Lofors & Sundquist, 2007). Although one Dutch study found no notable effect of social capital (Drukker et al., 2006), studies in the UK and Sweden have reported linear relationships between social capital (measured via a proxy of voter turnout at elections) and risk of schizophrenia (Kirkbride et al., 2007; Lofors & Sundquist, 2007). By contrast, a subsequent study in the UK, using validated measurements of social capital, demonstrated a non-linear relationship with schizophrenia, whereby both neighbourhoods with low and high levels of social capital had raised rates compared with those areas with intermediate values (Kirkbride et al., 2008b). One explanation for this nonlinear relationship is that while individuals living in neighbourhoods with low social capital may have fewer social resources to counteract the negative effects of city living, particular subgroups of the population in neighbourhoods with 'high' social capital may actually be excluded from accessing the 'available' social capital, consequently increasing stressful experiences, and possibly, subsequent risk of schizophrenia.

Findings showing an association between ethnic density and psychosis incidence are potentially consistent with the thesis that greater social support buffers stressful experiences and, in turn, is protective against psychosis. For example, ethnic density may provide greater *bonding* social capital, strengthening communities' resilience and providing social support and protective effects against mental distress. Indeed, the role for ethnic density on risk of psychosis is remarkably consistent across most (Faris & Dunham, 1939; Mintz & Schwartz, 1964), though not all (Cochrane & Bal, 1988) older studies, as well as in more contemporary studies (Boydell et al., 2001; Kirkbride et al., 2014; Veling, 2006; Becares et al., 2017; Dykxhoorn et al., 2019). Other aspects of neighbourhood ethnic composition have also been studied. For example, the effect of *ethnic fragmentation*—the extent to which different ethnic groups live in segregated or integrated patterns with the rest of the community in a given neighbourhood—has also been associated with risk of schizophrenia, though this may differ by ethnic group (Kirkbride, Morgan, et al., 2007; Kirkbride et al., 2014). In East London, people of Black African ethnic backgrounds were at greater risk of schizophrenia in neighbourhoods when they were more isolated from people of their own ethnic group (Kirkbride et al., 2014). By contrast, for people of Black Caribbean descent, a lack of integration with the white majority population was a more important determinant of risk (Kirkbride et al., 2014). More recently, in the rural east of England, higher levels of neighbourhood ethnic *diversity* were correlated with lower rates of non-affective psychotic disorders, broadly suggesting that greater ethnic integration may be protective against psychosis in rural areas (Richardson et al., 2018). Together, these findings suggest that the ethnic composition of neighbourhoods can influence the risk of psychosis, although the exact direction of this effect may differ between ethnic groups, and the mechanisms of action also remain to be fully elucidated. It is also still unclear whether these effects matter with regard to the risk of psychosis in the majority population, and at what thresholds ethnic composition factors exert their effects.

Current limits to causal inference

Historical and contemporary epidemiological studies in Western Europe and North America repeatedly show an urban (or at least socially and spatially patterned) gradient with the incidence of non-affective psychotic disorders. This has been observed across different settings, over a period spanning more than 90 years, and when exposure to adverse social environments is measured at different periods (birth, upbringing, adulthood) over the life course. These associations are relatively robust, remaining present after controlling for a number of different confounding factors, including age, sex, ethnicity (Kirkbride et al., 2006; Kirkbride et al., 2014), immigrant status (Sundquist et al., 2004), cannabis use (Lewis et al., 1992), and family history of psychotic disorders (Byrne et al., 2004; Lewis et al., 1992; Mortensen et al., 1999; Pedersen & Mortensen, 2001; for a review, see Kelly et al., 2010). Furthermore, these associations have persisted as the methodological rigour of epidemiological studies has improved, beginning with Faris and Dunham's study (1939) of crude hospital admission rates, through to longitudinal, nationwide register studies with more precise control for confounding (Mortensen et al., 1999; Pedersen & Mortensen, 2001; Pedersen & Mortensen, 2006).

Despite these advances, understanding whether these robust associations are also *causal* remains an important and contested space within the mental health research community. At one level, knowledge of the inequitable spatial distribution should serve as an important resource for mental healthcare planning (see 'Primary and secondary prevention'), as recently demonstrated in England (McDonald et al., 2021; Kirkbride et al., 2013), regardless of whether this patterning is a cause or consequence of the onset and manifestation of psychotic disorders. But from a public health perspective, it is important—for the common goal of preventing the onset of psychotic disorders—to establish whether or not specific environments cause psychosis.

In this section we outline several criticisms of the current epidemiological literature, devoting most attention to the issue of *social drift* versus *social causation*. If the propensity to live in a particular type of environment is it-self influenced by the prodromal phase of psychotic disorders (*social drift*), it is possible that people with paranoid beliefs, disordered thoughts, or social withdrawal may move into environments which are more socially fragmented, affording greater anonymity and tolerance of atypical behaviours, or environ-ments which have historically offered cheaper rents in the face of difficulties maintaining education, employment, and social contacts. Paradoxically, it is often densely populated inner-city areas with low levels of social cohesion and historically cheaper rents which offer such spaces. Alternatively, but resulting in the same non-causal association between the urban environment and risk of psychosis, families with someone in the early stages of psychosis may choose to relocate to live nearer specialist psychiatric services, often located in more urban settings. Both are examples of so-called *intra-generational* social drift, where the change in social environments occurs during an individual's life, typ-ically during (and as a result of) the prodromal phase of psychosis or following onset. A third non-causal mechanism may explain associations between urban environments and psychosis risk, that of so-called *inter-generational* social drift, or selection. That is, the change in social environments occurs prior to the prodromal phase of disorder in childhood or before the proband's birth as a result of increased familial risk through exposure to greater genetic and/or en-vironmental exposures for psychosis. These issues are discussed further below.

Under either scenario, the association between adverse social environments and psychosis would not be causal, but a consequence of reverse causation, or *social selection* into more urban areas (Lapouse et al., 1956). At the population level, these processes may be further exacerbated by upward social mobility among unaffected families and individuals more likely to remain in education and employment, and move out of deprived inner-city areas, leaving a residual population in the city with a higher risk of psychotic disorders, described pre-viously as the *social residue* hypothesis (Freeman, 1994).

The extent to which social drift explains the association between urban envir-onments and risk of psychosis is yet to be fully quantified. Data from Quebec, Canada shows that 34.5% of patients diagnosed with a first-episode psychosis move to residential locations in the six years following their diagnosis (Ngui et al., 2013). But this movement is not exclusively downwards. For example, in the study by Ngui et al. (2013), net downward migration towards more de-prived areas was limited to low single-digit percentages. Further research from Denmark has found similar patterns (Pedersen, 2015); the majority of people with schizophrenia spectrum disorder remained in the same degree of urban-ization (defined by the authors according to settlement size) five years after onset, 16.5% moved to a higher degree of urbanization, while 14% moved to less urban areas. Together, these findings indicate that residential mobility after psychosis onset is unlikely to be unidirectional; moves to less deprived areas may, in part, be precipitated by people returning to live with family after psychosis onset. Further, social drift and causation are not mutually exclusive; both processes may operate simultaneously, either on different individuals, or on the same individual who initially drifts into more socially adverse environments only to be exposed to further stressors as a result of those environments. More work here is required to understand longitudinal exposure to such social adversities and the decisions which underlie and precipitate residential moves in the run up to, and following, psychosis. Residential instability itself—particularly in childhood and adolescence—has also been shown to be an independent risk factor for schizophrenia onset in longitudinal samples (Price et al., 2018; Paksarian et al., 2015). Recent research from England suggests those people who are considered to have at-risk mental states (a high-risk group for psychosis, based on early prodromal symptoms or genetic liability) already live in environments which are more similar to the environments at onset of people with psychosis than they are to controls (Kirkbride et al., 2014), which is inconsistent with a solely drift-based explanation for these associations.

Studies which demonstrate that urban birth and upbringing are associated with risk of psychosis (Lewis et al., 1992; Marcelis et al., 1998; Mortensen et al., 1999; Pedersen & Mortensen, 2001) provide evidence against the former, *intragenerational* social drift—social movement throughout one's lifespan—as the sole explanation for greater risk of psychosis in urban areas. However, these findings do not preclude the possibility that a more nuanced *intergenerational* drift still accounts for excess rates of psychotic disorders in more urban populations. Here, the intergenerational drift hypothesis posits that individuals who are at increased risk of psychosis (either due to genetic liability or exposure to environmental adversities) gradually drift into inner-city areas over successive generations (Marcelis et al., 1998), even though the phenotypic expression of psychotic disorder may remain dormant for several generations. If, for example, greater genetic liability to psychosis is associated with neurocognitive impairments (Germine et al., 2016; Kendler et al., 2014; Liebers et al., 2016; Toulopoulou et al., 2007; van Os et al., 2017), at a population level this may result in reduced educational attainment, employment prospects, and housing opportunities, in addition to the possible effects of increased social withdrawal or isolation. Thus, greater genetic liability for psychosis may progressively lead families into more urban, deprived, or isolated environments over successive generations. On the one hand, when psychotic disorder emerges in a given individual, the association between urban birth and psychosis (i.e. the intragenerational association) would appear causal, although it may really be driven by intergenerational drift resulting from increased genetic liability for psychosis over successive generations. Adjustment for family history of psychotic disorders may control for some intergenerational social drift, but family history will only capture a limited proportion of variance in genetic liability (Yang et al., 2010) (a similar limitation also applies to current polygenic risk scores for different mental health outcomes, including schizophrenia).

The current empirical evidence for intergenerational social drift remains equivocal. Earlier studies, reliant on indirect inferences, found mixed evidence. For example, Pedersen and Mortensen (2001) observed that people who moved from urban to rural environments during childhood subsequently had a reduced risk of psychosis, a finding which appears inconsistent with intergenerational drift. If the association between urban birth and later risk of psychosis is entirely a consequence of increased genetic liability accumulated over generations, movement away from an urban environment after birth should have no bearing on subsequent risk. As van Os and colleagues (van Os et al., 2010) state, this appears to suggest that the urbanicity-psychosis association is not a non-causal by-product of intergenerational drift. Nonetheless, in further analysis of similar data, Pedersen and Mortensen have also shown that some of the urban–rural differences in schizophrenia rates were due to a family's urban residence predating the individual's birth (Pedersen & Mortensen, 2006), which the authors suggested could be accounted for by selective migration into cities by families who shared unknown traits or genetic liability for schizophrenia, which also precipitated such migration. Interestingly, synergistic effects (a combined effect of two factors greater than the sum of each) between urbanicity and family history of schizophrenia—as a proxy for genetic risk—have been found in a Danish cohort; the effect of family history as a predictor for schizophrenia was stronger in more urban populations (van Os et al., 2004).

More recently, epidemiological studies have begun to leverage more detailed familial and genetic data, in combination with advances in causal inference methods in epidemiology, to test whether genetic risk factors explain associations between environmental risk factors and later psychosis. In one such study, Sariaslan and colleagues (Sariaslan et al., 2015) investigated the role of neighbourhood population density and deprivation at age 15 on the subsequent risk of schizophrenia (and depression) in a cohort of over 2 million people in Sweden. Like previous studies in Scandinavian population registers (Mortensen et al., 1999; Pedersen & Mortensen, 2001; Pedersen & Mortensen, 2006), they found strong evidence of an association between population density, deprivation, and risk of schizophrenia in the full sample. However, further analyses showed these effects were attenuated, and subsequently disappeared, when controlling for genetic risk by restricting the sample to first-degree cousins and siblings, respectively (Sariaslan et al., 2015). The authors interpreted this as evidence of a non-causal relationship between the urban environment and risk of schizophrenia, and argued that previous observations were driven by shared familial factors (either environmental or genetic). In a smaller follow-up study, Sariaslan et al. (2016) utilized polygenic risk scores (PRS), based on 22 known genetic loci for schizophrenia from available genome-wide association studies (GWAS) at the time (at least 145 such loci have subsequently been identified (Pardinas et al., 2018), to show that genetic liability for schizophrenia predicted residency in more deprived neighbourhoods in adulthood. This has been recently replicated in other samples (Conde et al., 2017; Paksarian et al., 2018; Newbury et al., 2020; Solmi et al., 2020). Together these results suggest that some of the association between urban residency and later risk of psychosis may be—at least partially—shaped by (genetic or familial) intergenerational selection into certain environments over time. Nevertheless, these findings are currently still insufficient to preclude a causal role for the social environment. In a recent Danish study, adjustment for PRS for schizophrenia did not confound the relationship between schizophrenia and urbanicity at birth, only resulting in slight attenuation of the urban residency effect in adolescence (Paksarian et al., 2018). This is supported by recent findings from the ALSPAC birth cohort in Bristol, UK, showing that control for both PRS for schizophrenia and maternal history of mental health problems did not confound the association between birth in more deprived environments and later risk of positive psychotic experiences (Solmi et al., 2020). This finding has been recently replicated in another longitudinal birth cohort in England (Newbury et al., 2020). Similar findings have been reported with respect to parental socioeconomic status at birth and risk of schizophrenia (Agerbo et al., 2015). Nonetheless, these findings have largely been restricted to European samples and may not generalize to other groups, particularly given that PRS are sensitive to ethnic background (Curtis, 2018).

One further critical limitation of this field also deserves attention here. Almost all the studies reviewed in this chapter—and in the field to date—have been conducted in high-income countries in the Global North. Whether or not there are higher rates of psychotic disorder in other urban settings is unclear, but of paramount importance to inform both global public mental health and our understanding of the aetiology of psychotic disorders around the world. If urbanicity is a ubiquitous causal risk factor for psychotic symptoms or disorders, then the expected rapid urbanization of modern society, particularly in LMIC contexts, would have huge implications for the provision of mental health services for people with a psychotic disorder. However, if rural–urban differences in risk of psychosis were not universally found, this would provide important clues for aetiology.

Data are beginning to emerge from contexts where psychosis epidemiology has historically received less attention, as noted in parts above. For example, the recent multinational comparison of incidence rates across 17 centres in six countries (Jongsma et al., 2018) found only limited support for rural–urban differences in risk outside of the UK and the Netherlands. Here, incidence rates in Spanish, Italian and Brazilian settings were much lower than those reported in northern European settings (see also, for example, Mulè et al., 2017), with no evidence of high rates in Southern European or Brazilian urban settings. One further previous incidence study from Sao Paulo, Brazil, also found lower than expected incidence rates for a city of its size, though did not formally analyse rural–urban differences in risk (Menezes et al., 2007). Few studies of urban–rural differences in psychosis rates have been conducted in the Global South (see Solmi et al., 2017 for a recent review), and among those that have there are some methodological caveats which presently limit causal inference (Morgan et al., 2016; Kirkbride et al., 2018). For example, the recent international study of 42 countries found no overall association between urban residence and the prevalence of psychotic experiences and psychotic disorders in a large sample of adults from the Global South (DeVylder et al., 2018), using cross-sectional self-report survey data from the WHO's World Health Survey. Interestingly, there was a high degree of international heterogeneity when these results were pooled across low (I^2=63.6%, a measure of heterogeneity used in meta-analysis, where heterogeneity greater than 50% indicate substantial heterogeneity) and middle-income countries (I^2=59.8%). This indicates that in some countries the prevalence of psychotic experiences was higher in urban settings (i.e. Laos, Mali, Estonia, Morocco, Mexico), while in some countries higher in rural settings (i.e. Nepal, Vietnam, the Czech Republic, Hungary, South Africa). In most (N=32) countries, however, no evidence of a difference was detectable in the samples available. Unfortunately, the survey was not designed to test whether urban–rural differences in the incidence of psychotic disorders existed (Kirkbride et al., 2018), and no data were available from large nations such as China.

Interestingly, in China (a middle-income country), a review of the recent literature suggested that, as the country underwent rapid urbanization over two decades, the lifetime prevalence of schizophrenia in urban areas doubled between 1990 and 2010, while rural rates remained the same (Chan et al., 2015). Similarly, a cross-sectional survey in Chengdu, China, reported higher levels of psychotic experiences in men born in urban areas (Coid et al., 2017). While these data suggests that rural–urban differences in schizophrenia may exist in some areas in the Global South, these studies have largely been cross-sectional, and are largely subject to the same challenges of causal inference as those outlined here (Kirkbride et al., 2018), including the reliance on cross-sectional measures of prevalence. New incidence studies in the Global South hold promise in addressing some of these issues (Morgan et al., 2016; Morgan et al., 2023), but a challenge for the field will be to implement a set of comparable, prospective studies of the epidemiology of psychotic disorders in different settings to fully understand whether city living is a risk factor or consequence.

A further important limitation of the literature concerns the often crude (inexact) measurement of exposure to various environmental factors in the city and beyond. Most studies have used administrative units as a proxy for ecological neighbourhoods (Boydell et al., 2001; Hare, 1956; Kirkbride et al., 2007; Kirkbride et al., 2014), but these may be crude proxies, given they may not be socially or economically homogenous, nor coterminous with neighbourhoods as perceived by their inhabitants. Moreover, most studies have ignored other potential levels of causation relevant to mental health, including the role of the family (although, see earlier with regard to using family-based designs to control for shared familial effects) or the school. Here, Zammit and colleagues (2010) provide a notable exception, and previously found that for young people, school-level social fragmentation was a stronger predictor of risk of psychosis than its neighbourhood level construct (Zammit et al., 2010). This underlines the importance of recognizing how different putative levels of causation may have stronger or weaker effects on risk of psychosis at different points over the life course (March et al., 2008). For children and young adolescents, neighbourhoods may be less causally relevant than family or school-based environments, the former only attaining salience as they emerge into later adolescence and young adulthood. Relatively limited research has explored how cumulative exposure to different levels of organization (families, schools, communities, neighbourhoods) affects risk of psychosis over the life course. While studies across all these levels are missing, Pedersen and colleagues have reported a greater risk of schizophrenia with more years lived in higher degrees of urbanization, indicating a role for constant, cumulative, or repeated exposures frequently observed in urban areas (Pedersen & Mortensen, 2001). Further data from a recent longitudinal study of parents and children in the UK have also demonstrated that prolonged exposure to adverse social experiences, such as repeated neighbourhood conflict during childhood, is associated with increased odds of developing psychotic symptoms in late adolescence (Solmi et al., 2017).

Further research is also required to unpick whether the various socioeconomic characteristics associated with the risk of psychosis—deprivation, inequality, social fragmentation, social isolation, ethnic density, and so forth—hold any specificity to psychosis, or whether they are better conceptualized as tapping into a common latent construct of general social adversity which may predict psychosis (Padmanabhan et al., 2017). Conceptualizing these as individual risk factors may not be consistent with how they coalesce in urban environments. Moreover, like any study of higher-order effects, studies examining socioeconomic determinants of risk of psychosis are inevitably susceptible to ecological fallacy, whereby individual-level outcomes such as psychosis or schizophrenia are attributed to population level exposures such as income inequality and social cohesion (Allardyce et al., 2005; Boydell et al., 2001; Drukker et al., 2006; Kirkbride et al., 2007; Kirkbride et al., 2008a; Kirkbride et al., 2014, Solmi et al., 2018).

Potential mechanisms

There is substantial evidence to support the hypothesis that non-affective psychotic disorders occur more commonly in urban than rural areas, but the extent to which this is driven by exposure to environmental adversities, as a result of the confluence of socio-genetic drift over many generations, or the interplay of both processes remains to be fully elucidated. While we urgently need further investment in applied causal inference (see earlier) in epidemiology to address these issues, it is becoming clear that the brains of people who are born and grow up in more urban environments respond differently to social stressors than the brains of those who grow up in more rural environments. Emerging neuroscientific findings with participants without psychotic disorders show an association between urban upbringing and stress responses in the perigenual anterior cingulate cortex (Pacc, involved in modulating stress regulation), and between current urban residence and stress responses in the amygdala (involved in evaluating environmental threats) (Lederbogen et al., 2011). The same research group found deficits in grey matter volumes among healthy volunteers exposed to urban environments (Haddad et al., 2015), while another recent study from Germany found reduced cortical thickness among participants brought up in urban environments compared with rural controls (Besteher et al., 2017). All of these areas have been implicated in schizophrenia, but the studies themselves did not include individuals with a diagnosis of psychotic disorder. Studies using virtual reality have also demonstrated greater levels of subclinical psychotic symptoms such as paranoia in response to densely populated environments (Broome et al., 2013; Veling et al., 2016). To ascertain whether these mechanisms might explain the increased risk of psychosis in urban environments, research is needed involving people at high risk of, or diagnosed with psychotic disorder. It should also be noted that these neuroscientific findings may also be affected by the process of intergenerational drift described earlier.

Primary and secondary prevention

Regardless of cause—genetic, environmental, or both—the overrepresentation of psychotic disorders in more urban, more deprived, or more socially isolated environments merits a public health response which minimizes mental health inequalities faced by some populations. We can separate the approaches aimed at reducing these inequalities into those which seek to alleviate suffering following the onset of psychotic disorders (i.e. the prevention of downstream adverse physical, mental, and social outcomes) and those which seek to prevent the onset of psychotic disorder in the first place.

By understanding that urban populations will experience greater rates of psychosis (regardless of whether the environment is causally generating those rates) we can better plan service provision according to the likely needs of those populations. For example, by providing specialist mental healthcare services, such as Early Intervention in Psychosis [EIP] services, where they are most needed (i.e. in communities with greater concentrations of deprivation, young people, or ethnic minority groups, all risk factors for psychosis), we can more efficiently allocate finite resources within a system to improve population health based on where that need is likely to arise (Vassos et al., 2012; Kirkbride & Jones, 2014; Kirkbride, 2015; McDonald et al., 2021). For example, we have previously used epidemiological data on the incidence of psychotic disorders to influence psychosis service policy and provision in the context of EIP services in England (Department of Health, 2014; Rethink Mental Illness, 2014; NHS England, 2023). In theory, this improved allocation of resources should allow services to deliver a mandated package of EIP care to more people who require it, which in turn should prevent more negative downstream (physical, mental, and social) outcomes following the first episode of psychosis. This may also help minimize further downward social drift among those experiencing psychosis, preventing exacerbation of inequalities in health and social outcomes for people with psychosis. Extensions and refinements to the model are underway, and advocacy for similar tools in other settings is underway (Csillag et al., 2018; McGrath et al., 2018).

The prevention of the excess risk of psychotic disorders observed in populations exposed to urban environments is a more difficult issue, and will of course depend on what the causal determinants of this association prove to be. Previous studies have suggested that, if we could identify and remove all factors associated with excess risk in urban populations, we could prevent between 20–35% of cases of schizophrenia and other psychotic disorders (Kirkbride et al., 2010; Marcelis et al., 1998; Mortensen et al., 1999). In moving towards the identification of these targets, greater interdisciplinary efforts will be required to fully elucidate the roles of genetic and environmental factors in the aetiology of psychotic disorders, acknowledging that a cascade of pathways, potentially incorporating downward intergenerational drift, and subsequent exposure to a range of negative environmental sequelae, may be involved. Our preventative response will depend on the exact interplay of such factors. If future studies conclusively demonstrate that the association between urban birth, upbringing, and adult life and later psychotic disorders is solely under genetic control, this may favour universal prevention strategies solely focused on the identification of genetically high-risk individuals in the population. Alternatively, gene-environment interplay may advocate for more indicated prevention strategies, seeking to minimize subsequent exposure to socioenvironmental adversities among those at high risk for psychosis in urban populations. Finally, two key priorities for the field are to identify whether urban living is associated with increased risk of psychotic experiences or disorder in contexts in the Global South, and second, where such evidence is found, to determine whether this association is causal. Given rapid global urbanization, if urban living—or the underlying social adversities which inform this construct—independently increases risk of psychosis, then selected prevention strategies, targeting populations within highly urbanized, deprived, or isolated communities may be most effective in preventing a substantial proportion of the burden of psychotic disorders which unevenly afflict those who live in cities.

Acknowledgements

This work was supported by a Sir Henry Dale Fellowship held by James B. Kirkbride, jointly funded by the Wellcome Trust and the Royal Society (grant number: 101272/Z/13/Z).

References

Agerbo, E., et al. (2015). Polygenic risk score, parental socioeconomic status, family history of psychiatric disorders, and the risk for schizophrenia: a Danish population-based study and meta-analysis. *JAMA Psychiatry*, *72*(7), 635–641.

Allardyce, J., et al. (2005). Social fragmentation, deprivation and urbanicity: relation to first-admission rates for psychoses. *Br J Psychiatry*, *187*, 401–406.

Bastien, R., et al. (2023). The incidence of non-affective psychotic disorders in low and middle-income countries: a systematic review and meta-analysis. *Soc Psychiatry Psychiatr Epidemiol*, *58*, 523–536.

Becares, L., Dewey, M., & Das Munshi, J. (2017). Ethnic density effects for adult mental health: systematic review and meta-analysis of international studies. *Psychol Med*, *48*(12), 2054–2072.

Besteher, B., et al. (2017). Associations between urban upbringing and cortical thickness and gyrification. *J Psychiatr Res*, *95*, 114–120.

Bhugra, D., et al. (1996). First-contact incidence rates of schizophrenia in Trinidad and one-year follow-up. *Br J Psychiatry*, *169*(5), 587–592.

Binbay, T., et al. (2012). Testing the psychosis continuum: differential impact of genetic and nongenetic risk factors and comorbid psychopathology across the entire spectrum of psychosis. *Schizophr Bull*, *38*, 992–1002.

Boydell, J., et al. (2001). Incidence of schizophrenia in ethnic minorities in London: ecological study into interactions with environment. *BMJ*, *323*(7325), 1336–1338.

Broome, M. R., et al. (2013). A high-fidelity virtual environment for the study of paranoia. *Schizophr Res Treatment*, *2013*, 1–7.

Burns, J. K. & Esterhuizen, T. (2008). Poverty, inequality and the treated incidence of first-episode psychosis: an ecological study from South Africa. *Soc Psychiatry Psychiatr Epidemiol*, *43*(4), 331–335.

Burns, J. K., Tomita, A., & Kapadia, A. S. (2014). Income inequality and schizophrenia: increased schizophrenia incidence in countries with high levels of income inequality. *Int J Soc Psychiatry*, *60*(2), 185–196.

Byrne, M., et al. (2004). Parental socio-economic status and risk of first admission with schizophrenia—a Danish national register based study. *Soc Psychiatry Psychiatr Epidemiol*, *39*(2), 87–96.

Cannon, M. (2002). Obstetric complications and schizophrenia: historical and meta-analytic review. *Am J Psychiatry*, *159*(7), 1080–1092.

Chan, K. Y., et al. (2015). Prevalence of schizophrenia in China between 1990 and 2010. *J Glob Health*, *5*(1), 010410.

Cochrane, R. & Bal, S. S. (1988). Ethnic density is unrelated to incidence of schizophrenia. *Br J Psychiatry*, *153*(3), 363–366.

Coid, J. W., et al. (2017). Urban birth, urban living, and work migrancy: differential effects on psychotic experiences among young Chinese men. *Schizophr Bull*, *44*(5), 1123–1132.

Conde, L. C., et al. (2017). Higher genetic risk for schizophrenia is associated with living in urban and populated areas. *Eur Neuropsychopharmacol*, *27*(Supplement 3), S488.

Croudace, T. J., et al. (2000). Non-linear relationship between an index of social deprivation, psychiatric admission prevalence and the incidence of psychosis. *Psychol Med*, *30*(1), 177–185.

Csillag, C., et al. (2018). Early intervention in psychosis: from clinical intervention to health system implementation. *Early Interv Psychiatry*, *12*(4), 757–764.

Curtis, D. (2018). Polygenic risk score for schizophrenia is more strongly associated with ancestry than with schizophrenia. *Psychiatr Genet*, *28*(5), 85–89.

Curtis, S., et al. (2006). The ecological relationship between deprivation, social isolation and rates of hospital admission for acute psychiatric care: a comparison of London and New York City. *Health Place*, *12*(1), 19–37.

Department of Health (2014). Annual report of the chief medical officer 2013: public mental health priorities: assessing the evidence. London. Retrieved from https://www.gov.uk/government/publications/chief-medical-officer-cmo-annual-report-public-mental-health

DeVylder, J. E., et al. (2018). Association of urbanicity with psychosis in low- and middle-income countries. *JAMA Psychiatry, 75*(7), 678–686.

Di Forti, M., et al. (2019). The contribution of cannabis use to variation in the incidence of psychotic disorder across Europe (EU-GEI): a multicentre case-control study. *Lancet Psychiatry, 6*(5), 427–436.

Drukker, M., et al. (2006). Social disadvantage and schizophrenia. A combined neighbourhood and individual-level analysis. *Soc Psychiatry Psychiatr Epidemiol, 41*(8), 595–604.

Dykxhoorn, J., Hollander, A-C., Lewis, G., Dalman, C., & Kirkbride, J. (2019). Family networks during migration and risk of non-affective psychosis: a population-based cohort study. *Schizophr Research, 208*, 268–275.

Dykxhoorn, J., Lewis, G., Hollander, A-C., Kirkbride, J., & Dalman, C. (2020). Association of neighbourhood migrant density and risk of non-affective psychosis: a national, longitudinal cohort study. *Lancet Psychiatry, 7*(4), 327–336.

Eaton, W. W., Mortensen, P. B., & Frydenberg, M. (2000). Obstetric factors, urbanization and psychosis. *Schizophr Res, 43*(2–3), 117–123.

Faris, R. & Dunham, H. (1939). *Mental disorders in urban areas: an ecological study of schizophrenia and other psychoses.* Chicago/London: University of Chicago Press.

Fearon, P., et al. (2006). Incidence of schizophrenia and other psychoses in ethnic minority groups: results from the MRC AESOP Study. *Psychol Med, 36*(11), 1541–1550.

Freeman, H. (1994). Schizophrenia and city residence. *Br J Psychiatry Suppl,* (23), 39–50.

Germine, L., et al. (2016). Association between polygenic risk for schizophrenia, neurocognition and social cognition across development. *Transl Psychiatry, 6*(10), e924.

Giggs, J. (1973). The distribution of schizophrenics in Nottingham. *Trans Inst Br Geogr, 59*(59), 55–76.

Giggs, J. A. (1986). Mental disorders and ecological structure in Nottingham. *Soc Sci Med, 23*(10), 945–961.

Giggs, J. A. & Cooper, J. E. (1987). Ecological structure and the distribution of schizophrenia and affective psychoses in Nottingham. *Br J Psychiatry, 151*, 627–633.

Goldberg, E. & Morrison, S. (1963). Schizophrenia and social class. *Br J Psychiatry, 109*, 785–802.

Grech, A., Van Os, J., & Investigators, G. (2017). Evidence that the urban environment moderates the level of familial clustering of positive psychotic symptoms. *Schizophr Bull, 43*, 325–331.

Gureje, O., Olowosegun, O., Adebayo, K., & Stein, D. J. (2010). The prevalence and profile of non-affective psychosis in the Nigerian Survey of Mental Health and Wellbeing. *World Psychiatry, 9*, 50–55.

Haddad, L., et al. (2015). Brain structure correlates of urban upbringing, an environmental risk factor for schizophrenia. *Schizophr Bull, 41*(1), 115–122.

Hare, E. H. (1956). Mental illness and social conditions in Bristol. *J Mental Sci, 102*, 349–357.

Haukka, J., et al. (2001). Regional variation in the incidence of schizophrenia in Finland: a study of birth cohorts born from 1950 to 1969. *Psychol Med*, *31*(6), 1045–1053.

Heinz, A., Deserno, L., & Reininghaus, U. (2013). Urbanicity, social adversity and psychosis. *World Psychiatry*, *12*, 187–197.

Hickling, F. W. & Rodgers-Johnson, P. (1995). The incidence of first contact schizophrenia in Jamaica. *Br J Psychiatry*, *167*, 193–196.

Hollingshead, A. & Redlich, F. C. (1954). Social stratification and schizophrenia. *Am Socio Rev*, *19*(3), 302–306.

Jablensky, A., et al. (1992). Schizophrenia: manifestations, incidence and course in different cultures. A World Health Organization ten-country study. *Psychol Med Monogr Suppl*, *20*, 1–97.

Jongsma, H. E., et al. (2018). Treated incidence of psychotic disorders in the multinational EU-GEI study. *JAMA Psychiatry*, *75*(1), 36–46.

Kebede, D., Alem, A., Shibre, T., Negash, A., Deyassa, N., & Beyero, T. 2004. The sociodemographic correlates of schizophrenia in Butajira, rural Ethiopia. *Schizophr Res*, *69*, 133–141.

Kelly, B. D., et al. (2010). Schizophrenia and the city: a review of literature and prospective study of psychosis and urbanicity in Ireland. *Schizophr Res*, *116*(1), 75–89.

Kendler, K. S., et al. (2014). IQ and schizophrenia in a Swedish national sample: their causal relationship and the interaction of IQ with genetic risk. *Am J Psychiatry*, *172*(3), 259–265.

Kirkbride, J. B. (2015). Epidemiology on demand: population-based approaches to mental health service commissioning. *BJPsych Bull*, *39*(5), 242–247.

Kirkbride, J. B. & Jones, P. B. (2014). Parity of esteem begins at home: translating empirical psychiatric research into effective public mental health. *Psychol Med*, *44*(8), 1569–1576.

Kirkbride, J. B., et al. (2006). Heterogeneity in incidence rates of schizophrenia and other psychotic syndromes: findings from the 3-center AeSOP study. *Arch Gen Psychiatry*, *63*(3), 250–258.

Kirkbride, J. B., et al. (2008a). Psychoses, ethnicity and socio-economic status. *Br J Psychiatry*, *193*(1), 18–24.

Kirkbride, J. B., et al. (2008b). Testing the association between the incidence of schizophrenia and social capital in an urban area. *Psychol Med*, *38*(08), 1083–1094.

Kirkbride, J. B., et al. (2012). Incidence of schizophrenia and other psychoses in England, 1950–2009: a systematic review and meta-analyses. *PLoS ONE*, *7*(3), e31660.

Kirkbride, J. B., et al. (2013). A population-level prediction tool for the incidence of first-episode psychosis: translational epidemiology based on cross-sectional data. *BMJ Open*, *3*(2), e001998.

Kirkbride, J. B., et al. (2014). Social and spatial heterogeneity in psychosis proneness in a multilevel case–prodrome–control study. *Acta Psychiatr Scand*, *132*(4), 283–292.

Kirkbride, J. B., et al. (2014). Social deprivation, inequality, and the neighborhood-level incidence of psychotic syndromes in East London. *Schizophr Bull*, *40*(1), 169–180.

Kirkbride, J. B., et al. (2017). The epidemiology of first-episode psychosis in early intervention in psychosis services: findings from the Social Epidemiology of Psychoses in East Anglia [SEPEA] study. *Am J Psychiatry*, *174*(2), 143–153.

Kirkbride, J. B., et al. (2012). Incidence of schizophrenia and other psychoses in England, 1950–2009: a systematic review and meta-analyses. *PLoS One, 7,* e31660.

Kirkbride, J. B., et al. (2010). Translating the epidemiology of psychosis into public mental health: evidence, challenges and future prospects. *J Public Ment Health, 9*(2), 4–14.

Kirkbride, J. B., et al. (2007). Neighbourhood variation in the incidence of psychotic disorders in Southeast London. *Soc Psychiatry Psychiatr Epidemiol, 42*(6), 438–445.

Kirkbride, J. B., Keyes, K. M., & Susser, E. (2018). City living and psychotic disorders— implications of global heterogeneity for theory development. *JAMA Psychiatry, 75*(12), 1211–1212.

Kirkbride, J. B., Morgan, C., Fearon, P., Dazzan, P., Murray, R. M., & Jones PB. (2007). Neighbourhood-level effects on psychoses: re-examining the role of context. *Psychol Med, 37*(10), 1413–1425.

Lapouse, R., Monk, M. A., & Terris, M. (1956). The drift hypothesis and socioeconomic differentials in schizophrenia. *Am J Public Health Nations Health, 46*(8), 978–986.

Lasalvia, A., et al. (2014). First-contact incidence of psychosis in north-eastern Italy: influence of age, gender, immigration and socioeconomic deprivation. *Br J Psychiatry, 205*(2), 127–134.

Lederbogen, F., et al. (2011). City living and urban upbringing affect neural social stress processing in humans. *Nature, 474*(7352), 498–501.

Lewis, G., et al. (1992). Schizophrenia and city life. *Lancet, 340*(8812), 137–140.

Liebers, D. T., et al. (2016). Polygenic risk of schizophrenia and cognition in a population-based survey of older adults. *Schizophr Bull, 42*(4), 984–991.

Lofors, J. & Sundquist, K. (2007). Low-linking social capital as a predictor of mental disorders: a cohort study of 4.5 million Swedes. *Soc Sci Med, 64*(1), 21–34.

Marcelis, M., et al. (1998). Urbanization and psychosis: a study of 1942–1978 birth cohorts in the Netherlands. *Psychol Med, 28*(4), 871–879.

March, D., et al. (2008). Psychosis and place. *Epidemiol Rev, 30*(1), 84–100.

Mashaphu, S. & Mkize, D. L. (2007). HIV seropositivity in patients with first-episode psychosis. *S Afr J Psychiatr, 13*(3), 90–94.

Maylaih, E., Weyerer, S., & Hafner, H. (1989). Spatial concentration of the incidence of treated psychiatric disorders in Mannheim. *Acta Psychiatr Scand, 80*(6), 650–656.

McDonald, C., et al. (2001). Number of older siblings of individuals diagnosed with schizophrenia. *Schizophr Res, 47*(2–3), 275–280.

McDonald, K., et al. (2021). Using epidemiological evidence to forecast population need for early treatment programmes in mental health: a generalisable Bayesian prediction methodology applied to and validated for first-episode psychosis in England. *Br J Psychiatry, 219*(1), 383–391.

McGrath, J. (1999). Hypothesis: is low prenatal vitamin D a risk-modifying factor for schizophrenia?. *Schizophr Res, 40*(3), 173–177.

McGrath, J., et al. (2004). A systematic review of the incidence of schizophrenia: the distribution of rates and the influence of sex, urbanicity, migrant status and methodology. *BMC Med, 2*(1), 13.

McGrath, J. J., Mortensen, P. B., & Whiteford, H. A. (2018). Pragmatic psychiatric epidemiology—if you can't count it, it won't count. *JAMA Psychiatry, 75*(2), 111–112.

McGrath, J. J., et al. (2015). Psychotic experiences in the general population: a cross-national analysis based on 31,261 respondents from 18 countries. *JAMA Psychiatry, 72,* 697–705.

McKenzie, K., Whitley, R., & Weich, S. (2002). Social capital and mental health. *Br J Psychiatry, 181*(4), 280–283.

Menezes, P. R., et al. (2007). Incidence of first-contact psychosis in São Paulo, Brazil. *Br J Psychiatry, 191*(Suppl. 51), 2–7.

Menezes, P. R., et al. (2007). Incidence of first-contact psychosis in Sao Paulo, Brazil. *Br J Psychiatry Suppl, 51,* s102–s106.

Mintz, N. L. & Schwartz, D. T. (1964). Urban ecology and psychosis: community factors in the incidence of schizophrenia and manic-depression among Italians in greater Boston. *Int J Soc Psychiatry, 10*(2), 101–118.

Morgan, C., et al. (2016). The incidence of psychoses in diverse settings, INTREPID (2): a feasibility study in India, Nigeria, and Trinidad. *Psychol Med, 46*(09), 1923–1933.

Morgan, C., et al. (2023). Epidemiology of Untreated Psychoses in 3 Diverse Settings in the Global South: the International Research Program on Psychotic Disorders in Diverse Settings (INTREPID II). *JAMA Psychiatry, 80*(1), 40–48.

Mortensen, P. B., et al. (2003). Individual and familial risk factors for bipolar affective disorders in Denmark. *Arch Gen Psychiatry, 60*(12), 1209–1215.

Mortensen, P., et al. (1999). Effects of family history and place and season of birth on the risk of schizophrenia. *N Engl J Med, 340,* 603–608.

Mulè, A., et al. (2017). Low incidence of psychosis in Italy: confirmation from the first epidemiological study in Sicily. *Soc Psychiatry Psychiatr Epidemiol, 52*(2), 155–162.

Newbury, J., et al. (2022). Association between genetic and socioenvironmental risk for schizophrenia during upbringing in a UK longitudinal cohort. *Psychol Med, 52*(8), 1527–1537.

Ngui, A. N., et al. (2013). Does elapsed time between first diagnosis of schizophrenia and migration between health territories vary by place of residence? A survival analysis approach. *Health Place, 20*(Supplement C), 66–74.

NHS England (2023). *Implementing the early intervention in psychosis access and waiting time standard.* London: NHS England. https://www.england.nhs.uk/mentalhealth/wp-content/uploads/sites/29/2016/04/eip-guidance.pdf

Nuevo, R., Chatterji, S., Verdes, E., Naidoo, N., Arango, C., & Ayuso-Mateos, J. L. (2012). The continuum of psychotic symptoms in the general population: a cross-national study. *Schizophr Bull, 38,* 475–485.

Padmanabhan, J. L., et al. (2017). The 'polyenviromic risk score': aggregating environmental risk factors predicts conversion to psychosis in familial high-risk subjects. *Schizophr Res, 181,* 17–22.

Paksarian, D., et al. (2015). Childhood residential mobility, schizophrenia, and bipolar disorder: a population-based study in Denmark. *Schizophr Bull, 41*(2), 346–354.

Paksarian, D., et al. (2018). The role of genetic liability in the association of urbanicity at birth and during upbringing with schizophrenia in Denmark. *Psychol Med, 48*(2), 305–314.

Pardinas, A. F., et al. (2018). Common schizophrenia alleles are enriched in mutation-intolerant genes and in regions under strong background selection. *Nat Genet, 50*(3), 381–389.

Pedersen, C. B. (2015). Persons with schizophrenia migrate towards urban areas due to the development of their disorder or its prodromata. *Schizophr Res, 168*(1–2), 204–208.

Pedersen, C. B. & Mortensen, P. B. (2001). Evidence of a dose-response relationship between urbanicity during upbringing and schizophrenia risk. *Arch Gen Psychiatry, 58*(11), 1039–1046.

Pedersen, C. B. & Mortensen, P. B. (2006). Urbanicity during upbringing and bipolar affective disorders in Denmark. *Bipolar Disord, 8*(3), 242–247.

Perälä, J., et al. (2008). Geographic variation and sociodemographic characteristics of psychotic disorders in Finland. *Schizophr Res, 106*(2–3), 337–347.

Price, C., Dalman, C., Zammit, S., & Kirkbride, J. (2018). Association of residential mobility over the life course with nonaffective psychosis in 1.4 million young people in Sweden. *JAMA Psychiatry, 75*(11), 1128–1136.

Rethink Mental Illness (2014). Lost generation: why young people with psychosis are being left behind, and what needs to change. Retrieved from https://www.rethink.org/media/2628/lost-generation-rethink-mental-illness-report.pdf

Richardson, L., et al. (2018). Association of environment with the risk of developing psychotic disorders in rural populations: findings from the social epidemiology of psychoses in East Anglia study. *JAMA Psychiatry, 75*(1), 75–83.

Sariaslan, A., et al. (2015). Does population density and neighborhood deprivation predict schizophrenia? A nationwide Swedish family-based study of 2.4 million individuals. *Schizophr Bull, 41*(2), 494–502.

Sariaslan, A., et al. (2016). Schizophrenia and subsequent neighborhood deprivation: revisiting the social drift hypothesis using population, twin and molecular genetic data. *Transl Psychiatry, 6*(5), e796.

Scully, P. J., et al. (2004). Schizophrenia, schizoaffective and bipolar disorder within an epidemiologically complete, homogeneous population in rural Ireland: small area variation in rate. *Schizophr Res, 67*(2–3), 143–155.

Sham, P. C., et al. (1992). Schizophrenia following pre-natal exposure to influenza epidemics between 1939 and 1960. *Br J Psychiatry, 160*, 461–466.

Silver, E., Mulvey, E. P., & Swanson, J. W. (2002). Neighborhood structural characteristics and mental disorder: Faris and Dunham revisited. *Soc Sci Med, 55*(8), 1457–1470.

Solmi, F., et al. (2018). Trajectories of neighborhood cohesion in childhood, and psychotic and depressive symptoms at age 13 and 18 years. *J Am Acad Child Adolesc Psychiatry, 56*(7), 570–577.

Solmi, F., et al. (2020). Neighbourhood characteristics at birth and positive and negative psychotic symptoms in adolescence: findings from the ALSPAC birth cohort. *Schizophr Bull, 46*(3), 581–591.

Solmi, F., Dykxhoorn, J., & Kirkbride, J. B. (2017). Urban–rural differences in major mental health conditions. In Okkels, N., Kristiansen, C. B., & Munk-Jorgensen, P. (eds) *Mental health and illness in the city.* Singapore: Springer Singapore, 1–106.

Soosay, I., et al. (2012). Trauma exposure, PTSD and psychotic-like symptoms in post-conflict Timor Leste: an epidemiological survey. *BMC Psychiatry, 12*, 229.

Sundquist, K., Frank, G., & Sundquist, J. (2004). Urbanisation and incidence of psychosis and depression: follow-up study of 4.4 million women and men in Sweden. *Br J Psychiatry, 184*, 293–298.

Supanya, S., Morgan, C., & Reininghaus, U. (2016). Systematic review and meta-analysis of the prevalence of psychotic experiences in countries outside of North America, Europe, and Australasia. *NPJ Schizophrenia, 2*, 53.

Szöke, A., et al. (2014). Rural–urban variation in incidence of psychosis in France: a prospective epidemiologic study in two contrasted catchment areas. *BMC Psychiatry, 14*(1), 78.

Toulopoulou, T., et al. (2007). Substantial genetic overlap between neurocognition and schizophrenia: genetic modeling in twin samples. *Arch Gen Psychiatry, 64*(12), 1348–1355.

United Nations Department of Economic and Social Affairs (2019). World urbanization prospects: the 2018 revision. New York. Retrieved from https://population.un.org/wup/Publications/Files/WUP2018-Report.pdf

van Os, J., et al. (2017). Evidence that polygenic risk for psychotic disorder is expressed in the domain of neurodevelopment, emotion regulation and attribution of salience. *Psychol Med, 47*(14), 2421–2437.

van Os, J., Kenis, G., & Rutten, B. P. F. (2010). The environment and schizophrenia. *Nature, 468*, 203.

van Os, J., Pedersen, C. B., & Mortensen, P. B. (2004). Confirmation of synergy between urbanicity and familial liability in the causation of psychosis. *Am J Psychiatry, 161*(12), 2312–2314.

Vassos, E., et al. (2012). Meta-analysis of the association of urbanicity with schizophrenia. *Schizophr Bull, 38*(6), 1118–1123.

Vassos, E., Pedersen, C. B., Murray, R. M., Collier, D. A., & Lewis, C. M. (2012). Meta-analysis of the association of urbanicity with schizophrenia. *Schizophr Bull, 38*(6), 1118–1123.

Veling, W. A. (2006). Ethnic density and incidence of schizophrenia in ethnic minorities in the Netherlands. *Schizophr Res, 81*, 174.

Veling, W., et al. (2016). Environmental social stress, paranoia and psychosis liability: a virtual reality study. *Schizophr Bull, 42*(6), 1363–1371.

Wainwright, N. W. J. & Surtees, P. G. (2004). Area and individual circumstances and mood disorder prevalence. *Br J Psychiatry, 185*(3), 227 LP–232.

Wicks, S., et al. (2005). Social adversity in childhood and the risk of developing psychosis: a national cohort study. *Am J Psychiatry, 162*(9), 1652–1657.

Yang, J., Visscher, P. M., & Wray, N. R. (2010). Sporadic cases are the norm for complex disease. *Eur J Hum Genet, 18*(9), 1039–1043.

Zammit, S., et al. (2010). Individuals, schools, and neighborhood: a multilevel longitudinal study of variation in incidence of psychotic disorders. *Arch Gen Psychiatry, 67*(9), 914–922.

2

Psychosis across persons 1: Minority ethnic groups and migration

Els van der Ven

Background

Human migration is the process of forced or voluntary movement of people across borders with the goal of settling for a temporary or indefinite amount of time. It is an innate characteristic of humans. Reasons for migration may vary between a search for better economic circumstances, work or school opportunities, or reunification with loved ones. It may also be an escape from unsafe situations including war, persecution, human rights violations, natural disasters, or the effects of climate change. The conditions in which a person migrates, combined with the expectations and the—sometimes ambivalent—attitude towards migration in the host country shape experiences in the host environment.

In 2019, the United Nations estimated global migration at nearly 300 million international migrants or about 3.5% of the world population, a number that has been steadily increasing. Europe and Asia each hosted more than 80 million international migrants (~55% of the total), North America hosted around 60 million (~20%), and Africa, Latin America and the Caribbean, and Oceania hosted the smallest numbers, with percentages of 10 or less. Given the growing mobility of populations, the health of migrants is a critical public health issue. In light of this, it is concerning that migrants experience higher rates of mental health problems. In particular, there is a long history of research showing that certain migrant and minority populations have a higher risk of developing a psychotic disorder compared with host populations.

In this chapter we provide an overview of evidence on and candidate explanations for variations in the incidence of psychotic disorder and in the prevalence of psychotic experiences by, as relevant, migrant status, region of origin, and ethnic group. We conclude by considering the implications of the evidence to date.

Concepts of migration, ethnicity, and race

This chapter includes different concepts used to describe and categorize migrant, ethnic, and racial groups. The terms 'immigrant' (often simply referred to as 'migrant') and 'emigrant' are used to designate a person who moves into a country, either permanently or for a prolonged period of time, and someone who moves out of a country to another, respectively. Internal migrants are individuals who move to a different region within a country. Most research on migrants has focused on foreign-born, that is, first-generation migrants who have a personal history of migration. Children of migrants and subsequent generations are sometimes referred to as second (or third and so on) generation migrants, even though they have no personal history of migration.

Ethnicity usually relates to a sense of belonging and identification resulting from a variety of factors, such as birth region, language, religion, ancestry, and physical features (Bhopal & Rankin, 1999). People have also been demarcated according to visible minority status or skin colour to investigate the impact of discrimination. In various countries with long migration histories, including the US and Brazil, people are also classified by race. While historically used as a means to justify oppression based on a biological feature, race is a social construct that is closely linked to racism, i.e. to 'the systematic oppression of a racial group to the social, economic and political advantage of another' (Hathaway, 2021; Merriam-Webster.com, 2021).

The epidemiology of psychoses in the context of migration and ethnicity

Driven by the influential 10-country study of the World Health Organization, which reported little variation in the incidence of schizophrenia in different cultures across the world (Jablensky et al., 1992), there was—until recently—a belief within the scientific community that 'contrary to almost any other common condition, the incidence of schizophrenia is independent of the environment and a characteristic of human populations' (Crow, 2000). This assumption of universality has been challenged by various epidemiological findings that demonstrate large variation in incidence across places and populations (McGrath, 2006; McGrath, 2007). Most notably, there is extensive literature reporting an increased incidence of psychotic disorder among various migrant and minority ethnic minority populations in high-income countries.

The first empirical study in this field dates back to 1932. The Norwegian psychiatrist Ødegaard found a twofold increase in rates of first hospital admission for psychosis among Norwegian migrants to Minnesota, compared with native Minnesotans and Norwegians living in Norway. While in the US the social emphasis on the aetiology of psychosis largely disappeared during the twentieth century, British researchers rekindled interest in the field from the 1980s onwards. Several subsequent studies have reported strikingly high incidence rates for non-affective psychotic disorder (NAPD) among the Black Caribbean population in the UK (Cochrane & Bal, 1989; Harrison et al., 1988). These findings are reinforced by an elevated incidence among other migrant and minority ethnic groups in Europe, including in the Moroccan and Surinamese populations in the Netherlands (Veling et al., 2006), various migrant groups from low- and high-income countries in Scandinavia (Cantor-Graae et al., 2003; Leao et al., 2006), and, most recently, African migrants in Australia (O'Donoghue et al., 2021).

Several meta-analyses suggest that the incidence of psychotic disorders in all minority ethnic populations combined is about two times that of majority populations. However, these overall estimates mask substantial variation (Bourque et al., 2011; Morgan et al., 2019). For example, recent studies from the UK have reported a six- to fourfold increased incidence in Black Caribbean and Black African populations, respectively, while rates in other minority ethnic groups in the UK were either not, or only modestly, increased (Coid et al., 2008). In the Netherlands, studies have reported an elevated incidence for migrants from Morocco, Surinam, and the Netherlands Antilles, but less so for Turkish migrants (Veling et al., 2006).

Variations are also evident by place of migration (Selten et al., 2020), by host region (Termorshuizen et al., 2022), by gender (van der Ven & Selten, 2018), and by refugee status (Hollander et al., 2016). For instance, several studies indicate that there is no elevated incidence of psychosis in migrants to Canada or Israel (Anderson et al., 2015; Weiser et al., 2008). Interestingly, in the case of migration to Israel, Jewish immigrants may be moving from a minority position in their country of birth to a majority position in the host environment.

To add further complexity to these patterns of incidence, results from the multinational EU-GEI study indicated that incidence may also vary by host region (Jongsma et al., 2018). That is, the extent to which rates were elevated in minority ethnic populations in this study was dependent on the host region, with generally higher rates in urban areas in Northern Europe than in any included area in Southern Europe. For instance, the standardized incidence rate for all ethnic minority groups in Paris and London was more than 75 per 100,000 person-years while that for ethnic minority groups in Barcelona, Valencia, and Santiago was less than 15 per 100,000 person-years.

Variations by gender have been reported in the UK, where in one study an elevated incidence was observed specifically among Bangladeshi and Pakistani women. In the Netherlands, a higher incidence of psychotic disorder has been reported among minority ethnic men from the Maghreb relative to women from the same region, with a ratio of 5:1.

Lastly, there is meta-analytic evidence that the incidence of psychotic disorders may be particularly high among refugees relative to other migrants (i.e. IRR of 2.4 for refugees vs. 1.9 for other migrants) (Brandt et al., 2019). Importantly, the evidence suggests that variation is the norm. This is not surprising given the vast diversity in cultural heritage, migratory histories, and social positions of minority ethnic populations.

Other migrant, minority ethnic, and racialized populations

An issue with the epidemiological evidence, to date, is that most studies have been conducted in Northern Europe—in fact, in the UK and the Netherlands—with some studies in Southern Europe, the US, Canada, Australia, and Israel. In the US, the most convincing evidence of a disparity between Black and white Americans comes from a prospective cohort study of pregnant women in California (Bresnahan et al., 2007). All women receiving prenatal care at the Alameda County Kaiser Permanente Medical Care Plan Clinics between 1959 and 1966 were enrolled in the study and, among their children, Black individuals were over twice as likely to receive a schizophrenia spectrum diagnosis compared with white individuals (risk ratio = 2.28, 95% CI = 1.39–3.76). Furthermore, this relationship was not attenuated by indicators of socioeconomic status (SES) or by including a range of other putative confounders (e.g. maternal pre-pregnancy body mass index, paternal age).

There is a dearth of research on the incidence or prevalence of psychotic disorder among international migrants in the Global South. In most places, there are no reliable population databases or censuses with data on international migrants to support such research. One subpopulation of migrants in the Global South that has been studied are refugees staying temporarily or for prolonged periods in refugee camps. In 90 refugee camps across 15 low- and middle-income countries (LMIC), Kane et al. (2014) found that the second largest proportion of visits for mental, neurological, and substance use problems in primary healthcare was attributable to psychotic disorder (22.7%). In the Burj el-Barajneh camp, a protracted refugee setting in Lebanon, researchers found a lifetime prevalence of psychosis of 3.3% (95% CI 1.0–5.5), which is similar to what has been reported in general population samples. In conclusion, studies on the prevalence of psychosis among refugees in LMIC are inconclusive and warrant new studies with rigorous methodology.

We also have much to learn about incidence among internal migrants. Research from the Hunan Province in China suggests that migrant workers who migrated from rural to urban areas were 1.5 times more likely to be acutely admitted to hospital with schizophrenia compared with the general population (Zhu et al., 2018). A recent study from Bologna, Italy, reported a twofold increased risk of psychosis for internal and external migrants compared with Italians from Emilia Romagna, the region surrounding Bologna. Most of these internal migrants moved from southern Italy, where rates of unemployment and poverty are higher (Tarricone et al., 2016).

Minority ethnic populations that are severely marginalized but without recent migration history include indigenous people, populations that occupied a land before colonization. Although the quality of studies varies, there is some evidence of elevated incidence and prevalence of schizophrenia among the New Zealand Māori compared with the non-Māori (Kake et al., 2008; Tapsell et al., 2018). Further, Lynge and Jacobsen (1995) found high first admission rates for schizophrenia among Greenlandic, primarily Inuit, men compared with Danish men. Together, these findings warrant more investigation, yet they add to the body of evidence suggesting that the increased risk of psychosis may be due to marginalization and social disadvantage rather than a direct effect of migration.

Methodological considerations

In interpreting these findings, it is important to consider methodological artefacts such as bias and confounding.

Diagnostic bias

A conspicuous explanation for these findings has been disproportional misdiagnosis. Various early studies from the US and the UK suggested that clinicians tend to misinterpret and misattribute the phenomenology presented especially by Black individuals, resulting in the overdiagnosis of schizophrenia and underdiagnosis of affective disorders (Adebimpe, 1981; Littlewood & Lipsedge, 1997; Mukherjee et al., 1983), a finding replicated even in recent studies (Gara et al., 2019). This body of literature suggests that systemic racism and its sequelae inflate the perception of psychopathology among primarily Black individuals where there is more cultural and social distance from the predominant culture (Metzl, 2009).

Even though diagnostic bias is a serious issue, there are several lines of reasoning and evidence that suggest it cannot entirely account for consistent evidence of variations in incidence across ethnic groups. For instance, in several studies efforts were made to minimize diagnostic bias, for instance by including relatives in the diagnostic process or by ethnic blinding, i.e. assigning a diagnosis while remaining blind to a person's ethnic background. These approaches did not have a strong attenuating effect on rates of psychosis among minority ethnic groups. Another study found no substantive difference in the number of Black Caribbean patients diagnosed with a psychotic disorder by either a Jamaican or British psychiatrist (Hickling et al., 1999). Further, two studies used vignettes to investigate racial stereotyping in diagnosis. Neither found strong evidence that psychiatrists were more likely to diagnose schizophrenia when the ethnicity of individuals was described in case vignettes as Black. Importantly, more recent studies focus on all psychotic disorders, not just schizophrenia, and tend to report high rates for psychotic disorders as one category. This is not, then, an issue of specifically mis- or overdiagnosis of schizophrenia.

Outcomes

It has been suggested that an excess of brief psychoses in response to social stress causes a high incidence in Black minorities (Littlewood & Lipsedge, 1997). However, studies on outcomes from the UK do not support this. Results from AESOP-10, a 10-year follow-up study in the UK, indicated that the trajectory of first-episode psychosis (FEP) in Black Caribbean patients showed a more continuous course of illness and lower rates of recovery compared with white British patients. Both Black Caribbean and Black African patients had worse social functioning and service use outcomes over the 10-year follow-up, including a higher likelihood of compulsory admission and police involvement (Morgan et al., 2017). In the GAP-5 study, reporting on the 5-year outcome of FEP patients in South London, similar ethnic disparities in service use outcomes were found, that is, more compulsion and longer hospital admissions in Black African and Black Caribbean patients, but no ethnic differences in functional disability, recovery rates, or illness severity during the follow-up period (Ajnakina et al., 2017). Importantly, neither study provides evidence for a more benign course of illness among Black minorities in the UK.

Sampling bias

In the city of The Hague, Netherlands, a first-contact incidence study was conducted, while at the same time a psychiatric register was operational. Researchers compared the two sampling methods and found that the first-contact approach had a tendency to miss older Dutch patients who were treated for another disorder before the onset of psychosis. On the basis of register data, the incidence of schizophrenia among migrant groups was slightly attenuated, yet still notably increased, compared with the first-contact method (Hogerzeil et al., 2017). Irrespective of the study design, sampling bias is probably present in most studies and affects the extent to which the reported incidence resembles the true incidence of psychotic disorder in migrant and minority ethnic groups. However, the consistency of the findings across study designs suggests that its influence is unlikely to change the overall incidence pattern.

Selective migration

According to the notion of selective migration, individuals with a genetic predisposition for psychosis are more likely to emigrate. In a thought-provoking thought experiment, Selten and colleagues (2002) imagined that the entire Surinamese population migrated to the Netherlands and recalculated incidence rates among the Surinamese population in the Netherlands. When doing this, the incidence remained increased compared with the Dutch majority population. Another study investigated the prevalence of previously identified risk factors for psychosis among Swedish men who emigrated later in life. Prospective emigrants had better social adjustment and intellectual ability. Overall, this study found no evidence of a predisposition for psychosis among prospective emigrants.

In short, while it is important to remain vigilant regarding the presence of bias and confounding effects, there is limited evidence that the observed increased incidence of psychotic disorders in migrant and minority ethnic groups can be fully explained by methodological artefacts.

Variations in psychotic experiences by migrant and ethnic group

In addition to variations in psychotic disorder, recent reports also suggest ethnic differences in the prevalence of low-level psychotic experiences in general population samples.

Low-level psychotic experiences (e.g. infrequent, non-distressing hallucinations; paranoia; etc.) are highly prevalent in the general population (approximately 5–10%; Linscott & van Os, 2013; van Os et al., 2009) and evidence suggests that they exist on a continuum with psychotic disorders. Several studies have found that these experiences are more prevalent in minority ethnic groups, including Black populations in the UK (e.g. Morgan et al., 2009), Turkish and Moroccan individuals in the Netherlands (Vanheusden et al., 2008), and in Latin people in the US (e.g. Paksarian et al., 2016). In a recent systematic review and meta-analysis, Tortelli and colleagues (2018) identified 19 studies of adults (age 16 or over) that have reported data on psychotic experiences in migrant or minority ethnic groups. The most consistent finding was that people from Black groups, compared with majority groups, more often reported psychotic experiences, both current (from 7 studies with 26 effect sizes: odds ratio, OR = 1.8, 95% CI: 1.4–2.3) and lifetime (from 4 studies with 9 effect sizes: pooled OR = 1.3, 95% CI: 1.1–1.6).

The interpretation of these experiences varies by ethnocultural context. For instance, in some minority ethnic individuals, these experiences have been interpreted as dissociative experiences and an adaptive response to extremely stressful situations. Similarly, in Black groups, increased suspiciousness has been considered 'healthy cultural mistrust' in response to unsafe and hostile living environments (Wilson et al., 2016). Nonetheless, psychological theories of the origins of hallucinations and delusions suggest that even endorsement of adaptive quasi-psychotic experiences may—in the event of exposure to further risks—develop into more persistent, severe, and distressing psychotic symptoms (Freeman, 2016), suggesting that ethnic variations in the prevalence of psychotic experiences may be related to such variations at the level of clinical disorder. If this is so, in populations with high rates of disorder, we would also expect psychotic experiences to be more prevalent. To date, the pattern of findings suggests that this is indeed the case.

Candidate explanatory factors: (1) Biological

Several biological candidates have been proposed to account for high rates of psychosis in certain migrant and minority ethnic groups. Even though often categorized as biological factors, suggesting a purely biological pathway towards psychopathology, they may have genetic or environmental root causes.

Obstetric complications

A meta-analysis found a small but 'statistically' significant effect of complications during pregnancy or delivery and elevated risk of psychosis in offspring (Cannon et al., 2002). There is abundant evidence in the US showing that Black women are at substantially increased risk for many obstetric complications, spanning preterm delivery, reduced foetal growth, and increased infection rates. Importantly, findings indicate that access to prenatal care and a variety of sociodemographic factors (e.g. income) do not explain racial disparities in birth outcomes (e.g. Wang et al., 2020). Neighbourhood- and individual-level factors appear to impact the disparity in these outcomes. A recent study revealed that exposure to environmental contaminants (e.g. air pollution, heat exposure) is linked to higher rates of preterm birth and low birth weight differentially in Black mothers compared with other mothers in the US, possibly due to an interaction between prenatal stress and contaminants (Bekkar et al., 2020). In addition, psychological distress related to perceived neighbourhood crime levels and breakdown of order and social control have also been linked to preterm birth in Black mothers, and Black women show higher levels of other stress biomarkers compared with white women of the same SES in mid- to late-pregnancy, including particular inflammatory markers (e.g. C-reactive protein) and adrenocorticotropic hormone (Giurgescu et al., 2012). Overall, these findings suggest that ethnic disparities in the rates of obstetric complications, in conjunction with contextual stressors, could contribute to a developmental trajectory towards psychosis among Black and other minority ethnic groups. That is, one pathway between socioeconomic and ethnic inequalities and psychoses may be via increased risk of obstetric complications. However, very few studies have directly examined this and those that have (e.g. in the UK) suggest that Black Caribbean patients with psychosis have fewer obstetric complications than white British patients with a psychotic disorder (Hutchinson et al., 1997).

Vitamin D

Prenatal and chronic postnatal hypovitaminosis D has also been proposed as a potential risk for psychosis in migrant and minority ethnic populations, especially individuals from the Global South who live in cooler climates with less sunlight, the most important source for vitamin D (McGrath, 2011). Studies in rats have demonstrated that a lack of vitamin D may alter dopaminergic activity in the brain lending some face validity to this hypothesis. However, it does not correspond to findings of increased incidence of psychosis among migrants moving to similar or even warmer climates, for instance, migrants from the former Soviet Union migrating to Israel (Weiser et al., 2008) and Finns migrating to Sweden (Leao et al., 2006). Along similar lines, it does not correspond with patterns of risk in the UK, where Asians have the highest rates of vitamin D deficiency and lower rates of psychosis than Black Caribbeans (Morgan et al., 2010).

Candidate explanatory factors: (2) Cannabis use

There is substantial evidence that cannabis use, especially forms with high concentrations of tetrahydrocannabinol, is associated with an increased risk of psychotic disorder (Di Forti et al., 2009; Di Forti et al., 2019). Cannabis use was therefore initially considered a potential candidate to explain high psychosis rates primarily in Black Caribbeans in the UK (Sharpley et al., 2001). However, in clinical studies, the reported prevalence of cannabis use was similar in ethnic minority patients compared with the majority group in the Netherlands (Veen et al., 2002; Veling et al., 2008a) and in the UK (Mazzoncini et al., 2010).

Candidate explanatory factors: (3) Individual social environment

Ethnic identity and acculturation

One social factor that is believed to play a role at the individual level is the style of 'acculturation', the extent to which an individual holds on to their ethnic identity after going through a cultural change. Findings on ethnic identity in relation to psychosis are equivocal. In a case–control study by Veling and colleagues (2010), ethnic identity (i.e. subjective feelings and ideas about one's own ethnic background) was associated with risk of psychosis. Specifically, individuals with psychosis were more likely to have an assimilated identity and less likely to have a separated identity or positive association with their ethnic group compared with hospital controls and siblings. Findings among Black minority ethnic groups in the UK, however, suggest an opposite pattern: an increased odds for psychosis corresponding to higher levels of ethnic identification with own ethnic group. Perceived discrimination mediated this association (Reininghaus et al., 2010).

In recent analyses of case–control data from the EU-GEI study, concerning a large cohort with a first episode psychosis and controls from sites in five European countries and Brazil, researchers found that the relationship between migrant or minority group status and odds of psychosis no longer remained when adjusted for a measure of linguistic distance. Importantly, there were differences between generations in the nature of the association. While linguistic distance had the strongest confounding effect in first-generation migrants, social disadvantage was more important in second and subsequent generations (Jongsma et al., 2021).

Social disadvantage, discrimination, and hostility

At the level of individual experience, there is evidence that more frequent exposure to social adversities over the life course, particularly discrimination, may be important. For example, research in a general population sample demonstrated that perceived discrimination was, independent of its source (appearance, sexual orientation, handicap), associated with subclinical, delusional ideas (Janssen et al., 2004). In the UK, studies have indicated that adverse social circumstances such as parental separation, household discord, housing instability, and financial difficulties are associated with odds of psychosis and more common in ethnic minority groups, in particular Black Caribbeans (Morgan et al., 2007). The same applies to markers of social and economic disadvantage in adulthood (Morgan et al., 2008). However, the measures in these studies are crude and do not provide much information about the underlying mechanism. In addition, SES alone does not appear to explain much of the variance in risk of psychosis across ethnic minority groups.

Several studies have examined the potential role of discrimination and perceived disadvantage. For instance, research using the Fourth National Survey of Ethnic Minorities in the UK, indicated an association between the estimated annual prevalence of psychosis and reports of experienced racism, verbal abuse, and racial attacks (Karlsen & Nazroo, 2002). It is notable that the strongest effect was for experiences involving physical threat and violence (racial attacks). Veling et al. (2008b), in the Netherlands, reported that the highest incidence rates were among those populations known to experience the highest levels of discrimination (i.e. Moroccan: IRR = 4.8). These findings are reinforced by recent systematic reviews of perceived discrimination that found overall support for an association with psychosis at the symptom and disorder level (Pearce et al., 2019). Together, these findings point to discrimination and perceived disadvantage as potentially important factors among minority ethnic groups.

Structural racism

One underlying construct tying various strings together is that of structural racism. This concept is defined by the social policies and norms that lead to inequities in access to important resources, such as education and healthcare, exposure to environmental toxins, and stressors. As mentioned, the neighbourhood and social context may hold a significant portion of the relative contribution of risk for psychosis. Evidence from the US further supports the notion that this may occur through individual-level discrimination as well as through collective trauma at the community level (e.g. police violence) (Anglin et al., 2021). Experimental studies suggest that repeated exposure to discrimination may have lasting neurodevelopmental and neurobiological effects, especially regarding long-term changes in neural circuits responsible for pairing threat cues to neutral stimuli (Harnett, 2020). Social and environmental stressors connected to structural racism (e.g. neighbourhood disadvantage, collective trauma, discrimination) that are disproportionately experienced by migrant and minority ethnic groups, could therefore contribute to psychosis risk in these populations.

Candidate explanatory factors: (4) Broader social environment

Studies from various contexts have found that the greater the proportion of the own ethnic group in the neighbourhood, the lower the risk of psychotic disorder (Faris & Dunham, 1939; Kirkbride et al., 2008; Veling et al., 2008c) and psychotic experiences (Das-Munshi et al., 2012). For instance, in The Hague the incidence of psychosis was highest for Turkish, Moroccan, and Surinamese migrants living in areas with low own-group density (Veling et al., 2008c). In highly ethnically dense areas, the risk was similar to that for non-migrant Dutch, even though the level of deprivation is highest in areas where immigrants constitute a large proportion of the population (Veling et al., 2008c). It has therefore been suggested that ethnic density, perhaps as a proxy for social cohesion, mitigates the pathogenic effects of minority stress, including discrimination and chronic strains (Veling & Susser, 2011). Most recently, Swedish registry data indicated that lower own-region migrant density was associated with an increased risk of psychotic disorders among migrants and children of migrants, in particular for migrants from Asia and sub-Saharan Africa (Dykxhoorn et al., 2020). The ethnic density effect has also been replicated at school level; that is, non-migrant, Swedish children attending schools with a high proportion of foreign-born children had an increased risk for developing psychosis later in life and vice versa (Zammit et al., 2010).

This line of research may coincide with identified individual-level exposures of importance such as increased exposure to discrimination and hostility. In addition, places with high ethnic density may promote resilience and provide more resources and social support for minority groups. However, it is unclear whether these individual- and region-level exposures are directly related to psychotic disorder.

Underlying mechanisms

Stress sensitivity

One proposed mechanism for linking the environment to psychosis is that of 'sensitization'. This occurs when repeated exposure to adversity leads to a progressively greater response to new stressors. There is evidence that people with an increased risk for psychosis demonstrate a sensitized response over time, which may be expressed at the cognitive (e.g. incorrectly perceiving neutral facial expressions as angry), behavioural (e.g. psychotic hyper-reactivity to stressors), and neural levels (e.g. increased reactivity in social-emotional circuitry) (Morgan et al., 2019). Given the high prevalence of social adversity in minorities, it is conceivable that their increased likelihood of developing psychosis is the result of a sensitized stress response. However, Gevonden et al. (2016) examined reactivity to daily stress in a sample of Moroccan and Dutch men, using experience sampling and an experimental exposure to social peer evaluations, and found no evidence that reactivity to stressors was more pronounced among Moroccan men.

There has been some research trying to connect the social environment to structural and functional alterations in the brain (Meyer-Lindenberg & Tost, 2012). Identifying the neurobiological correlates of social adversities among minorities may provide a direct link with psychotic disorder. The major advantage of this approach is that it circumvents reporting biases and measurement error inherent to observational studies. There is tentative evidence for increased functional connectivity of the anterior cingulate cortex in response to stress among minorities. However, this line of work is still in its infancy.

A sociodevelopmental pathway to psychosis

It has been suggested that a sociodevelopmental pathway may account for the high rates of psychosis in many migrant and minority populations (Morgan et al., 2010; Morgan et al., 2019). This model proposes that cumulative disadvantage in early life may impact neurobiological function and lead to the development of an enduring liability to psychosis among individuals with underlying genetic risk. This liability may be initially expressed by low-level psychotic experiences, which may evolve into full-blown disorder in the context of exposures to new stressors and/or high-potency cannabis. A key element of the model is that for a proportion of individuals social contextual factors are the primary drivers of the onset of psychotic illness. As a consequence, in populations where such exposures are more common it is expected that rates of psychosis will be higher. It may be this, then, that explains, for example, high rates in certain migrant and ethnic minority populations.

Implications and future directions

Although there is accumulating evidence suggesting a role of the social context in the excess risk of psychosis among migrant and ethnic minority populations, many questions remain. Migration and ethnicity are not risk factors in themselves and the evidence suggests they are proxies for exposures that modify the risk of psychosis. Future research needs to elucidate the underlying mechanisms so that the origins of psychotic illness can be better understood and more effective interventions can be designed and implemented. Given the drastic lack of diversity in this line of research, new studies should expand to more geographical and sociocultural contexts, especially in the Global South.

References

Adebimpe, V. R. (1981). Overview: white norms and psychiatric diagnosis of Black patients. *Am J Psychiatry, 138*(3), 279–285.

Ajnakina, O., et al. (2017). Patterns of illness and care over the 5 years following onset of psychosis in different ethnic groups; the GAP-5 study. *Soc Psychiatry Psychiatr Epidemiol, 52*(9), 1101–1111.

Anderson, K. K., et al. (2015). Incidence of psychotic disorders among first-generation immigrants and refugees in Ontario. *CMAJ, 187*(9), E279–E286.

Anglin, D. M., et al. (2021). From womb to neighborhood: a racial analysis of social determinants of psychosis in the United States. *Am J Psychiatry, 178*(7), 599–610.

Bekkar, B., et al. (2020). Association of air pollution and heat exposure with preterm birth, low birth weight, and stillbirth in the US: a systematic review. *JAMA Netw Open, 3*(6), e208243.

Bhopal, R., & Rankin, J. (1999). Concepts and terminology in ethnicity, race and health: be aware of the ongoing debate. *Br Dent J, 186*(10), 483–484.

Bourque, F., van der Ven, E., & Malla A. (2011). A meta-analysis of the risk for psychotic disorders among first- and second-generation immigrants. *Psychol Med, 41*(5), 897–910.

Brandt, L., et al. (2019). Risk of psychosis among refugees: a systematic review and meta-analysis. *JAMA Psychiatry, 76*(11), 1133–1140.

Bresnahan, M., et al. (2007). Race and risk of schizophrenia in a US birth cohort: another example of health disparity? *Int J Epidemiol, 36*(4), 751–758.

Cannon, M., Jones, P. B., & Murray, R. M. (2002). Obstetric complications and schizophrenia: historical and meta-analytic review. *Am J Psychiatry, 159*(7), 1080–1092.

Cantor-Graae, E., et al. (2003). Migration as a risk factor for schizophrenia: a Danish population-based cohort study. *Br J Psychiatry, 182*, 117–122.

Cochrane, R. & Bal, S. S. (1989). Mental hospital admission rates of immigrants to England: a comparison of 1971 and 1981. *Soc Psychiatry Psychiatr Epidemiol, 24*(1), 2–11.

Coid, J. W., et al. (2008). Raised incidence rates of all psychoses among migrant groups: findings from the East London first episode psychosis study. *Arch Gen Psychiatry, 65*(11), 1250–1258.

Crow, T. (2000). Schizophrenia as the price that *Homo sapiens* pays for language: a resolution of the central paradox in the origin of the species. *Brain Res Brain Res Rev, 31*, 118–129.

Das-Munshi, J., et al. (2012). Ethnic density as a buffer for psychotic experiences: findings from a national survey (EMPIRIC). *Br J Psychiatry, 201*(4), 282–290.

Di Forti, M., et al. (2009). High-potency cannabis and the risk of psychosis. *Br J Psychiatry, 195*(6), 488–491.

Di Forti, M., et al. (2019). The contribution of cannabis use to variation in the incidence of psychotic disorder across Europe (EU-GEI): a multicentre case-control study. *Lancet Psychiatry, 6*(5), 427–436.

Dykxhoorn, J., et al. (2020). Association of neighbourhood migrant density and risk of non-affective psychosis: a national, longitudinal cohort study. *Lancet Psychiatry, 7*(4), 327–336.

Faris, R. & Dunham, H. (1939). *Mental disorders in urban areas*. Chicago, IL: University of Chicago Press.

Freeman, D. (2016). Persecutory delusions: a cognitive perspective on understanding and treatment. *Lancet Psychiatry, 3*(7), 685–692.

Gara, M. A., et al. (2019). A naturalistic study of racial disparities in diagnoses at an outpatient behavioral health clinic. *Psychiatr Serv, 70*(2), 130–134.

Gevonden, M., et al. (2016). Reactivity to social stress in ethnic minority men. *Psychiatry Res, 246*, 629–636.

Giurgescu, C., et al. (2012). Relationships among neighborhood environment, racial discrimination, psychological distress, and preterm birth in African American women. *J Obstet Gynecol Neonatal Nurs, 41*(6), E51–E61.

Harnett, N. G. (2020). Neurobiological consequences of racial disparities and environmental risks: a critical gap in understanding psychiatric disorders. *Neuropsychopharmacology, 45*(8), 1247–1250.

Harrison, G., Owens, D., Holton, A., Neilson, D., & Boot, D. (1988). A prospective study of severe mental disorder in Afro-Caribbean patients. *Psychol Med, 18*, 643–657.

Hathaway, Y. (2021). "They Made us into a Race. We Made Ourselves into a People": a corpus study of contemporary Black American Group identity in the non-fictional writings of Ta-Nehisi Coates. *Corpus Pragmatics, 5*(3), 313–334.

Hickling, F. W., McKenzie, K., Mullen, R., & Murray, R. (1999). A Jamaican psychiatrist evaluates diagnoses at a London psychiatric hospital. *Br J Psychiatry, 175*, 283–286.

Hogerzeil, S. J., et al. (2017). Incidence of schizophrenia among migrants in the Netherlands: a direct comparison of first contact longitudinal register approaches. *Soc Psychiatry Psychiatr Epidemiol, 52*(2), 147–154.

Hollander, A. C., et al. (2016). Refugee migration and risk of schizophrenia and other non-affective psychoses: cohort study of 1.3 million people in Sweden. *BMJ, 352*, i1030.

Hutchinson, G., et al. (1997). The increased rate of psychosis among African-Caribbeans in Britain is not due to an excess of pregnancy and birth complications. *Br J Psychiatry, 171*, 145–147.

Jablensky, A., et al. (1992). Schizophrenia: manifestations, incidence and course in different cultures: a World Health Organization ten-country study. *Psychol Med, 20*(Supplement 20), 1–97.

Janssen, I., et al. (2004). Childhood abuse as a risk factor for psychotic experiences. *Acta Psychiatr Scand, 109*(1), 38–45.

Jongsma, H. E., et al. (2021). Social disadvantage, linguistic distance, ethnic minority status and first-episode psychosis: results from the EU-GEI case-control study. *Psychol Med, 51*(9), 1536–1548.

Jongsma, H. E., et al. (2018). Treated incidence of psychotic disorders in the multinational EU-GEI study. *JAMA Psychiatry, 75*(1), 36–46.

Kake, T. R., Arnold, R., & Ellis, P. (2008). Estimating the prevalence of schizophrenia among New Zealand Maori: a capture-recapture approach. *Aust N Z J Psychiatry, 42*(11), 941–949.

Kane, J. C., et al. (2014). Mental, neurological, and substance use problems among refugees in primary health care: analysis of the Health Information System in 90 refugee camps. *BMC Med, 12*, 228.

Karlsen, S. & Nazroo, J. (2002). Relation between racial discrimination, social class and health among ethnic minority groups. *Am J Public Health, 92*, 624–631.

Kirkbride, J. B., et al. (2008). Testing the association between the incidence of schizophrenia and social capital in an urban area. *Psychol Med, 38*(8), 1083–1094.

Leao, T. S., et al. (2006). Incidence of schizophrenia or other psychoses in first- and second-generation immigrants: a national cohort study. *J Nerv Ment Dis, 194*(1), 27–33.

Linscott, R. J. & van Os, J. (2013). An updated and conservative systematic review and meta-analysis of epidemiological evidence on psychotic experiences in children and adults: on the pathway from proneness to persistence to dimensional expression across mental disorders. *Psychol Med, 43*(6), 1133–1149.

Littlewood, R. & Lipsedge, M. (1997). *Aliens and alienists: ethnic minorities and psychiatry*, 3rd edition. London; New York: Routledge, xvi, 352.

Lynge, I. & Jacobsen, J. (1995). Schizophrenia in Greenland: a follow-up study. *Acta Psychiatr Scand, 91*(6), 414–422.

Mazzoncini, R., et al. (2010). Illicit substance use and its correlates in first episode psychosis. *Acta Psychiatr Scand, 121*(5), 351–358.

McGrath, J. (2011). Migrant status, vitamin D and risk of schizophrenia. *Psychol Med, 41*(4), 892–893; author reply 894.

McGrath, J. J. (2007). The surprisingly rich contours of schizophrenia epidemiology. *Arch Gen Psychiatry, 64*(1), 14–16.

McGrath, J. J. (2006). Variations in the incidence of schizophrenia: data versus dogma. *Schizophr Bull, 32*(1), 195–197.

Metzl, J. (2009). *The protest psychosis: how schizophrenia became a Black disease*. Boston, MA: Beacon Press, xxi, 246.

Meyer-Lindenberg, A. & Tost, H. (2012). Neural mechanisms of social risk for psychiatric disorders. *Nat Neurosci, 15*(5), 663–668.

Morgan, C., et al. (2008). Cumulative social disadvantage, ethnicity and first-episode psychosis: a case-control study. *Psychol Med, 38*(12), 1701–1715.

Morgan, C., et al. (2017). Ethnicity and long-term course and outcome of psychotic disorders in a UK sample: the AESOP-10 study. *Br J Psychiatry, 211*(2), 88–94.

Morgan, C., et al. (2009). Ethnicity, social disadvantage and psychotic-like experiences in a healthy population based sample. *Acta Psychiatr Scand, 119*(3), 226–235.

Morgan, C., et al. (2010). Migration, ethnicity, and psychosis: toward a sociodevelopmental model. *Schizophr Bull, 36*(4), 655–664.

Morgan, C., et al. (2007). Parental separation, loss and psychosis in different ethnic groups: a case-control study. *Psychol Med, 37*(4), 495–503.

Morgan, C., Knowles, G., & Hutchinson, G. (2019). Migration, ethnicity and psychoses: evidence, models and future directions. *World Psychiatry, 18*(3), 247–258.

Mukherjee, S., et al. (1983). Misdiagnosis of schizophrenia in bipolar patients: a multiethnic comparison. *Am J Psychiatry, 140*(12), 1571–1574.

O'Donoghue, B., et al. (2021). Risk of psychotic disorders in migrants to Australia. *Psychol Med, 51*(7), 1192–1200.

Paksarian, D., et al. (2016). Racial-ethnic disparities in empirically-derived subtypes of subclinical psychosis among a US sample of youths. *Schizophr Res, 170*(1), 205–210.

Pearce, J., et al. (2019). Perceived discrimination and psychosis: a systematic review of the literature. *Soc Psychiatry Psychiatr Epidemiol, 54*(9), 1023–1044.

Reininghaus, U., et al. (2010). Ethnic identity, perceptions of disadvantage, and psychosis: findings from the AESOP study. *Schizophr Res, 124*(1–3), 43–48.

Selten, J. P., van der Ven, E., & Termorshuizen, F. (2020). Migration and psychosis: a meta-analysis of incidence studies. *Psychol Med, 50*(2), 303–313.

Selten, J. P., et al. (2002). Odegaard's selection hypothesis revisited: schizophrenia in Surinamese immigrants to The Netherlands. *Am J Psychiatry, 159*(4), 669–671.

Sharpley, M., et al. (2001). Understanding the excess of psychosis among the African-Caribbean population in England. Review of current hypotheses. *Br J Psychiatry Suppl, 40,* s60–s68.

Tapsell, R., Hallett, C., & Mellsop, G. (2018). The rate of mental health service use in New Zealand as analysed by ethnicity. *Australas Psychiatry, 26*(3), 290–293.

Tarricone, I., et al. (2016). Risk of psychosis and internal migration: results from the Bologna First Episode Psychosis study. *Schizophr Res, 173*(1–2), 90–93.

Termorshuizen, F., et al. (2022). The incidence of psychotic disorders among migrants and minority ethnic groups in Europe: findings from the multinational EU-GEI study. *Psychol Med, 52*(7), 1376–1385.

Tortelli, A., et al. (2018). Subclinical psychosis in adult migrants and ethnic minorities: systematic review and meta-analysis. *BJPsych Open, 4*(6), 510–518.

van der Ven, E. & Selten, J. P. (2018). Migrant and ethnic minority status as risk indicators for schizophrenia: new findings. *Curr Opin Psychiatry, 31*(3), 231–236.

van Os, J., et al. (2009). A systematic review and meta-analysis of the psychosis continuum: evidence for a psychosis proneness-persistence-impairment model of psychotic disorder. *Psychol Med, 39*(2), 179–195.

Vanheusden, K., et al. (2008). Associations between ethnicity and self-reported hallucinations in a population sample of young adults in The Netherlands. *Psychol Med, 38*(8), 1095–1102.

Veen, N., et al. (2002). Use of illicit substances in a psychosis incidence cohort: a comparison among different ethnic groups in the Netherlands. *Acta Psychiatr Scand, 105*(6), 440–443.

Veling, W. & Susser, E. (2011). Migration and psychotic disorders. *Expert Rev Neurother, 11*(1), 65–76.

Veling, W., et al. (2008a). Cannabis use and genetic predisposition for schizophrenia: a case-control study. *Psychol Med, 38*(9), 1251–1256.

Veling, W., et al. (2008b). Discrimination and the incidence of psychotic disorders among ethnic minorities in The Netherlands. *Int J Epidemiol, 36*(4), 761–768.

Veling, W., et al. (2008c). Ethnic density of neighbourhoods and incidence of psychotic disorder among immigrants. *Am J Psychiatry, 165,* 66–73.

Veling, W., et al. (2010). Ethnic identity and the risk of schizophrenia in ethnic minorities: a case-control study. *Schizophr Bull, 36*(6), 1149–1156.

Veling, W., et al. (2006). Incidence of schizophrenia among ethnic minorities in the Netherlands: a four-year first-contact study. *Schizophr Res, 86*(1–3), 189–193.

Wang, E., et al. (2020). Social determinants of pregnancy-related mortality and morbidity in the United States: a systematic review. *Obstet Gynecol, 135*(4), 896–915.

Weiser, M., et al. (2008). Elaboration on immigration and risk for schizophrenia. *Psychol Med, 38*(8), 1113–1119.

Wilson, C., et al. (2016). Context matters: the impact of neighborhood crime and paranoid symptoms on psychosis risk assessment. *Schizophr Res, 171*(1–3), 56–61.

Zammit, S., et al. (2010). Individuals, schools, and neighborhood: a multilevel longitudinal study of variation in incidence of psychotic disorders. *Arch Gen Psychiatry, 67*(9), 914–922.

Zhu, Y., et al. (2018). Association between migrant worker experience, limitations on insurance coverage, and hospitalization for schizophrenia in Hunan Province, China. *Schizophr Res, 197*, 93–97.

3

Psychosis across persons 2: Poverty, trauma, and sociodevelopment

Charlotte Gayer-Anderson,
Stephanie Beards, and Ulrich Reininghaus

Introduction

This chapter will critically review current research on, and models of, the aetiology of psychosis, paying particular attention to the limited research on social risk factors in settings beyond North America, Europe, and Australia (herein the 'Global North'). Our understanding of the risk architecture for psychoses has transformed in recent years due to a number of developments in genetics, neuroscience, and epidemiology. It is now evident, for example, that the complex confluence of factors that influence onset includes environmental factors, both social (e.g. trauma) and non-social (e.g. infection), operating at both area and individual levels over the life course. The two primary questions this chapter will address are: What is known about socioenvironmental risk factors for psychosis in the 'Global South', and how does this depart from the knowledge base in the Global North? What is the value, and the methodological and logistical challenges, of extending research to more diverse settings where the distribution of risk factors differs (e.g. poverty, trauma, substance use, etc.)? The effects of poverty and trauma, their association with *psychotic experiences*, will also be considered in this chapter, given that these have been reported to be (phenomenologically and temporarily) continuous with psychotic disorder, reflecting an extended psychosis phenotype. In addition, psychotic experiences are known to share some of the same demographic, environmental, and psychopathological risk factors with psychotic disorders (Linscott & van Os, 2013; van Os & Linscott, 2012), and therefore provide a useful foundation from which to examine the aetiology of psychosis.

Contemporary models of psychosis seek to explain onset through the integration of biological, social, and psychological mechanisms (Reininghaus

& Morgan, 2014). According to Howes and Murray's (2014) latest aetiological model of psychosis, the three predominant theories (dopamine, neurodevelopmental, cognitive), can be thought to co-exist under one uniting framework. It is now proposed that neurodevelopmental changes due to genetic variation, prenatal and perinatal hazards, and exposure to childhood adversity sensitize the dopamine system in the brain, and can result in increased dopamine synthesis and release. Alongside this, experiences of social adversity can bias an individual's cognitive schema to view themselves and the world around them in a more negative and threatening light. When an individual experiences further stress, this activates the dopamine system which may cause the misattribution of salience to certain stimuli, and an interpretation based on biased cognitive processes. For some individuals, these experiences can lead to psychotic symptoms such as paranoia and hallucinations, which in turn cause further stress and confusion. The experience of these early symptoms is proposed to lead to a vicious cycle, and the excess strain on the dopamine system can contribute to development of psychotic symptoms that eventually become hardwired and resistant to change (Howes & Murray, 2014). It is important to note that this integrated aetiological model was developed mostly based on research from North America, Europe, and Australia. This chapter aims to assess how these ideas may need to be modified in light of research from the Global South.

Neurodevelopmental and non-social risk factors

There is evidence that obstetric complications, such as prenatal exposure to infection (e.g. influenza, rubella, poliovirus, and toxoplasmosis) and perinatal hazards (e.g. low birthweight, caesarean section, hypoxia), are associated with an increased risk of schizophrenia in offspring in countries in the Global North (Brown & Derkits, 2010; Cannon et al., 2002; Khandaker et al., 2013). Nutritional deficiency in pregnancy has also been found to be associated with an increased risk of schizophrenia in offspring (van Os & Reininghaus, 2017). A twofold increase in the risk of schizophrenia was reported in the children of mothers who were exposed to the Dutch famine during early gestation (Susser et al., 1996). Further, an excess of markers of altered neurodevelopment, early cognitive impairment, and social problems in childhood have been linked to an increased risk of schizophrenia (Bramon et al., 2005; Jones et al., 1994; Reichenberg et al., 2010). Given that neurodevelopmental risk factors such as infectious diseases and nutritional deficiencies are common in many countries in the Global South (Darnton-Hill & Mkparu, 2015; Gomwalk &

Ahmad, 1989), these need to be considered as potentially important factors that confer risk.

Lambo first noted an increased risk of psychotic disorders in offspring exposed to obstetric complications in Nigeria in the mid-1950s (Lambo, 1960). Similar associations between obstetric complications and risk of psychosis have also been observed in later Nigerian studies by Gureje et al. (1994) and Ibukun et al. (2015). This latter study further reported a lag in the attainment of developmental milestones in early onset psychosis patients. Nutritional deficiencies in pregnancy have been found in studies of the Chinese famine of 1959–1961 that reported prenatal exposure to famine to be associated with an increased risk of schizophrenia in later life (St Clair et al., 2005; Wang & Zhang, 2017; Xu et al., 2009). These putative neurodevelopmental risk factors all require further replication in the Global South, but are potential targets for preventive interventions (van Dyke, 2013). Chapter 4 will provide a detailed review of these factors in the context of genetic and other biological risk factors.

Childhood adversity and family functioning

Research on the impact of childhood adversity (e.g. sexual abuse, physical abuse, neglect, bullying, parental separation) in the development of psychosis has been extensively studied in Western Europe, Australia, and, to a lesser extent, North America (e.g. Varese et al., 2012; Matheson et al., 2013), though there remain some methodological limitations impeding any inferences on possible causal associations (Morgan & Gayer-Anderson, 2016). Studies of these associations in the Global South remain scarce, despite assertions that considerations of cultural influence should be required when interpreting findings of any research on childhood adversity and mental health outcomes (e.g. Korbin, 1991). For instance, there is evidence to suggest that family structure, functioning, and relationships can differ across contexts and geographical locations (Punch, 2016). Differences may include the value placed on connectedness, interdependence, and group cohesion, which—while clearly an oversimplification to divide the world into two camps on the basis of GDP—may be reduced, on average, in high-income societies compared with the rest of the world. High-income settings in the Global North are also typically characterized by the more limited availability of extended family than in the majority of the world (Kim et al., 2001; Social Trends Institute, 2015), although clearly there is variation within and between countries of the Global South. Such environments could plausibly buffer, or conversely compound, the effects of specific traumatic events or adverse environments in childhood. On the other hand, it has been argued that children in many cultures in the Global South (e.g. Arab, Asian, African) will more likely judge an authoritarian style of punishment and discipline as a normative duty of parents and teachers (e.g. Saif Al Dawla, 2001). This could conceivably affect associations if it is the subjective emotional impact (both immediate and longer-term reflections on the event), as opposed to the act of perpetration, that is implicated in the aetiology of psychosis.

A few studies would appear to corroborate this latter standpoint. In one such study conducted in Kenya (Mamah et al., 2016), there was no difference in reported physical abuse or sexual abuse between a group of secondary school students identified as being at high risk of psychosis (n 135) and those considered at low risk (n 142). By contrast, more negative relationships with family members, death or separation from someone in the family, and perceived loneliness were more common in individuals considered to be at risk of psychosis. Similarly, in a South African sample of first-episode psychosis patients (n 77) and matched controls (n 52), no differences were found between the two groups in the prevalence of various types of childhood abuse (physical, sexual, emotional) or neglect (physical, emotional) (as measured by the Childhood Trauma Questionnaire—CTQ) (Kilian et al., 2017). The authors explained this difference due to high overall adversity in both patients and controls compared with other similar studies, which is consistent with a recent meta-analysis of 189 studies that found childhood trauma to be much more prevalent in low- and middle-income countries (LMICs) compared with high-income countries (HICs) (according to World Bank criteria, 2013) (Viola et al., 2016).

By contrast, other studies from the Global South provide evidence that appear to be consistent with the majority of findings from countries in the Global North. Binbay et al. (2012), in Izmir, Turkey, found evidence of a linear association between adversity in childhood (death of a parent, divorce, and separation from parents) and varying levels of symptoms, from subclinical to disorder, while Şahin et al. (2013) reported more frequent emotional and physical neglect, and emotional and physical abuse in both a group of individuals with ultra-high risk of psychosis (n 41) and with a first-episode psychosis (n 83), compared with a control group (n 69) in Istanbul, Turkey. In a study of 284 undergraduate men in Durbin, South Africa, contact forms of sexual abuse were associated with higher paranoid ideation and psychoticism traits compared with no abuse (Collings, 1995). No differences were found in these measures between those who reported non-contact forms of sexual abuse and no abuse. Similarly, in a sample of 1,672 adolescents from South Korea, scores of psychoticism and paranoid ideation were found to be higher in young people who reported incestuous experiences compared with their non-victimized counterparts (Kim & Kim, 2005). Finally, Li et al. (2014a) found psychoticism to be associated with emotional and sexual abuse, and emotional and physical neglect, but not physical abuse. The authors attribute the negative finding for physical abuse to commonly used proverbs in China, such as 'No beating, no success' and 'Spare the rod, spoil the child', thus potentially predisposing young people to being tolerant to harsh forms of physical discipline.

An analysis of Global School-based Student Health Survey (GSHS) data from 19 LMICs (n 104,614 students) found the prevalence of bullying to vary markedly across cultures, with generally lower rates in Asian countries (8% to 28%) and higher in Africa (26% to 61%) (Fleming & Jacobsen, 2009). However, studies exploring the impact of bullying on psychosis are lacking. Experiences of bullying were found to be higher in high-school students deemed at ultra-high risk of psychosis compared with 'healthy' controls in a cross-sectional survey conducted in South Korea (Kang et al., 2012), as well as Chinese adolescents who scored highly on measures of paranoid ideation and psychosis proneness (Li et al., 2014b).

Very few studies have considered cross-cultural differences in the association between childhood adversity and psychosis. One notable study by McGrath and colleagues (2017), using the WHO World Mental Health surveys comprising a sample of 23,998 adults across 18 countries, compared the associations between individual childhood adversities (e.g. family violence, physical abuse, sexual abuse, neglect, separation from or death of a parent) and psychotic experiences across low-, middle-, and high-income countries (according to World Bank criteria, 2003). The authors found no differential impact of individual adversities on reports of psychotic experiences across the three different country groups. In addition, Wüsten & Lincoln (2017) found no difference in the effect of family support during childhood, and satisfaction with family relationships, on psychosis proneness between community samples of individuals living in some countries in the Global South (Chile, Columbia, Indonesia; n 1000) versus those living in Germany or the USA (n 317). By contrast, high criticism among family members was more strongly associated with psychosis proneness in the Global South countries. Further investigation is required to ascertain whether the effects of childhood abuse and adversity are consistent in settings outside the Global North, with particular attention given to the conceptualization of, and attitude towards, abuse and adversity in childhood across different social and religious backgrounds.

Social disadvantage

There has been considerable interest in the complex associations between social disadvantage (e.g. income, unemployment, education level, social status) and mental health outcomes, including the development of psychotic disorders, in the Global North (e.g. Kessler et al., 2005; Jenkins et al., 2008; Read, 2010). However, these associations have been investigated to a far lesser extent in the Global South. While reviews exist for the association between poverty and poverty alleviation interventions and common mental disorders (e.g. Lund et al., 2011; Patel & Kleinman, 2003), investigations into the association between social disadvantage and psychosis in the Global South remain scarce. Of the small number of studies that have considered the impact of social disadvantage on the development of psychosis, findings include those from a large community survey conducted in Tehran, Iran (n 2158) in which unemployment rates were correlated with self-reported psychotic symptoms (Sharifi et al., 2012). An ecological study from South Africa also found higher rates of unemployment in people with first-episode psychosis (n 160) compared with population levels (78% vs. 41%) (Burns & Esterhuizen, 2008).

However, contrary to previous research, some markers of social disadvantage have not been found to be associated with psychosis in the expected way. In the Sharifi et al. (2012) study, *higher* education level was associated with self-reported psychotic experiences, and hypothesized associations were not found for lower income levels. Similar findings have also been found in Uganda where higher education has been found to be associated with an increased prevalence of delusional ideation in a sample of 80 young adults aged between 18 and 30 years (Lundberg et al., 2004), and in a Tanzanian study (n 899), where those earning an income were more likely to report psychotic symptoms compared with those who were not, and also those living in rooms/flats were less likely to report psychotic symptoms compared with those living in a house (Jenkins et al., 2010).

A further study which compared Black Caribbean patients with first-onset schizophrenia recruited in London (n=38) compared with a similar sample recruited from Trinidad (n=46) found interesting differences in unemployment rates between the patient groups (Bhugra et al., 2000). The London sample had much higher rates of unemployment compared with the general population (80% in the patient group compared with 21.9% in the general population), whereas rates in Trinidad were broadly similar (unemployment rate for individuals aged 15–64 years in Trinidad was 18.5% compared with 14.8% in the patient group). One possible explanation for these findings may be that these markers (i.e. high unemployment, higher education levels, more cramped living conditions) represent a proxy for urban living, a risk factor which has shown strong links to psychosis (Vassos et al., 2012; see Chapter 1). It may be that the impact of city living on mental health outcomes poses even more of a risk for Global South societies due to rapidly increasing urban populations (Menezes, 2014). Moreover, the broader concept of social disadvantage and poverty varies widely not only across countries in the Global North and South, but even within low-resource settings (Maselko, 2017). As a consequence, the heterogeneous findings for the role of socioeconomic disadvantage are likely attributable to the weak, inconsistent, and culturally insensitive conceptualization and measurement of these factors.

Adult life events

Further, there is evidence of an association between stressful life events and psychosis from studies in the Global North. For example, a meta-analysis indicated around a threefold increase in risk after exposure to life events (Beards et al., 2013), albeit with some methodological limitations (e.g. cross-sectional studies with small sample sizes, inconsistent measurement of life events, mixed first-episode and non-first-episode samples, and absent or poorly selected control group). Although fewer research studies have investigated the association outside of Europe and North America, researchers have sporadically investigated cross-cultural variation over the past several decades. One of the early WHO-sponsored studies, conducted by Day and colleagues (Day et al., 1987), found an association between recent life events and psychosis in six out of nine international study settings, including sites within India, Japan, and Columbia, therefore providing some evidence for the cross-cultural replicability of the life events–psychosis relationship (Day et al., 1987). Despite the large sample size of this landmark study (n=386 first-episode psychosis patients), it is limited by the lack of a comparison group. However, support for this association has also been found in the Global South using a case–control design. A Saudi Arabian case–control study (cases n=48; controls n=62) found that people with first-episode psychosis reported more life events compared with controls in the immediate period prior to onset (Al Khani et al., 1986), and a more recent case–control study (n 367 first-episode cases and n 367 population controls matched for sex, age, and neighbourhood) conducted in Brazil also found that recent adverse life events were associated with an increased odds of developing a first episode of psychosis (Menezes, 2013).

There is also evidence to suggest that an association is present when considering psychotic-like experiences within the general population. A Tanzania-based study of 899 adults aged 15–59 years found an association between the number of stressful life events and prevalence of psychotic symptoms, with a fivefold increase for those reporting two or more stressful life events in the previous six months (Jenkins et al., 2010). Interestingly, associations were not found for those reporting just one life event, which is suggestive of a possible threshold effect. Similar effects have also been found in an Ethiopian study (n

2000) where the experience of six or more stressful life events in the past year was associated with a twofold increase in a high score on a measure of psychosis (Tafari et al., 1991), and a study conducted in an urban area in Iran also found an independent association between recent stressful life events and increased prevalence of self-reported paranoia and psychoticism (Sharifi et al., 2012). It is worth noting, however, that these studies, being cross-sectional, do not make it possible to test for temporal priority, making it difficult to discern whether psychotic symptoms were experienced before or after exposure to recent life events.

Further, findings are not always consistent. An early Nigerian study did not find any association between first-episode psychosis and recent life events (Gureje & Adewunmi, 1988). Intriguingly, it was the control subjects (n 50) who reported more life events than patients (n=42), which also matches findings from the early WHO study in their Nigerian site (Day et al., 1987). One possibility is that their life events measures were unable to capture issues related to the rapid societal changes occurring at that place and time, and this could partially explain the lack of association. Another study compared the recent life event history of those with an onset of acute and transient psychotic disorder (n 18) with those with bipolar disorder (n 20) in an Indian setting (Chakraborty et al., 2007), and similarly did not find evidence for an increased number of life events in those with recent onset psychosis. But these individuals did report experiencing more 'undesirable' events over which the individual had little control, which suggests that the contextual aspects of the life events may also play an important role.

Another important consideration is the type of events which could contribute to the development of psychosis. Child mortality may be more than twelve-times higher in LMICs compared with HICs (UNICEF, 2014), and researchers have begun to investigate the aetiological relevance of this type of exposure. Using self-report data from the World Health Survey and restricting the analysis to 44 LMICs (n 59,444 women aged 18–49 years), Koyanagi et al. (2017) found a higher prevalence of psychotic experiences (16% vs. 11.8%) in women who had experienced child death—arguably the most stressful and traumatic event that a parent can experience. In addition to this specific event, other stressful experiences (including those associated with poor health systems) during pregnancy, birth, and early infancy, may also further increase the risk of psychosis. The researchers also highlighted the important contribution of depressive symptoms, as the association between child death and psychosis was less marked after adjustment for depression, except for delusions of control. These findings suggest a complex interaction between psychosis and depression after exposure to stressful life events.

Racial discrimination

Evidence from the Global North has indicated an increase in psychosis across migrant groups, especially among individuals migrating from countries where the majority population is Black (e.g. Bourque et al., 2011; Kirkbride et al., 2012; see Chapter 2). However, research also suggests that migrants do not come from settings with particularly high rates of psychosis (Bhugra et al., 1996; Mahy et al., 1999). This suggests that it may be the social experience and conditions of being a migrant or belonging to a minority ethnic group that contributes to the increased risk of developing psychosis. However, what is not clear is whether individuals from ethnic minorities living in countries in the Global South have similarly higher rates of psychosis compared with the native-born population, perhaps as a result of increased ethnic or cultural discrimination. Limited research evidence suggests that ethnic discrimination could indeed increase the risk of mental illness in non-Western countries. So, for example, a national household survey conducted in South Africa (n 4351 adults aged 18 years and over) found experience of ethnic and non-ethnic discrimination to be associated with an increased risk of any DSM-IV disorder, including mood, anxiety, and substance use disorders, but the presence of psychotic disorders was not measured in this study (Moomal et al., 2009). It is worth noting that this association was notably attenuated when adjustment was made for other sources of social stress, including stressful life events, and interestingly, non-ethnic discrimination was found to be more strongly associated with mental health outcomes than ethnic discrimination. The authors consider the South African context in explaining these findings, and propose that their nation's long and complicated history of ethnic discrimination against Black groups may have increased coping and equipped individuals to better handle this type of discrimination (Moomal et al., 2009).

Social isolation, social networks, and support

While many have argued that dissatisfactory relationships are a consequence of psychosis and impending illness, there is evidence to suggest that social isolation and a lack of social support are implicated in the onset of psychosis (Gayer-Anderson & Morgan, 2013). Outside of high-income countries, the findings of the association between marital status, social network size, and perceived social support with psychosis are mixed.

Jenkins et al. (2015) carried out an epidemiological household survey to study the prevalence of psychotic symptoms and their risk factors in Nyanza province, Kenya (n 1158). Being single was associated with twofold increased odds of psychotic symptoms, while there was no association between size of social network, and results indicative of *higher* levels of social support being associated with the presence of at least one psychotic symptom. In a comparative study conducted in Tanzania's largest city, Dar es Salaam, in a household survey of 899 respondents, none of the indices of social isolation (marital status, social network size, and perceived social support) were associated with psychotic symptoms once adjusting for recent life events, past-year cannabis use, and common mental disorders (Jenkins et al., 2010). In a door-to-door survey of close to 68,500 individuals living in rural Ethiopia, individuals who had never been married, compared with those in a relationship, had almost three times the odds of non-affective psychosis, and over six times the odds for those who were widowed, divorced, or separated (Kebede et al., 2004). Moreover, interactions were found between marital status and sex, age, and area of residence, such that the observed joint effects of marital status was higher than the expected joint OR for men, those over the age of 35, and those living in more rural areas. In a representative general population survey (n 1,268) in Izmir, Turkey, Alptekin et al. (2009) found that low perceived support was associated with over a fourfold odds of reporting psychotic symptoms (OR=4.5, 95% CI 2.3–8.6), while no association was found for single marital status. However, in a larger, more recent survey of 4,011 residents from the Izmir population, a linear association was found between single marital status and the five groups of increasing clinical severity of psychosis (Binbay et al., 2012). As with research in the Global North, the vast majority of these studies are cross-sectional, thereby limiting the inferences that can be made on the direction of these effects. Nevertheless, these varied findings may be a consequence of the fact that the bearing of positive as well as negative aspects of social networks (e.g. support vs. shame) implicate themselves differently across different cultural settings. For example, as mentioned earlier, there is a higher prevalence of multigenerational and family households in many community-based cultures compared with those that are individual-focused, and therefore, it has been postulated that higher levels of support are expected and received from family members (Maselko, 2017). Conversely, the shame and stigma surrounding an individual's mental health may introduce difficulties in activating one's social network, or receiving help from one's network when needed. Within the context of Asian societies, Saw and Okazaki (2012) comment that psychosis signifies 'more than an individual affliction, and family members must conceal the individual's mental illness or shun him or her in order to maintain the social network'.

Finally, the use of information communication technology is rapidly evolving, and is now a routine part of individuals' daily lives, via the internet, mobile, or smartphone applications, social media networks, not only in HICs but also in LMICs. The WHO (2011) has commented that 'the penetration of mobile phone networks in many LMICs surpasses other infrastructure such as paved roads, and electricity, and dwarfs fixed internet deployment'. In contrast to findings from HICs, where mobile phone usage has been shown to be associated with higher stress levels (e.g. Thomée et al., 2011), studies in low-resource settings have shown mobile phone usage to be associated with better mental health (e.g. Pearson et al., 2017), particularly in contexts where families and significant others lived faraway. A new avenue of research would therefore be also beneficial to the question of whether ownership and use of information communication technology may be detrimental or protective in the context of psychosis onset in LMICs.

Substance use

Cannabis is the most widely used illicit substance in the world. Global prevalence estimates suggest around 3.9% of adults use cannabis on an annual basis, and there are substantial fluctuations in use across different parts of the world. The estimated percentage of adult cannabis consumption in the past year includes 1.9% in Asia, 2.3% in South and South-Eastern Europe, 5.9% in South America, and 7.5% in Africa (UNODC, 2015). Research studies from the Global North suggest strong links between cannabis use and psychosis, both experiences within the general population and in those with psychotic disorders (Di Forti et al., 2015; Van Gastel et al., 2014). Only a handful of studies have investigated this association in a Global South country, one being as long ago as 1896, when the psychiatrist T.S. Clouston observed that 40 of 253 individuals in a Cairo asylum had a psychotic-like illness attributable to the use of hashish (Clouston, 1896). Further, studies of early psychosis onset in adolescents across South Africa suggest an important role for cannabis (Lachman et al., 2012; Paruk et al., 2009), with 68.8% (n = 31) of people with first-episode psychosis reporting a history of lifetime cannabis use (Paruk et al., 2013). A community survey of adults in Tanzania (n 899) found higher rates of psychotic symptoms (odds ratio of 8.23) in those who had reported cannabis use in the preceding year (Jenkins et al., 2010). A similar community study of young adults in Trinidad (n 472 participants aged 12–23 years) also found a positive association between cannabis use and self-reported psychotic experiences (Konings et al., 2008). However, associations were only found in those who began smoking cannabis before the age of 14 years, suggesting evidence of developmental specificity, and the importance of documenting early onset of cannabis use. An additional qualitative study involving focus group discussions with caregivers, mental healthcare providers, alternative healers, and key informants, conducted in Trinidad, Nigeria, and India, provided results indicating that the use of cannabis was often cited as a cause of psychosis in the former two sites, but not in India (Cohen et al., 2016).

Another substance which has shown associations with psychotic symptoms is khat; a stimulant plant which produces amphetamine-like effects. It is widely consumed in parts of Africa and the Middle East, namely Somalia, Yeman, Ethiopia, and has been introduced to North America and Europe by migrants and refugees from these countries (Balint et al., 2009). In a large study of Somali combatants (n 8124), paranoid symptoms were found to be more frequent in those who reported using khat compared with non-khat users (8.9% vs. 2.6%), and the risk of paranoia was found to increase with higher khat use (Odenwald et al., 2009). As has been found for cannabis, it is early onset and excessive khat use that is associated with psychosis among Somalian patients (Odenwald et al., 2005). However, the evidence linking khat use and psychosis is still limited due to the small number of studies. The direction of causality remains unclear—is khat able to induce psychosis in those who have never experienced it previously, or does it only exacerbate pre-existing symptoms (Odenwald, 2014)?

War-related trauma and natural disasters

Very few studies have examined the role of exposure to the trauma of armed conflict in relation to psychosis in the Global South (Keraite et al., 2016; Soosay et al., 2012). Soosay et al. (2012), in a post-conflict area in Timor Leste, found a higher prevalence of psychotic experiences in individuals exposed to conflict-related trauma, as measured with the traumatic event inventory of the Harvard Trauma Questionnaire (assessing common traumatic experiences of conflict-affected and refugee populations). There was also some evidence of a dose-response relationship in this study, in that the odds of reporting psychotic experiences increased as the number of potentially traumatic events increased (Soosay et al., 2012). A similar pattern of findings was evident in a recent cross-sectional study in South Sudan, which also reported an increase in the odds of reporting psychotic experiences as the number of potentially traumatic events increased (Ayazi et al., 2016). In the first National Mental Health Survey conducted in Sri Lanka, exposure to one or more conflict-related events and loss or injury of a family member or friend through conflict were associated with increased odds of reporting psychotic experiences (Keraite et al., 2016). The results from this study further suggested that linked and cumulative exposure to conflict-related traumatic events (including exposure to interpersonal violence and threat) was associated with psychotic experiences (Keraite et al., 2016).

Another very important factor that may be relevant to the development of transient and more enduring psychotic experiences in countries in the Global

South is war-related migration including both internal displacement and emigration. There is some indirect evidence on the association between war-related emigration and psychosis from a recent Swedish register study of more than 1.3 million people that reported an increased incidence of schizophrenia and non-affective psychotic disorder in a cohort including migrants and refugees from LMICs, including those affected by various humanitarian crises resulting from conflict (e.g. Afghanistan, Iraq, Iran, various countries in central Africa) as well as famine (e.g. various countries in east Africa), compared with non-refugee migrants and the native-born Swedish population (Hollander et al., 2016). However, the association between war-related internal displacement and migration on the one hand, and psychosis on the other, has been under-researched and, overall, direct evidence on the role of war-related migration as a potential factor contributing to psychosis in the Global South remains scarce. A more detailed account of minority ethnic groups, migration, and psychosis in non-Western countries can be found in Chapter 2.

While several studies have reported that exposure to natural disasters is associated with an increased risk of developing non-psychotic disorders (Dorrington et al., 2014; Ekanayake et al., 2013; Meewisse et al., 2011; van der Velden et al., 2013), to date, only a small number of studies have investigated this exposure in relation to psychosis. Keraite et al. (2014) reported that psychotic experiences were more common in individuals directly exposed to the tsunami disaster of 2002 and in those who had a family member who died or was injured as a result of the tsunami in the Sri Lankan National Mental Health Survey. This finding is consistent with studies from high income countries that suggest parental death is associated with an increased risk of a psychotic disorder (Morgan et al., 2007). A high prevalence of psychotic experiences has also been reported in a sample drawn from the population affected by the 2005 earthquake in Northern Pakistan and Kashmir (Ayub et al., 2015). Living through a natural disaster and armed conflict have also been put forward as potential prenatal hazards that increase the risk of psychosis in the offspring of mothers, who experience significant levels of stress through exposure to such events (van Os & Reininghaus, 2017), which, however, requires further scrutiny in future research.

Conclusion

Environmental factors, operating at both area and individual levels, play a major role in the aetiology of psychosis, interacting with more proximal genetic and neurobiological factors across the life course. The current evidence base for the role of socioenvironmental factors in the onset of psychosis in the Global South is scarce, and much remains unknown. The examples explored in this review, outlined in Table 3.1, of neurodevelopmental factors, childhood trauma and family functioning, socioeconomic status, adult life events, substance use, urbanicity, and more distal life exposures (war-related trauma and natural disasters), suggest that while a considerable body of evidence does indeed translate from the Global North to the Global South, some findings do not.

While there are reassuring indications of a growing emphasis on the importance regarding these determinants on the risk of psychosis in settings outside of North America, Europe, and Australia, there is clearly a need for more high-quality and robust research. Unquestionably, this will benefit from cross-disciplinary collaborations between epidemiologists, psychologists, psychiatrists, anthropologists, and economists (Maselko, 2017). For example, the distribution of, the values placed upon, and connotations associated with, various specific social factors are likely to deviate quite substantially, not only between countries in the Global South, but also from what is observed in the Global North; anthropological work is vital in order to appreciate the differences and nuances of how and why social factors impact the onset of mental health problems in different populations. In addition, Amatrya Sen's Capabilities Approach (Sen, 1999) provides a framework for addressing factors (operating both proximally and distally) and improving social circumstances that are relevant to mental health and well-being. It has recently been used to inform how the global mental health and economic development agendas can be combined to stimulate positive social, cultural, economic, political, and environmental change in LMIC settings (White et al., 2016).

Finally, there is no evidence to suggest that the previously proposed aetiological models of psychosis would not be applicable globally, in broad outline at least. With Howes' and Murray's (2014) model in mind, neurodevelopmental changes as a consequence of genetic variations, in combination with potential prenatal and perinatal insults and exposure to stress in childhood, lead to increased sensitivity of the dopamine system. When compounded with stressful events in adulthood (e.g. threatening or intrusive interpersonal events, war-related trauma, natural disasters), or chronic difficulties (e.g. living in an urban environment, food insecurity and financial stress, or absence of support), this leads to elevated dopamine levels in some brain regions, which can be expressed behaviourally as psychotic experiences or disorder (Walker et al., 2008). There is no reason to believe that such biological mechanisms would behave differently across populations, yet the distribution and personal significance of specific stressors would appear to vary across nations to some degree. This has implications for public health and clinical strategies, and highlights the urgent need to elucidate how these vary across different populations in order to target these determinants more efficiently and effectively in different cultural settings.

Table 3.1 Summary of findings, and some conceptual and methodological considerations.

	Summary of findings	Conceptual and methodological considerations
Neurodevelopmental/Non-social risk factors	Limited amount of research suggests obstetric complications, delayed attainment of developmental milestones, and nutritional deficiencies may be relevant.	Putative neurodevelopmental risk factors require further replication using prospective designs.
Childhood trauma, family functioning	Fragmented relationships with family members (e.g. loss or separation from a parent) appear to more consistently be associated with psychosis in the Global South. Where the research diverges is the impact of various forms of contact abuse or neglect.	There is a need for more robust research exploring different types of adversity in children, as well as consideration of the severity of events. Qualitative and anthropological research may help to elucidate what are meaningful and harmful exposures in childhood in different settings.
Socioeconomic status, education level, poverty	Limited research suggests that markers of social disadvantage, including unemployment, education level, overcrowding may be relevant for psychosis onset. However, differences in the direction of effect may be influenced by level of urbanicity.	Longitudinal research is needed to help establish causal associations and direction of effects between social disadvantage and psychosis. This may help to identify which specific markers are associated with risk of psychotic disorders, as well as highlight factors which may help to reduce risk in those who face social adversity. It is also difficult to accurately assess income in informal low resource economies, and composite indexes of multiple deprivation may be better suited to addressing socioeconomic status and poverty.

(continued)

Table 3.1 Continued

	Summary of findings	Conceptual and methodological considerations
Adult life events & difficulties (including ethnic discrimination, social isolation)	Overall, it appears that, as in Global North, psychotic disorder and psychotic experiences may be preceded by the experience of stressful life events. However, they are clearly not sufficient or necessary for the causation of psychosis and they are likely to have their effects within a larger domain of difficult social circumstances.	Heterogeneity in terms of life events measurement—are studies measuring the same thing; are measures adapted to each cultural context? Need to better understand the context, both within individuals (what are the actual life events that might increase the risk for psychosis?) and the wider country setting (what are the cultural/societal changes that may impact on the types of events experienced?)
Substance use	Limited research suggests a similar association between cannabis use and psychosis to that widely reported in the Global North. Khat is another substance which may contribute to onset and is of particular relevance to certain African and Middle Eastern countries.	Current research in the Global South does not take into account the strength or strain of cannabis used, and whether this is an important consideration. Recent increases in THC-potency have been noted in many Global North countries (Cascini et al., 2012), and this is likely to be the case in some Global South countries. With many cannabis users also preferring high-THC strains (Morgan et al., 2012), the impact this could have on mental health is concerning.
War-related trauma, natural disasters, migration	A few studies have reported exposure to war-related traumatic events and natural disasters to be associated with an increased prevalence of psychotic experiences.	The role of war-related migration, internal displacement in particular, has been under-researched; incidence and case–control studies of first-episode psychosis are required to investigate the potential impact of exposure to war-related trauma, migration, and natural disasters further.

References

Al Khani, M. A. F., Bebbington, P. E., Watson, J. P., & House, F. (1986). Life events and schizophrenia: a Saudi Arabian study. *Br J Psychiatry, 148,* 12–22.

Alptekin, K., Ulas, H., Akdede, B. B., Tümüklü, M., & Akvardar, Y. (2009). Prevalence and risk factors of psychotic symptoms: in the city of Izmir, Turkey. *Soc Psychiatry Psychiatr Epidemiol, 44,* 905.

Ayazi, T., Swartz, L., Eide, A. H., Lien, L., & Hauff, E. (2016). Psychotic-like experiences in a conflict-affected population: a cross-sectional study in South Sudan. *Soc Psychiatry Psychiatr Epidemiol, 51,* 971–979.

Ayub, M., Saeed, K., Kingdon, D., & Naeem, F. (2015). Rate and predictors of psychotic symptoms after Kashmir earthquake. *Eur Arch Psychiatry Clin Neurosci, 265,* 471–481.

Balint, E. E., Falkay, G., & Balint, G. A. (2009). Khat–a controversial plant. *Wien Klin Wochenschr, 121,* 604–614.

Beards, S., Gayer-Anderson, C., Borges, S., Dewey, M.E., Fisher, H.L., & Morgan, C. (2013). Life events and psychosis: a review and meta-analysis. *Schizophr Bull, 39,* 740–747.

Bhugra, D., et al. (1996). First-contact incidence rates of schizophrenia in Trinidad and one-year follow-up. *Br J Psychiatry, 169,* 587–592.

Bhugra, D., et al. (2000). Factors in the onset of schizophrenia: a comparison between London and Trinidad samples. *Acta Psychiatr Scand, 101,* 135–141.

Binbay, T., et al. (2012). Testing the psychosis continuum: differential impact of genetic and nongenetic risk factors and comorbid psychopathology across the entire spectrum of psychosis. *Schizophr Bull, 38,* 992–1002.

Bourque, F., van der Ven, E., & Malla, A. (2011). A meta-analysis of the risk for psychotic disorders among first-and second-generation immigrants. *Psychol Med, 41,* 897–910.

Bramon, E., et al. (2005). Dermatoglyphics and schizophrenia: a meta-analysis and investigation of the impact of obstetric complications upon a-b ridge count. *Schizophr Res, 75,* 399–404.

Brown, A. S. & Derkits, E. J. (2010). Prenatal infection and schizophrenia: a review of epidemiologic and translational studies. *Am J Psychiatry, 167,* 261–280.

Burns, J. K. & Esterhuizen, T. (2008). Poverty, inequality and the treated incidence of first-episode psychosis: an ecological study from South Africa. *Soc Psychiatry Psychiatr Epidemiol, 43,* 331–335.

Cannon, M., Jones, P. B., & Murray, R. M. (2002). Obstetric complications and schizophrenia: historical and meta-analytic review. *Am J Psychiatry, 159,* 1080–1092.

Cascini, F., Aiello, C., & Di Tanna, G. (2012). Increasing delta-9-tetrahydrocannabinol (Δ-9-THC) content in herbal cannabis over time: systematic review and meta-analysis. *Curr Drug Abuse Rev, 5,* 32–40.

Chakraborty, R., Chatterjee, A., Choudhary, S., Singh, A. R., & Chakraborty, P. K. (2007). Life events in acute and transient psychosis—a comparison with mania. *Ger J Psychiatry, 10,* 36–40.

Clouston, T. S. (1896). The Cairo Asylum 2 Dr. Warnock on hasheesh insanity. *Br J Psychiatry, 42,* 790–795.

Cohen, A., et al. (2016). Concepts of madness in diverse settings: a qualitative study from the INTREPID project. *BMC Psychiatry, 16,* 388–400.

Collings, S. J. (1995). The long-term effects of contact and non-contact forms of child sexual abuse in a sample of university men. *Child Abuse & Negl, 16*, 1–6.

Darnton-Hill, I. & Mkparu, U. C. (2015). Micronutrients in pregnancy in low- and middle-income countries. *Nutrients, 7*, 1744–1768.

Day, R., et al. (1987). Stressful life events preceding the acute onset of schizophrenia: a cross-national study from the World Health Organization. *Cult Med Psychiatry, 11*, 123–205.

Di Forti, M., et al. (2015). Proportion of patients in south London with first-episode psychosis attributable to use of high potency cannabis: a case–control study. *Lancet Psychiatry, 2*, 233–238.

Dorrington, S., et al. (2014). Trauma, post-traumatic stress disorder and psychiatric disorders in a middle-income setting: prevalence and comorbidity. *Br J Psychiatry, 205*, 383–389.

Ekanayake, S., Prince, M., Sumathipala, A., Siribaddana, S., & Morgan, C. (2013). 'We lost all we had in a second': coping with grief and loss after a natural disaster. *World Psychiatry, 12*, 69–75.

Fleming, L. C., & Jacobsen, K. H. (2009). Bullying among middle-school students in low and middle income countries. *Health Promot Int, 25*, 73–84.

Gayer-Anderson, C., & Morgan, C. (2013). Social networks, support and early psychosis: a systematic review. *Epidemiol Psychiatr Sci, 22*, 131–146.

Gomwalk, N. E. & Ahmad, A. A. (1989). Prevalence of rubella antibodies on the African continent. *Rev Infect Dis, 11*, 116–121.

Gureje, O. & Adewunmi, A. (1988). Life events and schizophrenia in Nigerians a controlled investigation. *Br J Psychiatry, 153*, 367–375.

Gureje, O., Bamidele, R. & Raji, O. (1994). Early brain trauma and schizophrenia in Nigerian patients. *Am J Psychiatry, 151*, 368–371.

Hollander, A. C., Dal, H., Lewis, G., Magnusson, C., Kirkbride, J. B., & Dalman, C. (2016). Refugee migration and risk of schizophrenia and other non-affective psychoses: cohort study of 1.3 million people in Sweden. *BMJ, 352*, i1030.

Howes, O. D., & Murray, R. M. (2014). Schizophrenia: an integrated sociodevelopmental-cognitive model. *Lancet, 383*, 1677–1687.

Ibukun, A. I., Olubunmi, B. A., Cecilia, O. O., & Temitayo, I. G. (2015). Clinical Profile of Early Onset Psychosis in a Nigerian Sample. *Int Neuropsychiatr Dis J, 4*, 66–74.

Jenkins, R., et al. (2008). Debt, income and mental disorder in the general population. *Psychol Med, 38*, 1485–1493.

Jenkins, R., Mbatia, J., Singleton, N., & White, B. (2010). Prevalence of psychotic symptoms and their risk factors in urban Tanzania. *Int J Environ Res Public Health, 7*, 2514–2525.

Jenkins, R., et al. (2015). Adult psychotic symptoms, their associated risk factors and changes in prevalence in men and women over a decade in a poor rural district of Kenya. *Int J Environ Res Public Health, 12*, 5310–5328.

Jones, P., Rodgers, B., Murray, R., & Marmot, M. (1994). Child development risk factors for adult schizophrenia in the British 1946 birth cohort. *Lancet, 344*, 1398–1402.

Kang, N. I., Park, T. W., Yang, J. C., Oh, K. Y., Shim, S. H., & Chung, Y. C. (2012). Prevalence and clinical features of thought–perception–sensitivity symptoms: results from a community survey of Korean high school students. *Psychiatry Res, 198*, 501–508.

Kebede, D., Alem, A., Shibre, T., Negash, A., Deyassa, N., & Beyero, T. (2004). The sociodemographic correlates of schizophrenia in Butajira, rural Ethiopia. *Schizophr Res*, *69*, 133–141.

Keraite, A., Sumathipala, A., Siriwardhana, C., Morgan, C., & Reininghaus, U. (2016). Exposure to conflict and disaster: a national survey on the prevalence of psychotic experiences in Sri Lanka. *Schizophr Res*, *171*, 79–85.

Kessler, R.C., Chiu, W.T., Demler, O., & Walters, E.E. (2005). Prevalence, severity, and comorbidity of 12-month DSM-IV disorders in the National Comorbidity Survey Replication. *Arch Gen Psychiatry*, *62*, 617–627.

Khandaker, G. M., Zimbron, J., Lewis, G., & Jones, P. B. (2013). Prenatal maternal infection, neurodevelopment and adult schizophrenia: a systematic review of population-based studies. *Psychol Med*, *43*, 239–257.

Kilian, S., et al. (2017). Factors moderating the relationship between childhood trauma and premorbid adjustment in first-episode schizophrenia. *PLoS ONE*, *12*, 1–14

Kim, M. S., Aune, K. S., Hunter, J. E., Kim, H. J., & Kim, J. S. (2001). The effect of culture and self-construals on predispositions toward verbal communication. *Hum Commun Res*, *27*, 382–408.

Kim, H. S. & Kim, H. S. (2005). Incestuous experience among Korean adolescents: prevalence, family problems, perceived family dynamics, and psychological characteristics. *Public Health Nurs*, *22*, 472–482.

Kirkbride, J. B., et al. (2012). Incidence of schizophrenia and other psychoses in England, 1950–2009: a systematic review and meta-analyses. *PLoS ONE*, *7*, e31660.

Konings, M., Henquet, C., Maharajh, H. D., Hutchinson, G., & Van Os, J. (2008). Early exposure to cannabis and risk for psychosis in young adolescents in Trinidad. *Acta Psychiatr Scand*, *118*, 209–213.

Korbin, J. E. (1991). Cross-cultural perspectives and research directions for the 21st century. *Child Abuse Negl*, *15*, 67–77.

Koyanagi, A., Oh, H., Haro, J. M., Hirayama, F., & DeVylder, J. (2017). Child death and maternal psychosis-like experiences in 44 low-and middle-income countries: the role of depression. *Schizophr Res*, *183*, 41–46.

Lachman, A., Nassen, R., Hawkridge, S., & Emsley, R. A. (2012). A retrospective chart review of the clinical and psychosocial profile of psychotic adolescents with co-morbid substance use disorders presenting to acute adolescent psychiatric services at Tygerberg Hospital. *S Afr J Psychiatry*, *18*, 53–60.

Lambo, T. A. (1960). Further neuropsychiatric observations in Nigeria, with comments on the need for epidemiological study in Africa. *Br Med J*, *2*, 1696–1704.

Li, X., Wang, Z., Hou, Y., Wang, Y., Liu, J., & Wang, C. (2014a). Effects of childhood trauma on personality in a sample of Chinese adolescents. *Child Abuse Negl*, *38*, 788–796.

Li, E., et al. (2014b). The roles of victimization experiences, paranoia and salience misattribution in predicting psychosis proneness: the Twinsscan China Study. *Schizophr Res*, *153*, S339.

Linscott, R. J. & van Os, J. (2013). An updated and conservative systematic review and meta-analysis of epidemiological evidence on psychotic experiences in children and adults: on the pathway from proneness to persistence to dimensional expression across mental disorders. *Psychol Med*, *43*, 1133–1149.

Lund, C., et al. (2011). Poverty and mental disorders: breaking the cycle in low-income and middle-income countries. *Lancet, 378*, 1502–1514.

Lundberg, P., Cantor-Graae, E., Kabakyenga, J., Rukundo, G., & Östergren, P. O. (2004). Prevalence of delusional ideation in a district in southwestern Uganda. *Schizophr Res, 71*, 27–34.

Mahy, G. E., Mallett, R., Leff, J., & Bhugra, D. (1999). First-contact incidence rate of schizophrenia on Barbados. *Br J Psychiatry, 175*, 28–33.

Mamah, D., et al. (2016). Characterizing psychosis risk traits in Africa: a longitudinal study of Kenyan adolescents. *Schizophr Res, 176*, 340–348.

Maselko, J. (2017). Social epidemiology and global mental health: expanding the evidence from high-income to low-and middle-income countries. *Curr Epidemiol Rep, 4*, 166–173.

Matheson, S. L., Shepherd, A. M., Pinchbeck, R. M., Laurens, K. R., & Carr, V. J. (2013). Childhood adversity in schizophrenia: a systematic meta-analysis. *Psychol Med, 43*, 225–238.

McGrath, J. J., et al. (2017). The association between childhood adversities and subsequent first onset of psychotic experiences: a cross-national analysis of 23 998 respondents from 17 countries. *Psychol Med, 47*, 1230–1245.

Meewisse, M. L., Olff, M., Kleber, R., Kitchiner, N. J., & Gersons, B. P. (2011). The course of mental health disorders after a disaster: predictors and comorbidity. *J Trauma Stress, 24*, 405–413.

Menezes, P. R. (2013). Epidemiology of schizophrenia in Brazil. *Schizophr Bull, 39*, S70.

Menezes, P. R. (2014). Commentary: epidemiological mental health research: contribution from low-and middle-income countries is essential. *Int J Epidemiol, 43*, 301–303.

Moomal, H., et al. (2009). Perceived discrimination and mental health disorders: the South African Stress and Health study. *S Afr Med J, 99*, 383–389.

Morgan, C. J. A., et al. (2012). Sub-chronic impact of cannabinoids in street cannabis on cognition, psychotic-like symptoms and psychological well-being. *Psychol Med, 42*, 391–400.

Morgan, C. & Gayer-Anderson, C. (2016). Childhood adversities and psychosis: evidence, challenges, implications. *World Psychiatry, 15*, 93–102.

Morgan, C., et al. (2007). Parental separation, loss and psychosis in different ethnic groups: a case–control study. *Psychol Med, 37*, 495–503.

Odenwald, M. (2014). Mental health problems associated with the use and abuse of khat (Catha edulis). In Bentivoglio, M., Cavalheiro, E., Kristensson, K., & Patel, N. (eds) *Neglected tropical diseases and conditions of the nervous system.* New York: Springer New York, 293–305.

Odenwald, M., et al. (2005). Khat use as risk factor for psychotic disorders: a cross-sectional and case–control study in Somalia. *BMC Med, 3*, 1.

Odenwald, M., et al. (2009). Use of khat and posttraumatic stress disorder as risk factors for psychotic symptoms: a study of Somali combatants. *Soc Sci Med, 69*, 1040–1048.

Paruk, S., Ramlall, S., & Burns, J. K. (2009). Adolescent-onset psychosis: a 2-year retrospective study of adolescents admitted to a general psychiatric unit. *S Afr J Psychiatry, 15*(4), 86–92.

Paruk, S., Burns, J. K., & Caplan, R. (2013). Cannabis use and family history in adolescent first episode psychosis in Durban, South Africa. *J Child Adol Ment Health, 25*, 61–68.

Patel, V. & Kleinman, A. (2003). Poverty and common mental disorders in developing countries. *Bull World Health Organ, 81*, 609–615.

Pearson, A. L., Mack, E., & Namanya, J. (2017). Mobile phones and mental wellbeing: initial evidence suggesting the importance of staying connected to family in rural remote communities in Uganda. *PLoS ONE, 12*, 11.

Punch, S. (2016). Cross-world and cross-disciplinary dialogue: a more integrated, global approach to childhood studies. *Glob Stud Child, 6*, 352–364.

Read, J. (2010). Can poverty drive you mad? Schizophrenia, socio-economic status and the case for primary prevention. *NZ J Psychol, 39*, 7–19.

Reichenberg, A., et al. (2010). Static and dynamic cognitive deficits in childhood preceding adult schizophrenia: a 30-year study. *Am J Psychiatry, 167*, 160–169.

Reininghaus, U. & Morgan, C. (2014). Integrated models in psychiatry: the state of the art. *Soc Psychiatry Psychiatr Epidemiol, 49*, 1–2.

Şahin, S., et al. (2013). The history of childhood trauma among individuals with ultra high risk for psychosis is as common as among patients with first-episode schizophrenia. *Early Interv Psychiatry, 7*, 414–420.

Saif Al Dawla, A. (2001). Social factors affecting women's mental health in the Arab region. In Okasha, A., Maj, M. (eds) *Images in psychiatry: an Arab perspective.* Cairo (Egypt): WPA Publications, 207–223.

Saw, A., & Okazaki, S. (2012). What is the psychology of Asians. In E. C. Chang (ed.) *Handbook of adult psychopathology in Asians: theory, diagnosis and treatment.* Oxford: Oxford University Press, 15–29.

Sen, A. (1999). *Development as freedom.* New York: Random House.

Sharifi, V., et al. (2012). Self-reported psychotic symptoms in the general population: correlates in an Iranian urban area. *Psychopathology, 45*, 374–380.

Social Trends Institute (2015). An international report from the Social Trends Institute. Retrieved from http://sustaindemographicdividend.org/wp-content/uploads/2012/07/SDD-2011-Final.pdf

Soosay, I., et al. (2012). Trauma exposure, PTSD and psychotic-like symptoms in post-conflict Timor Leste: an epidemiological survey. *BMC Psychiatry, 12*, 229.

St Clair, D., et al. (2005). Rates of adult schizophrenia following prenatal exposure to the Chinese famine of 1959–1961. *JAMA, 294*, 557–562.

Susser, E., et al. (1996). Schizophrenia after prenatal famine. Further evidence. *Arch Gen Psychiatry, 53*, 25–31.

Tafari, S., Aboud, F. E., & Larson, C. P. (1991). Determinants of mental illness in a rural Ethiopian adult population. *Soc Sci Med, 32*, 197–201.

Thomée, S., Härenstam, A., & Hagberg, M. (2011). Mobile phone use and stress, sleep disturbances, and symptoms of depression among young adults—a prospective cohort study. *BMC Public Health, 11*, 66.

UNICEF (2014). Level and trends in child mortality. Retrieved from https://data.unicef.org/resources/levels-trends-child-mortality-report-2014/

UNODC World Drug Report (2015). Vienna: United Nations office on drugs and crime. Retrieved from http://www.unodc.org/documents/wdr2015/World_Drug_Report_2015.pdf

van der Velden, P. G., Wong, A., Boshuizen, H. C., & Grievink, L. (2013). Persistent mental health disturbances during the 10 years after a disaster: four-wave longitudinal comparative study. *Psychiatry Clin Neurosci, 67*, 110–118.

van Dyke, C. (2013). Research policies for schizophrenia in the global health context. *Int J Mental Health, 42*, 51–76.

Van Gastel, W. A., Vreeker, A., Schubart, C. D., MacCabe, J. H., Kahn, R. S., & Boks, M. P. M. (2014). Change in cannabis use in the general population: a longitudinal study on the impact on psychotic experiences. *Schizophr Res, 157*, 266–270.

van Os, J. & Linscott, R. J. (2012). Introduction: the extended psychosis phenotype—relationship with schizophrenia and with ultrahigh risk status for psychosis. *Schizophr Bull, 38*, 227–230.

van Os, J. & Reininghaus, U. (2017). *Comprehensive textbook of psychiatry (Kaplan & Sadock's).* (B. Sadock, Sadock, V., Ruiz, P. eds) Baltimore, MD: Lippincott Williams & Wilkins.

Varese, F., et al. (2012). Childhood adversities increase the risk of psychosis: a meta-analysis of patient-control, prospective-and cross-sectional cohort studies. *Schizophr Bull, 38*, 661–671.

Vassos, E., Pedersen, C. B., Murray, R. M., Collier, D. A., & Lewis, C. M. (2012). Meta-analysis of the association of urbanicity with schizophrenia. *Schizophr Bull, 38*, 1118–1123.

Viola, T. W., Salum, G. A., Kluwe-Schiavona, B., Sanvicente-Vieiraa, B., Levandowski, M. L., & Grassi-Oliveira, R. (2016). The influence of geographical and economic factors in estimates of childhood abuse and neglect using the childhood trauma questionnaire: a worldwide meta-regression analysis. *Child Abuse Negl, 51*, 1–16

Walker, E., Mittal, V., & Tessner, K. (2008) Stress and the hypothalamic pituitary adrenal axis in the developmental course of schizophrenia. *Annu Rev Clin Psychol, 4*, 189–216.

Wang, C. & Zhang, Y. (2017). Schizophrenia in mid-adulthood after prenatal exposure to the Chinese Famine of 1959–1961. *Schizophr Res, 184*, 21–25.

White, R. G., Imperiale, M. G., & Perera, E. (2016). The Capabilities approach: fostering contexts for enhancing mental health and wellbeing across the globe. *Global Health, 12*, 16.

World Health Organization (WHO) (2011). mHealth: new horizons for health through mobile technologies: second global survey on eHealth. Retrieved from https://apps. who.int/iris/bitstream/handle/10665/44607/9789241564250_eng.pdf?sequence= 1&isAllowed=y

Wüsten, C. & Lincoln, T. M. (2017). The association of family functioning and psychosis proneness in five countries that differ in cultural values and family structures. *Psychiatry Res, 253*, 158–164.

Xu, M. Q., et al. (2009). Prenatal malnutrition and adult schizophrenia: further evidence from the 1959–1961 Chinese famine. *Schizophr Bull, 35*, 568–576.

4

Psychosis across persons 3: Genes, biology, and neurodevelopment

Giulia Segre, Conrad Iyegbe, Sarah Tosato, Geraldo Busatto, and Paola Dazzan

Introduction

Our understanding of the aetiology of psychoses has advanced in recent years, and the broad consensus is that psychoses emerge as a consequence of complex interactions between genes, other biological factors, and environmental factors. Here, we review current evidence specifically on genes and other biological risks and mechanisms. In the context of this book, what is most notable is that most—in fact, almost all—of the evidence is derived from studies conducted in select centres in a few high-income countries (e.g. the US, parts of western Europe) with next to no evidence from the Global South. Thus, while the existing evidence points to a complex and dynamic pathophysiological model of psychosis, there is clearly much to be learned by expanding research to a greater variety of populations across the world.

The (false) Kraepelinian dichotomy

For the last 100 years, psychotic symptoms occurring in the absence of an organic brain disorder have been mostly classified into two main categories corresponding to the modern diagnostic equivalents of schizophrenia and bipolar disorders (O'Donovan et al., 2009; Williams et al., 2011). Both the Diagnostic and Statistical Manual of Mental Disorders (DSM-5, American Psychiatric Association, 2013) and the International Classification of Disease (ICD-10, World Health Organization, 1993) consider schizophrenia and bipolar disorder as two separate diagnostic entities. However, research increasingly suggests that the boundaries between these nosological entities are, at best, blurred. A multitude of genetic, neuroimaging, and neurocognitive studies point to overlaps in risks and possibly a shared biological basis for these disorders (Pearlson, 2015). For instance, clear evidence of an overlap can be seen in the familial co-aggregation of both schizophrenia and bipolar disorder (Maier et al., 2005; Mortensen et al., 2003). To take one example, a large twin study found that monozygotic (i.e. sharing the same DNA sequence) co-twins of individuals with schizophrenia had an increased risk of mania (8.2%) as well as schizophrenia (40.8%) and that monozygotic co-twins of individuals with mania had an increased risk of schizophrenia (13.6%) as well as mania (36.4%) (Cardno et al., 2002). Furthermore, in the same study the monozygotic co-twins of individuals with a diagnosis of schizoaffective disorder had the same increased risk for schizophrenia and mania (26.1%) (Cardno et al., 2002). However, it nonetheless remains that much of the current evidence on the genetics and neurobiology of psychoses is derived from samples constructed to include individuals meeting the criteria for a diagnosis of either schizophrenia or bipolar disorder. This is changing, but it points to an important limitation of the current evidence base.

Genetics

Developments in genetic studies of schizophrenia and bipolar disorder

In recent years there has been a clear, and important, shift in understandings of— and therefore approaches to studying—the architecture of genetic risk for psychoses. For some time, the expectation was that the genetic risk for schizophrenia and bipolar disorder was likely to be due to a small number of susceptibility genes. For a period, there was considerable excitement about reports linking specific genes with schizophrenia and bipolar disorder. However, even for the most 'promising' genes, such as Neuregulin 1 (NRG1) (Tosato et al., 2005) and dysbindin (DTNBP1) (O'Donovan et al., 2009), there has been a remarkable failure to replicate the same markers and haplotypes across studies, and a lack of consistency in implicating particular alleles in the development of psychosis (Sanders et al., 2008; Sullivan, 2008). This, along with technological advances, led to a shift from studies of candidate genes to genome-wide association studies (GWAS), which provide a framework for interrogating the relationship between common genetic variants distributed across the human genome and risk of disorder.

The Psychiatric Genomics Consortium (PGC) has assumed field-level responsibility for these efforts for mental disorders. It was created in 2007 with the specific goal of conducting GWAS studies in schizophrenia and bipolar disorder by bringing together psychiatric GWAS from around the world to enable adequately powered analyses. By centralizing analyses under a consortium umbrella, the PGC overcame the challenges of harmonizing quality control procedures, analytic methods, and phenotype definitions to enable meta and mega-analyses (Sullivan, 2010). It is through such initiatives that it has been possible to examine the effects of large numbers of genes, and the evidence that has emerged has contributed to a fundamental shift in putative models of the genetic basis for psychoses. The broad consensus now is that susceptibility is a function of the presence of large numbers of genes of small effect. Further, these studies have provided further evidence of overlap between schizophrenia and bipolar disorder. One, for example, reported a correlation coefficient of around 0.68 (Lee et al., 2013) (compared with 0.43 for schizophrenia and major depression). Subsequent studies have either reproduced these estimates (Stahl et al., 2019) or have advanced the field by localizing specific genes that may underlie these joint effects on risk (Smoller, 2013; Yao et al., 2021).

Genetic findings in schizophrenia

Many genetic variants spanning a wide distribution of effect sizes and frequencies have been implicated in schizophrenia. This includes, for example, genes expressed in the post-synaptic density (specialized junctions between neurons) that facilitate neuronal connectivity and signalling. These include members of the voltage-dependent calcium channel family of proteins *(CACNA1C, CACNB2,* and *CACNA1I)* and genes involved in glutamatergic neurotransmission and synaptic plasticity (such as for example *GRM3, GRIN2A, SRR,* and *GRIA1)* (Schizophrenia Psychiatric Genome-Wide Association Study (GWAS) Consortium, 2011; Owen et al., 2016). Other candidates include genes whose encoded products (proteins) are therapeutic targets for antipsychotic medications (for example, *DRD2)* (Schizophrenia Working Group of the Psychiatric Genomics Consortium, 2014). From a statistical perspective, the single most important genetic association for schizophrenia seems to originate from the Multi-Histocompatibility Complex (MHC) on chromosome 6*p*, which points to an important contribution of infection or autoimmunity. Similarly, pathway-level evidence has implicated gene transcriptional mechanisms known to be important in a group of antibody-producing (B) immune cells (Schizophrenia Working Group of the Psychiatric Genomics Consortium, 2014). These findings have been reinforced by the discovery of functional variation of the *C4* MHC gene that causes the derailment of synaptic pruning in early brain development (Sekar et al., 2016). Recent studies estimate that common alleles, captured by GWAS arrays, explain between one-third and one-half of the genetic variance in the liability for schizophrenia (Purcell et al., 2009), depending on the population and method used (International Schizophrenia Consortium et al., 2009; Lee et al., 2013).

In addition to common variants, called single nucleotide polymorphisms (SNPs), rare variants such as copy number variations (CNVs), which are large-scale deletions or duplications of the genome, may explain a proportion of risk for schizophrenia and bipolar disorder (Malhotra & Sebat, 2012). The clearest evidence that CNVs are mechanistically important for psychosis can be found in people who carry chromosome 22q deletions, about a quarter of whom develop schizophrenia (Van et al., 2017). Some CNVs, such as those present on chromosome 16p11.2 (Walsh & Bracken, 2011) and the deletions of the *NRXN1* gene (Rujescu et al., 2009), when present, also confer a greater risk of developing schizophrenia than the risk conferred by common variants. Furthermore, CNVs and more common risk variants may act cooperatively to influence risk for schizophrenia (Bergen et al., 2019; Tansey et al., 2016) and, additionally, may converge on the same set of gene and pathway-level candidates (Legge et al., 2021).

Apart from sample size (a general constraint in GWAS; Dudbridge, 2013), other obstacles to the interpretation of GWAS signals include the inability to localize the source of causal variants with fine-scale precision. The first obstacle results from the extensive correlation structure in the European genomic map. Systematic patterns of correlation between distinct genetic loci, known as linkage disequilibrium (LD), follow population-specific profiles. While advantageous for the purpose of disease locus detection, this is also a limitation, given that it is not possible to distinguish true causal variants from those that simply 'piggyback' onto association signals by virtue of being correlated with true causal variants. To overcome this limitation, a method called LD regression has been developed to test whether or not genomic inflation in this context represents a polygenic risk component to disease or inflated significance due to the population substructure (Bulik-Sullivan et al., 2015). Meanwhile, it is often the case that variants that map to the non-coding genome also reflect complexity at the gene expression level (Hauberg et al., 2016; Huckins et al., 2019; Richards et al., 2012). Finally, as LD follows population-specific profiles, it is key to establish what the profiles are across non-European groups to advance knowledge.

Genetic findings in bipolar disorder

An interesting review on this topic has been recently published (Gordovez & McMahon, 2020). Typical effect sizes (i.e. odds ratios) of common variants for bipolar disorder range between 1.1 and 1.4, and cumulatively explain about 25% of the heritability for bipolar disorder. Many of the same genes and pathways identified by GWAS analyses for schizophrenia (such as *CACNA1C* and *GRIN2A*) have also been implicated in bipolar disorder, while genes such as *SHANK2* have been implicated in autism (Pinto et al., 2010; Zaslavsky et al., 2019). While the role of CNVs in bipolar disorder seems much less conspicuous than in schizophrenia, current technological limitations preclude the systematic interrogation of CNVs of less than 30 kilobases in size in GWAS cohorts. Still, CNVs have been identified in large case–control data sets for bipolar disorder at three CNV loci that are also associated with schizophrenia. The first was a de novo mutation on chromosome 16p11.2 detected in individuals with early onset bipolar disorder (Malhotra et al., 2011) and subsequently confirmed by a large meta-analysis (Green et al., 2016), which found this was the only locus to survive stringent multiple test correction procedures. Further loci on chromosomes 1q21.1 and 3q29 still await corroborating evidence (Torres et al., 2016).

Polygenic risk scores

More recently, polygenic risk scores (PRS) have been developed and have found many diverse applications in psychiatric research (Purcell et al., 2009; Wray et al., 2014). Early applications of promise include the identification of correlates of genetic liability in a certain population (Socrates et al., 2021) and stratification of patients by therapeutic outcome (Zhang et al., 2019). The PRS is an index of genetic risk which is calculated as the weighted sum of risk alleles in an individual genome. The method reflects the fact that psychiatric traits have a genetic architecture that is highly polygenic; this is to say that a substantial proportion of schizophrenia heritability is accounted for by genetic factors that have small effects and affect risk cumulatively.

The PRS for schizophrenia has been calculated from the latest genetic data from the Psychiatric Genomic Consortium (Schizophrenia Working Group of the Psychiatric Genomics Consortium, 2014) and was found to explain about 7% of the variance of schizophrenia in the general population, assuming a lifetime prevalence of schizophrenia of 1%. Even if this PRS is higher than that of other psychiatric disorders, and even if it was calculated based on the GWAS of schizophrenia which is characterized by clinical heterogeneity, it still cannot be used as a screening tool for psychosis in the general population (Schizophrenia Working Group of the Psychiatric Genomics Consortium, 2014).

Still, the PRS for schizophrenia has been found to provide good discrimination between Bipolar I Disorder and Bipolar II Disorder, and between bipolar disorder with and without psychotic symptoms (Stahl et al., 2019). The fact that this evidence was generated using estimation methods able to discriminate between the effects of genome-wide polygenicity and other major confounders related to population structure again points to the importance of evaluating different populations to improve generalizability (Bulik-Sullivan et al., 2015). The genetic correlation between schizophrenia and bipolar disorder I has been estimated to be 0.71, compared with 0.51 for schizophrenia and bipolar disorder II. Meanwhile, bipolar disorder II has been found to correlate more strongly with the genetics of major depression (0.69) than with that of bipolar disorder I (0.30) (Stahl et al., 2019). These findings make a compelling case for a biological distinction between the main nosological constructs used to define bipolar disorder. As much as 60% of the heritability ascribed to common genetic variation is enriched in genomic regions that exist in an 'open' chromatin formation within the central nervous system. This suggests that the accessibility of DNA to the molecular machinery that translates genes into proteins is an important mechanistic consideration relevant to the disease process. Moreover, PRSs can be used to study gene and environment correlations and interactions (Colodro-Conde et al., 2018; Murray & Vassos, 2020).

GWAS analyses have also considered components of a broader psychosis phenotype through the merger of data sets across multiple disorders (Ruderfer et al., 2018). These analyses have identified eight pathways that survived stringent multiple testing criteria (Ruderfer et al., 2018). Notable patterns of gene enrichment signatures endorse the involvement of neuronal projections, neurogenesis, synaptic plasticity, and post-synaptic signalling pathways. It is clear from this and other ongoing functional work that individual genome-wide loci can have opposing effects on the risk of schizophrenia and bipolar and that the involvement of the MHC in psychosis risk is heavily slanted towards schizophrenia and not towards bipolar disorder.

The limited global representativeness of genetic research

The limited global representativity in GWAS cohorts has not changed much since 2009, when the level of non-European participation in GWAS was at 8%. Although the figure had reached 20% by 2016, this mainly reflected the expansion of a single ancestry group (East Asian) rather than a fundamental shift in the scientific culture as it had previously been advocated (Popejoy & Fullerton, 2016).

An important landmark in psychiatric GWAS research has been the completion of the first multi-ethnic GWAS of schizophrenia by the Genomics of Psychiatry Consortium (GPC). This included a cohort of 10,070 of African ancestry (6,152 cases and 3,918 controls), 4,324 of Latino ancestry (1,234 cases and 3,090 controls) and 10,580 of European ancestry (6,046 case and 4,534 controls) (Bigdeli et al., 2020). It also leveraged summary statistics from the 2014 GWAS schizophrenia analysis, relating to ~34,000 cases and ~45,000 controls from 46 European and 3 East Asian cohorts (Schizophrenia Working Group of the Psychiatric Genomics Consortium, 2014). In this study (Bigdeli et al., 2020), the GWAS of the Latino cohort yielded a single genome-wide hit identifying an associated Single Nucleotide Polymorphism (SNP) (rs776877in *GALNT13* at 2q23.3), which had not been identified by the previous PGC GWAS analysis for schizophrenia. No genome-wide hits were identified in the African ancestry cohort. Population differences in the genetic correlation structure (or LD) were leveraged through the meta-analytic integration of PGC and GPC cohorts. This yielded significant improvements in fine-scale resolution at 22 loci, as well as the emergence of 4 newly significant loci. The best-performing PRS were those trained and applied within a single ancestry group for African ancestry ($R^2_{Liability}$>0.01), Latino ancestry ($R^2_{Liability}$=0.02), and European ancestry ($R^2_{Liability}$=0.03). For African and Latino populations, ancestrally matched PRS performed better (in terms of the maximum variance explained) than scores based on the much larger PGC2-SZ study. The use of a trans-ancestry training sample yielded PRS that explained more variance than those trained against a single ancestry group for African ancestry ($R^2_{Liability}$>0.02), Latino ancestry ($R^2_{Liability}$=0.02), and European ancestry ($R^2_{Liability}$=0.04). This evidence highlights the advantages of incorporating data from diverse human populations into genetic studies.

The GPC's schizophrenia cohorts of Latino and African ancestry have now been included in the most recent GWAS for schizophrenia (https://www.medr xiv.org/content/10.1101/2020.09.12.20192922v1) (PGC3-SZ). The inclusion of these cohorts has led to a significant drop in the rate of genome-wide discoveries, as evidenced by a reduction in the total number of hits and the low concordance between results when these ancestries are included and excluded from the joint European and East Asian analyses (https://www.medrxiv.org/ content/10.1101/2020.09.12.20192922v1). It is also clear that a PRS trained in a joint European and Asian ancestral base has low power to predict caseness in an African ancestral context ($R^2_{Liability}$ = 0.008) (https://www.medrxiv.org/cont ent/10.1101/2020.09.12.20192922v1). Population differences in genome-wide allele frequencies, LD, and estimated effect sizes explain the failure of the PGC PRS to maintain a consistent level of predictive ability across diverse population groups (Martin et al., 2020). A large proportion of explanatory power is lost by treating each factor as though it is independent of these other effects (Gaziano et al., 2016; Harvey et al., 2014). Interestingly, however, for almost all European and Asian samples, PRSs had more explanatory power when using risk alleles derived from the full combined ancestry GWAS than from the matched ancestry GWAS. PRSs explained more variance in liability in cohorts of European ancestry (likely a result of the ancestry composition of the GWAS) but also in samples which by ascertainment were likely to include the most severe cases (i.e. hospitalized patients including those treated with clozapine) (Lancaster et al., 2019). So, even considering these limitations, PRS can have many applications in research, for example in patient stratification, or for the identification of correlates of liability in population samples, although considerably more effort should be made to include samples of non-European ancestry in GWAS studies in order to calculate PRSs also for these populations.

New directions: the Millions Veteran Study of psychosis traits

A number of initiatives have been developed to meet the need for more diverse samples. Among these are the Million Veteran and Veterans Affairs Cooperative Studies programmes. These studies reflect a strategic effort to advance genomics research that improves long-term health outcomes for military service personnel and are funded by the Department of Veterans Affairs Cooperative Studies Program (CSP). Capitalizing on the largest integrated national health system in the United States of America (USA) and on a genetic cohort with the highest representation of ethnic minorities in the USA, a primary GWAS study of schizophrenia and bipolar disorder has been undertaken in 11,910 post-quality control (QC) cases (Harvey et al., 2014) and 50,436 post QC controls (Gaziano et al., 2016) from the Veterans Health Administration (VHA) (Bigdeli et al., 2021). The defining clinical features of this cohort include: (i) large representation of individuals of African ancestry for schizophrenia (~54%), bipolar disorder (~25%) and a corresponding profile in controls; (ii) an older age profile ranging 50–69 years; (iii) a later age of onset, considering that a good mental health is a prerequisite for study enrolment; (iv) a large preponderance of men (~90%); and (v) relatively longer illness duration.

The primary GWAS analysis of this data set has resulted in new and non-overlapping genome-wide associations for schizophrenia and bipolar disorder (1 per each disorder). Although the discovery was based on European ancestral background, findings remained genome-wide significant after African and European Million Veteran Program (MVP) cohorts had been combined meta-analytically (Bigdeli et al., 2021). In the African ancestry MVP schizophrenia cohort (Table 4.1), a PRS trained within the same ancestry outperformed the PGC+CLOZUK (the amalgamation of the CLOZUK and Psychiatric Genomic Consortium initiatives) cohort (Pardiñas et al., 2018) which, though numerically superior, is an ill fit due to the ancestral mismatch (African vs. European). The best-performing risk score in the African ancestry MVP sample was derived using a trans-ancestry base (i.e. African + East Asian + European ancestry) to calibrate PRS weights. In the European ancestry MVP schizophrenia data set, the performance of the ancestrally matched PGC+CLOZUK PRS far exceeded that of a cosmopolitan training sample by a factor of two. European ancestry

Table 4.1 Association of Polygenic Risk Scores (PRS) for schizophrenia in the Million Veterans Program (MVP) data set

Training Set	Sample size Case/control	MVP: African ancestry (1,683 cases, 4,669 controls)						MVP: European ancestry (1,200 cases, 45,767 controls)			
		P_T	R^2_{lia}	β	Std Err	P	P_T	$R^2_{liability}$	β	Std Err	P
AA-GPC (Bigdeli et al., 2020):	5,826/4,616	0.5	0.010	0.30	0.03	$3.75E^{-25}$	0.5	1.2×10^{-3}	0.09	0.03	1.4×10^{-3}
LA-GPC (Bigdeli et al., 2020):	1,234/3,090	0.5	4.2×10^{-4}	0.06	0.03	0.05	0.005	1.6×10^{-3}	0.11	0.03	2.0×10^{-4}
CLOZUK+PGC (Pardiñas et al., 2018):	4,0675/6,4643	0.5	8.7×10^{-3}	0.38	0.04	$1.94E^{-18}$	0.5	0.08	0.85	0.03	8.5×10^{-141}
PGC-SCZ (Ripke et al., 2014):	32,838/44,357	0.5	5.6×10^{-3}	0.31	0.05	$3.00E^{-12}$	0.5	0.07	0.78	0.03	1.6×10^{-124}
EAS (Lam et al., 2019):	22,778/35,362	0.05	1.3×10^{-4}	0.03	0.03	0.28	5.0×10^{-06}	2.4×10^{-3}	0.13	0.03	6.4×10^{-6}
PGC+EAS+GPC (trans-ancestry)	47,735/72,343	0.5	0.020	0.42	0.03	$8.01E^{-35}$	0.05	0.04	0.57	0.03	2.2×10^{-82}

PT is the *P*-value threshold that maximized the *R2* of the training set-derived PRS in the MVP sample. *R²* is adjusted for the proportion of cases (i.e. the liability scale) assuming a 1% population prevalence for both schizophrenia and bipolar disorders β and *SE* are the regression coefficient and its standard error. AA: African ancestry; LA: Latino ancestry; EAS: East Asian ancestry.

findings in the MVP-bipolar data set (Table 4.2) showed a similar trend. The European-trained PRS performed best overall, surpassing the R^2 achieved by the multi-ancestry score by more than twofold. The performance of the multi-ancestry trained MVP-BP PRS in the African ancestry cohort was attenuated compared with the MVP-SZ PRS; thus scores trained against a European base did better at predicting caseness in African Americans than the multi-ethnic PRS, although the best overall construct in this population used African ancestry as training. Genetic correlations (Table 4.3) were high both across disorders (SZ and BP) within-ancestry (r_g 0.82–1.00), as well as across-ancestry and within-disorder (r_g 0.81–1.00).

Longer-term prospects for genetic research

Maintaining a stable pipeline of new initiatives that can overcome existing biases inherent in GWAS research will require the long-term commitment and investment of funding agencies and governments. A number of high-profile research initiatives are underway for psychosis research (Table 4.4). One of these is NeuroGAP (Stevenson et al., 2019), a National Institute of Health (NIH)-funded initiative set in four African countries aiming to recruit 30,000 cases and controls. Studies that can successfully and ethically tap into the genetic diversity present within Africa will be especially beneficial for the field, given that African genomes have about a million extra genetic variants per genome (Pereira et al., 2021) and less extensive LD, which lends itself to a more accurate identification of genetic variants linked to disorder. The benefit of this can already be seen in the disproportionate number (equating to 7%) of genome-wide significant findings that are attributable to a relatively small number (2%) of individuals with African ancestry (Morales et al., 2018).

Thus, in the context of GWAS, a greater representation of individuals of African ancestry will allow the detection of variants linked to outcomes that predate human population expansion out of Africa, which are more likely to be shared across global populations. PRSs that leverage these variants will benefit from increased generalizability across global populations (Duncan et al., 2019; Martin et al., 2017). African ancestry studies also look set to become a similarly powerful framework for understanding the scale and impact of rare genetic variants for the risk of psychosis. A recent landmark study found significant enrichment of private damaging mutations in genes that were critical to synaptic plasticity and neural circuitry in a cohort that consisted of only about 1,800 individuals with schizophrenia and controls from a single African population (South African Xhosa) (Gulsuner et al., 2020).

Table 4.2 Association of Polygenic Risk Scores (PRS) for bipolar disorder in the Million Veterans Program (MVP) data set

Training Set	Sample size Case/control	African American ancestry (1,037 BIP, 4,669 controls)					European ancestry (3,080 BIP, 45,767 controls)				
		P_T	$R^2_{liability}$	β	Std Err	P	P_T	$R^2_{liability}$	β	Std Err	P
AA-GPC (new)	1,990/4,616	0.5	5.1×10^{-3}	0.19	0.03	2.6×10^{-8}	0.5	4.6×10^{-4}	0.06	0.02	1.9×10^{-3}
LA-GPC (new)	1,032/3,090	0.5	1.6×10^{-3}	0.11	0.04	1.8×10^{-3}	0.05	5.3×10^{-4}	0.06	0.02	9.0×10^{-4}
PGC-BIP (Stahl et al., 2019)	20,352/31,358	0.05	3.3×10^{-3}	0.19	0.04	7.2×10^{-6}	0.05	0.02	0.36	0.02	3.8×10^{-70}
PGC+GPC (trans-ancestry)	23,374/39,064	0.5	1.0×10^{-3}	0.35	0.05	8.7×10^{-15}	0.5	8.9×10^{-3}	0.26	0.02	3.4×10^{-42}

PT is the P-value threshold that maximized the $R2$ of the applied training set PRS in the MVP sample. R^2 is adjusted for the proportion of cases (i.e. the liability scale) assuming a 1% population prevalence for both bipolar disorder and schizophrenia. β and SE are the regression coefficient and its standard error. AA: African ancestry; LA: Latino ancestry.

Table 4.3 Cross-disorder and trans-ancestry genetic correlations in the Million Veterans Program (MVP) data set

Trait 1			Trait 2		Statistics		
N_{cases}	$N_{controls}$		N_{cases}	$N_{controls}$	Correlation rG	Standard Error	P-value
SZ(EA)	1,228	5,000	**BPD(EA)** 3,152	5,000	0.82	0.12	5.0×10^{-16}
SZ(AA)	1,729	2,935	**BPD(AA)** 1,064	2,934	1.00	0.60	9.7×10^{-5}
SZ(EA)	1,228	10,000	**SZ(AA)** 1,729	5,869	0.81	0.23	2.0×10^{-5}
BPD (EA)	3,152	10,000	**BPD(AA)** 1,064	5,869	1.00	0.40	1.6×10^{-6}

Note: Results of genetic correlation analysis across traits and ancestries. Numbers of cases and controls are given by N_{cases} and $N_{controls}$. r_G corresponds to the genetic correlation coefficient, with SE reflecting standard error and P reflecting its significance. EA: European ancestry; AA: African Ancestry. BPD: bipolar disorder, SZ: schizophrenia.

Beyond Africa, significant strides have been made in the effort to boost the inclusion of individuals from the entire Global South in neuropsychiatric genetic research. Major new investments have enabled genetic research activity in the field of psychosis across Pakistan, Mexico, Colombia, and Mexico (Table 4.4), with a protocol for a schizophrenia GWAS in a South-Indian population having been recently published (Roberts et al., 2020). While improving individual estimates of risk, these studies will also provide an opportunity to learn how readily the existing landscape of GWAS insights extends to different populations. A case in point is the MHC locus on chromosome 6 (which represents the strongest psychiatric association signal reported to date); recent studies, including the largest schizophrenia GWAS to date of the East Asian population, suggest this is an important factor delineating the molecular aetiology of schizophrenia in Europeans and East Asians (Corvin & Morris, 2014; Lam et al., 2019).

Future research is needed to derive a better understanding of how emerging insights in the field of genetics may be shaped by local and global environmental effects (Mostafavi et al., 2020; Roberts et al., 2020), ideally in partnership with social science and perhaps following the research template of the European Network of Schizophrenia Networks for the Study of Gene Environment Interactions (EU-GEI) (van Os et al., 2008).

Finally, just as important as enabling new initiatives such as those listed in Table 4.4, are the steps taken to ensure they leave an enduring legacy of research capacity and infrastructure that can serve the needs of future generations. A gold standard paradigm is the Global Initiative for Neuropsychiatric

Table 4.4 Ongoing initiatives for genetic research on psychosis traits in diverse populations

Initiative	Acronym	Region	Phenotype	Recruitment goals
African Ancestry Genomics of Psychiatry Consortium	AA-GPC	New York, Southern California, Other US states, Trinidad, Nigeria	Schizophrenia, Bipolar Disorder, Psychosis	SZ: 6,240 BPD: 6,640 Controls: 12,500
Latino Ancestry GPC	LA-GPC	New York, Southern California, Atlanta	Schizophrenia, Bipolar Disorder, Psychosis	SZ: 4,000 BPD: 4,000 Controls: 5,000
Neuropsychiatric Genetics in African Populations (PMID: 30782936)	NeuroGAP	Ethiopia, Uganda, Kenya, South Africa	Schizophrenia, Bipolar Disorder, Psychosis	Psychosis: 17,000 Controls: 17,000
Neuropsychiatric Genetics of Psychosis in Mexico Populations (PMID: 33237255)	NeuroMex	Mexico	Schizophrenia, Bipolar Disorder, Psychosis	Psychosis: 4,000 Controls: 4,000
Genetics of Severe Mental Illness (PMID: 3237255)	Paisa Study	Colombia (Paisa population)	Psychotic and Mood Disorders: Schizophrenia, Bipolar Disorder, Major Depressive Disorder	Cases: 8,000 Controls: 8,000
Genetics of schizophrenia in Pakistan	GEN-SCRIP	Pakistan	Schizophrenia	Cases: 10,000 Controls: 10,000
Genetics of bipolar disorder in Pakistan	GEN-BLIP	Pakistan	Bipolar Disorder	Cases: 10,000 Controls: 2,000

Genetics Education in Research (GINGER) programme (van der Merwe et al., 2018), a core component of the NeuroGAP research programme (Stevenson et al., 2019). Its cohort of training fellows is selected from the research centres participating in the NeuroGAP study. Training is provided in two-year cycles by faculty members of the Broad Institute of Massachusetts Institute of Technology and Harvard and the Harvard T H Chan School of Public Health. The training curriculum includes teaching on genetic analysis, psychiatric phenotyping, epidemiology, bioinformatics, biostatistics, ethics, and manuscript and grant writing. A large part of curriculum development relies on suggestions from the trainees themselves, their African mentors, and host institutions.

Neurobiology

In parallel with genetics, there are a number of other biological systems that have been implicated in the pathophysiology of psychosis, again with evidence mostly derived from studies conducted in select high-income countries. As with research on genetics, we first consider what is known in general and then consider specifically research in the Global South.

Neurobiological mechanisms of environmental risk

Among these systems, the physiological stress response has been implicated in the development of psychosis, although the biological mechanisms underlying its role remain unclear. The vulnerability-stress model of psychosis posits that predisposing biological factors increase the sensitivity of some individuals to stressors, making them more vulnerable to develop psychosis under stressful circumstances (Myin-Germeys & van Os, 2007; Pariante, 2008). This is supported by evidence that an excess of stressful life events precedes the onset of psychosis and relapse in patients with schizophrenia (Beards et al., 2013; Walker et al., 2008). In addition, earlier adversities such as childhood trauma are strongly associated with onset of psychosis (Morgan et al., 2014). Finally, that patients with psychosis may have a higher sensitivity to stress is also supported by data suggesting that they perceive daily hassles as more stressful than individuals without psychosis (Mondelli et al., 2010a; Myin-Germeys & van Os, 2007).

How can these environmental stressors increase the risk of psychosis? Several studies over the last few years have proposed that this may occur via effects on the hypothalamus–pituitary–adrenal (HPA) axis, the main stress response system (Belvederi Murri et al., 2012). Support for this model comes from evidence that first-episode psychosis patients show abnormalities in HPA axis activity, e.g. increased cortisol levels throughout the day, blunted cortisol awakening response (CAR), and decreased cortisol response to psychosocial stressors (Mondelli et al., 2010a). Interestingly, the blunted CAR and the reduced HPA axis reactivity to stress are also associated with the presence of more severe symptoms and worse cognitive function in patients with psychosis, suggesting a link with clinical presentation (Aas et al., 2011). Additional evidence that the blunted CAR is not normalized by antipsychotic treatment further indicates that this may represent a trait, rather than a state, biological feature of psychosis (Mondelli et al., 2010a).

There may also be a synergistic relationship between activation of the HPA axis and activation of dopaminergic circuits implicated in the onset of psychosis. Although the exact mechanisms remain to be clarified, evidence suggests that glucocorticoid secretion (GRs) increases dopamine activity in certain brain regions, particularly in the mesolimbic system (Van Winkel et al., 2008). A neurochemical sensitization of the mesolimbic dopamine system (dopamine sensitization) can result from repeated exposure to sensitizing life stressors, and progress into increased stress-associated neurochemical activation, mainly of HPA hormones and dopamine. During active periods of illness (such as the prodromal phase, initial episode, and subsequent re-lapses), the dopaminergic system may be hyper-responsive to environmental stimuli, so that exposure to even moderate levels of stress could induce exces-sive dopamine release, precipitating onset in vulnerable individuals or relapse (Mizrahi, 2010).

Another biological pathway involved in the response to stress and rele-vant to the pathophysiology of psychoses is the immune system, which when activated produces raised levels of circulating pro-inflammatory cytokines. Cytokines like tumour necrosis factor (TNF)-α and interleukin (IL)-6 are prominent candidates for mediating the association between inflammatory response and psychosis. The mechanisms through which inflammatory cyto-kines could mediate the onset of psychosis are also unclear, but could include interactions with multiple pathways such as monoamine metabolism, neuro-endocrine function, and synaptic plasticity, all possibly leading to alterations in brain function and structure (Zajkowska & Mondelli, 2014). For example, cytokines are key regulators of both immune responses to pathogens (Miller et al., 2013) and prenatal neurodevelopment (Ratnayake et al., 2013). Thus, alterations in cytokine levels resulting from immune activation may disrupt normative neural development (Deverman & Patterson, 2009) and increase the risk of developing psychosis (Miller et al., 2013). Buka et al. (2001) found that increased levels of TNF-α measured in maternal serum at the time of birth were associated with schizophrenia and related psychotic disorders in the offspring. Also, elevated maternal TNF-α has been associated with a his-tory of infection in the third trimester of pregnancy, suggesting maternal in-fections could trigger immune activation. Interestingly, Allswede et al. (2016) found that higher anti-inflammatory Th2 cytokines in maternal serum at the time of birth were associated with lower odds of developing psychosis in adulthood. This may point to a protective effect of anti-inflammatory cyto-kine exposure at birth.

Later in life, immune activation has been observed in young individuals meeting criteria for an ultra-high-risk (UHR) state for psychosis, even prior to illness onset. For example, Zeni-Graiff et al. (2016) found that UHR subjects showed increased IL-6 levels and decreased IL-17 levels in serum, suggestive of a pro-inflammatory activation. Even more consistently, evidence from our own group has shown the presence of immune activation in adult patients with a first episode of psychosis. This includes, for example, raised levels of the pro-inflammatory cytokines IL-6, TNF-α, and IL-1β in patients at their first episode of both an affective and a non-affective psychosis (Di Nicola et al., 2013). Interestingly, Mondelli et al. (2015) have also found that increased levels of these inflammatory markers, particularly IL-6 and interferon (IFN)-γ, are associated with poor treatment response. This suggests that inflammatory markers at the onset of psychosis characterize a sub-group of patients with a particular type of outcome. As such, they could be considered possible predictors of treatment response and be useful in stratification approaches for clinical trials, as well as potential targets for the development of novel therapeutic agents (Mondelli et al., 2015).

Brain structure and neurodevelopmental indicators

Studies of the biology of psychoses have also pointed to the presence of a set of alterations of possible neurodevelopmental origin that precede, and contribute to, the onset of the disorder later on in life. For example, structural magnetic resonance imaging studies (sMRI) have found that already at illness onset, and before starting treatment, patients with psychosis—compared with controls—have smaller grey matter volumes of frontal cortex, medial temporal areas such as hippocampus and amygdala, thalamus, and larger pallidum and lateral ventricle volumes (Fusar-Poli & Meyer-Lindenberg, 2016; Van Erp et al., 2015). Brain alterations have been reported not only in volumes but also in gyrification, a morphological brain feature that develops very early in life and that is thought to reflect aberrations in neurodevelopment (Palaniyappan et al., 2015). Interestingly, a reduced brain gyrification of frontal and temporal areas, present already at onset, has been associated with worse response to treatment, independent of diagnosis (Palaniyappan et al., 2015). This suggests that early neurodevelopmental alterations could again represent a marker of unfavourable prognosis across psychoses, irrespective of diagnostic boundaries.

Further support for a neurodevelopmental origin of the brain changes seen in psychosis comes from evidence that reductions of subcortical structures, such as the putamen, globus pallidus, and thalamus, and the associated motor dysfunction and difficulties in integrating information from different sensory modalities are already evident at onset (Dazzan et al., 2004; Dazzan et al., 2008). Indeed, studies that have investigated individuals at high-risk of psychosis suggest that at least some brain changes precede onset and may characterize those individuals destined to develop the disorder. For example, at least some of the cortical grey matter abnormalities mentioned earlier are already present several years before the first episode of psychosis (Borgwardt et al., 2007; Dazzan et al., 2012). Volume reductions in temporoparietal, bilateral prefrontal, and limbic cortex have thus been proposed as neuroanatomical correlates of an enhanced vulnerability to psychosis, with reductions in superior temporal and inferior frontal areas being particularly associated with a transition to disorder (Fusar-Poli et al., 2011).

Of all the brain structural changes reported in psychosis and discussed earlier, reductions in hippocampal volume are among the most common findings across the whole psychosis spectrum. Smaller hippocampal volumes have already been found in patients with first-episode psychosis (Buehlmann et al., 2010; Velakoulis et al., 2006; Witthaus et al., 2009), and in some (Mechelli et al., 2011) but not all (Velakoulis et al., 2006) studies of individuals at ultra-high risk for psychosis. Recently, the ENIGMA-SZ Consortium examined a sample totalling more than 2000 patients with schizophrenia and found that smaller subcortical volumes were in fact most significant in the hippocampal region (Van Erp et al., 2015). Studies in non-affected individuals from large extended families affected by schizophrenia support the presence of a moderate genetic heritability for hippocampal volume, suggesting this region could represent an acceptable endophenotype (Roalf et al., 2015). Relevant to what was discussed earlier, hippocampal volume reductions represent an important component of the stress-vulnerability model of psychosis. Stress, the activation of the HPA axis, and raised cortisol levels have been suggested to play a role in volumetric and functional changes of the hippocampus in both animal and human studies (Mondelli et al., 2010b). Our own data in first-episode psychosis patients have also shown a significant association between smaller left hippocampal volumes and higher cortisol levels. This negative correlation supports the hypothesis that the smaller hippocampal volume consistently reported in psychosis could result, at least in part, from the biological cascade triggered by stress-related processes in the brain (Mondelli et al., 2010b; Velakoulis et al., 2006).

Evidence from the Global South and other regions: (1) Neurobiological mechanisms

There are some studies from the Global South or in non-white populations that have also investigated the presence of neurobiological factors such as immune activation in groups of subjects with recent-onset schizophrenia or young individuals in the UHR state for psychosis. The largest of those studies were carried out in China, with samples of around 100 first-episode psychosis patients (Chen et al., 2021; Song et al., 2013; Xiu et al., 2014). Such studies have replicated findings of increased levels of peripheral pro-inflammatory cytokines (Song et al., 2013; Chen et al., 2021) and decreased levels of anti-inflammatory markers (Xiu et al., 2014) in individuals with first-episode psychosis. There have also been findings of significant decrements in Insulin-like Growth Factor 1 (IGF-1) levels after antipsychotic treatment (Chen et al., 2021). Results of additional studies involving Chinese samples of more modest size have been variable, with reports of both increased (He et al., 2020) or decreased (Zhu et al., 2018) levels of pro-inflammatory cytokines in patients with first-episode schizophrenia. A few studies of the same kind have been carried out in Brazil (Corsi-Zuelli et al., 2020; Noto et al., 2014; Noto et al., 2019), the most recent one involving a sample of more than one-hundred first-episode psychosis patients (Corsi-Zuelli et al., 2020). These studies on Brazilian samples have replicated previous findings of increased levels of pro-inflammatory cytokines in first-episode psychosis patients relative to controls (Corsi-Zuelli et al., 2020; Noto et al., 2014; Noto et al., 2019) and reversal of such findings after antipsychotic treatment (Noto et al., 2014; Noto et al., 2019). There is also one report on 12 Brazilian UHR subjects who had higher IL-6 levels and lower IL-17 levels relative to controls (Zeni-Graiff et al., 2016). Finally, in a study conducted in India involving patients with schizophrenia (n=62) with a mean duration of illness of 18 months, levels of two cytokines (IL-17 and IL-10) were higher in direct proportion to the severity of symptoms (Chenniappan et al., 2020).

Taken together, the findings from these studies suggest that immune activation is present in recent-onset psychosis across diverse populations. However, serum measurements of pro-inflammatory cytokines are highly variable, raising doubts about the reproducibility of findings when studies are conducted with modestly sized samples. Thus, to examine the robustness of the findings reviewed here, separate meta-analyses of data on inflammatory markers gathered in studies carried out outside North America, Western Europe, and Australia are warranted. Moreover, as noted earlier, the presence of immune activation may be associated with alterations in brain function and structure (Zajkowska & Mondelli, 2014). Therefore, there is an urgent need for studies investigating associations between neuroimaging abnormalities and levels of markers of inflammatory activity in the same samples of subjects with first-episode psychosis or during UHR states; no such studies have yet been reported from countries in Asia, Africa, or Latin America.

Evidence from the Global South and other regions: (2) Brain structure and neurodevelopmental indicators

Despite the consistent findings from the neuroimaging studies reviewed earlier, there is limited population diversity of samples, since most MRI investigations of psychosis to date have been carried out in North America, Western Europe, and Australia. This raises questions as to whether findings may be generalized to the rest of the world's populations.

Intersubject variability of imaging measurements in groups of patients with psychosis is often wide. Therefore, MRI studies carried out in the Global South or with non-white populations attempting to replicate established literature findings should involve large samples whenever possible, in order to afford sufficient statistical power to avoid false-negative findings. Four relatively large-sized structural MRI studies have been conducted to date, each comparing groups of approximately 100 to 150 individuals with first-episode psychosis or at UHR states with control groups of similar size. For example, in a study carried out in Sao Paulo, Brazil, a sample of patients with a first-episode psychosis (n= 122, 62 of whom with a diagnosis of schizophrenia or schizophreniform disorder) was compared with 94 next-door neighbours with no history of psychosis (Schaufelberger et al., 2007). The authors reported grey matter volume reductions among those with first-episode psychosis relative to controls in the hippocampus and the prefrontal, superior temporal, and insular cortices, in line with the results of previous studies that used similar image acquisition and analysis methods. More recently, a study in Cape Town, South Africa, involved 93 individuals with first-episode schizophrenia and 98 controls; the authors found reduced cortical thickness in frontal regions (Asmal et al., 2018) and widespread microstructural white matter abnormalities (as assessed using diffusion MRI imaging methods) (Asmal et al., 2017) in patients compared with controls. In Japan, a multicentre MRI study of UHR subjects combining data from four sites reported increased caudate and lateral ventricle volumes and abnormal surface morphological patterns in the orbitofrontal cortex (suggestive of neurodevelopmental aberrations) in UHR subjects (n=107 to n=125) compared with controls (n=104 to n=110) (Nakamura et al., 2019; Sasabayashi et al., 2020). In the recent Shanghai-At-Risk-for-Psychosis study conducted in China, reduced cortical thickness was detected in selected parietal, temporal and frontal regions in 152 subjects at UHR compared to 92 healthy controls (del Re et al., 2021).

In addition to the relatively large investigations earlier, several studies have been published using partially overlapping, single-site samples of more modest size (usually fewer than 60). These studies also reported findings that are, in general, consistent with the results of investigations conducted in North America, Western Europe, and Australia. These include reduced volumes of frontal, cingulate, insular, temporal and parietal cortical, fusiform, and hippocampal regions in patients with first-episode psychosis in China (Guo et al., 2015; Luo et al., 2019; Wu et al., 2018; Yue et al., 2016; Zhao et al., 2018), Japan (Iwashiro et al., 2012; Kawano et al., 2015; Nakamura et al., 2013; Ota et al., 2011; Takahashi et al., 2011; Takahashi et al., 2020), and South Korea (Kim et al., 2019); and reduced volume or thickness of frontal, cingulate, parietal, temporal, and parahippocampal cortices in UHR individuals in South Korea (Jung et al., 2011; Kwak et al., 2019) and Japan (Iwashiro et al., 2012). In terms of white matter microstructural changes and disrupted anatomical connectivity, assessed with diffusion MRI-based techniques, these have been reported in patients with first-episode psychosis in China (Deng et al., 2019; Zeng et al., 2016; Zhang et al., 2015; Zhou et al., 2017), Japan (Ota et al., 2011), South Korea (Cho et al., 2016), and Brazil (Serpa et al., 2017), and in UHR subjects from China (Tang et al., 2019), South Korea (Cho et al., 2016), and Japan (Katagiri et al., 2015; Ota et al., 2011; Saito et al., 2017). Finally, altered structural covariance (possibly reflecting disrupted neurodevelopmental coordination) of frontal and insular regions has been reported in patients with first-episode psychosis from Brazil (Zugman et al., 2015). Negative findings for a number of structural imaging measures have been reported in only a few single-site MRI studies using partially overlapping UHR samples in Japan (Nakamura et al., 2013; Sakuma et al., 2018; Takayanagi et al., 2020; Takahashi, Tsugawa et al., 2020).

The convergence of the MRI findings reviewed earlier with the results of studies carried out in North America, Western Europe, and Australia provides an indication that first-episode psychosis and UHR states may both have similar underlying neuroanatomic substrates across different countries and populations. It should also be noted that a proportion of the MRI data compiled in large, contemporary international consortia has been contributed by research groups based in Asia and Latin America (Van Erp et al., 2015; Vieira et al., 2021). However, meta- or mega-analyses disaggregating these samples by region have not been conducted in the context of those consortia. Nevertheless, one separate structural MRI study did inspect whether patterns of brain volume deficits between patients with first-episode schizophrenia and controls differed across four ethnically distinct samples (white, African-Caribbean, Japanese, and Chinese), each sample with up to 50 patients and 50 controls. The authors found volume reductions of the right insula in first-episode psychosis patients across all four samples, providing support for the view that there are similarities in the neuroanatomical signature of recent-onset schizophrenia across ethnically distinct populations (Gong et al., 2015). However, since volume abnormalities of the insula may be a transdiagnostic marker across several mental disorders (Goodkind et al., 2015), the findings of this cross-ethnic study may not be specific for schizophrenia.

Finally, when evaluating the results of neuroimaging studies conducted with samples recruited in low- and middle-income settings, it is critical to bear in mind that findings may be influenced by socioeconomic factors that may be more prevalent in some low-resource settings. This is illustrated in a recent multicentric structural MRI study conducted in Latin America, including 334 patients with schizophrenia and 262 controls recruited in six different cities. Significant direct correlations with socioeconomic status were found for global and frontal grey matter volumes only in controls and for the hippocampus only in patients with schizophrenia (Crossley et al., 2021). In future large-scale studies of neurobiology across different countries and ethnic backgrounds, it will be essential to take into account the potentially confounding influence of a wide range of environmental variables, such as those related to neighbourhood socioeconomic conditions, exposure to violence, and levels of air pollution, among others.

Conclusions

The onset of psychosis is currently conceptualized as most likely to result from an interaction between genetic, neurobiological, and environmental factors, which together confer an increased risk for disorder. The research reviewed in this chapter—mostly from high-income countries—supports this formulation and elaborates on it by providing clues to the specific biological pathways that may link external, environmental stressors with disorder. A key challenge for research from here on is to examine these putative risks and mechanisms in more diverse populations. Indeed, the inclusion of individuals from diverse populations, backgrounds, and identities in genomic, neuroimaging, and other biomarker studies, will be of tremendous value in further delineating risks for and pathways to psychosis and in clarifying the extent to which these are generalizable or vary across the world's populations.

References

Aas, M., et al. (2011). Abnormal cortisol awakening response predicts worse cognitive function in patients with first-episode psychosis. *Psychol Med*, *41*, 463–476.

Allswede, D. M., Buka, S. L., Yolken, R. H., Torrey, E. F., & Cannon, T. D. (2016). Elevated maternal cytokine levels at birth and risk for psychosis in adult offspring. *Schizophr Res*, *172*, 41–45.

American Psychiatric Association (2013). *Diagnostic and statistical manual of mental disorders (DSM-5°)*. Washington, DC: American Psychiatric Pub.

Asmal, L., du Plessis, S., Vink, M., Chiliza, B., Kilian, S., & Emsley, R. (2018). Symptom attribution and frontal cortical thickness in first-episode schizophrenia. *Early Interv Psychiatry, 12*(4), 652–659.

Asmal, L., du Plessis, S., Vink, M., Fouche, J. P., Chiliza, B., & Emsley, R. (2017). Insight and white matter fractional anisotropy in first-episode schizophrenia. *Schizophr Res, 183*, 88–94.

Cho, K. I., et al. (2016). Altered thalamo-cortical white matter connectivity: probabilistic tractography study in clinical-high risk for psychosis and first-episode psychosis. *Schizophr Bull, 42*(3), 723–731.

Beards, S., Gayer-Anderson, C., Borges, S., Dewey, M. E., Fisher, H. L., & Morgan, C. (2013). Life events and psychosis: a review and meta-analysis. *Schizophr Bul, 39*(4), 740–747.

Belvederi Murri, M., et al. (2012). Hypothalamic-pituitary-adrenal axis and clinical symptoms in first-episode psychosis. *Psychoneuroendocrinology, 37*, 629–644.

Bergen, S. E., et al. (2019). Joint contributions of rare copy number variants and common SNPs to risk for schizophrenia. *Am J Psychiatry, 176*(1), 29–35.

Bigdeli, T. B., et al. (2020). Contributions of common genetic variants to risk of schizophrenia among individuals of African and Latino ancestry. *Mol Psychiatry, 25*(10), 2455–2467.

Bigdeli, T. B., et al. (2021). Genome-wide association studies of schizophrenia and bipolar disorder in a diverse cohort of US veterans. *Schizophr Bull, 47*(2), 517–529.

Borgwardt, S. J., et al. (2007). Structural brain abnormalities in individuals with an at-risk mental state who later develop psychosis. *Br J Psychiatry, 191*, 69–75.

Buehlmann, E., et al. (2010). Hippocampus abnormalities in at risk mental states for psychosis? A cross-sectional high resolution region of interest magnetic resonance imaging study. *J Psychiatr Res, 44* (7), 7–53.

Buka, S. L., Tsuang, M. T., Torrey, E. F., Klebanoff, M. A., Bernstein, D., & Yolken, R. H. (2001). Maternal infections and subsequent psychosis among offspring. *Arch Gen Psychiatry, 58*(11), 1032–1037.

Bulik-Sullivan, B. K., et al. (2015). LD Score regression distinguishes confounding from polygenicity in genome-wide association studies. *Nat Genet, 47*(3), 291–295.

Cardno, A. G., Rijsdijk, F. V., Sham, P. C., Murray, R. M., & McGuffin, P. (2002). A twin study of genetic relationships between psychotic symptoms. *Am J Psychiatry, 159*, 539–545.

Chen, D., Li, H., Zhao, Q., Song, J., Lin, C., & Yu, J. (2021). Effect of risperidone treatment on insulin-like growth factor-1 and interleukin-17 in drug naïve first-episode schizophrenia. *Psychiatry Res, 297*, 113717.

Chenniappan, R., Nandeesha, H., Kattimani, S., & Nanjaiah, N. D. (2020). Interleukin-17 and interleukin-10 association with disease progression in schizophrenia. *Ann Neurosci, 27*(1), 24–28.

Colodro-Conde, L., et al. (2018). Association between population density and genetic risk for schizophrenia. *JAMA Psychiatry, 75*(9), 901–910.

Corsi-Zuelli, F., et al. (2020). Cytokine profile in first-episode psychosis, unaffected siblings and community-based controls: the effects of familial liability and childhood maltreatment. *Psychol Med*, *50*(7), 1139–1147.

Corvin, A., & Morris, D. W. (2014). Genome-wide association studies: findings at the major histocompatibility complex locus in psychosis. *Biol Psychiatry*, *75*(4), 276–283.

Crossley, N. A., et al. (2021). Structural brain abnormalities in schizophrenia in adverse environments: examining the effect of poverty and violence in six Latin American cities. *Br J Psychiatry*, *218*(2), 112–118.

Davies C, et al. (2020). Prenatal and perinatal risk and protective factors for psychosis: a systematic review and meta-analysis. *Lancet Psychiatry*, *7*(5), 399–410.

Dazzan, P., et al. (2012). Volumetric abnormalities predating the onset of schizophrenia and affective psychoses: an MRI study in subjects at ultrahigh risk of psychosis. *Schizophr Bull*, *38*(5), 1083–1091.

Dazzan, P., et al. (2008). Neurological abnormalities and cognitive ability in first-episode psychosis. *Br J Psychiatry*, *193*(3), 197–202.

Dazzan, P., et al. (2004). The structural brain correlates of neurological soft signs in ÆSOP first-episode psychoses study. *Brain*, *127*(1), 143–153.

Del Re, E. C., et al. (2021). Baseline cortical thickness reductions in clinical high risk for psychosis: brain regions associated with conversion to psychosis versus non-conversion as assessed at one-year follow-up in the shanghai-at-risk-for-psychosis (SHARP) study. *Schizophr Bull*, *47*(2), 562–574.

Deng, Y., et al. (2019). Tractography-based classification in distinguishing patients with first-episode schizophrenia from healthy individuals. *Prog Neuropsychopharmacol Biol Psychiatry*, *88*, 66–73.

Deverman, B. E. & Patterson, P. H. (2009). Cytokines and CNS development. *Neuron*, *64*, 61–78.

Di Nicola, M., et al. (2013). Serum and gene expression profile of cytokines in first-episode psychosis. *Brain Behav Immun*, *31*, 90–95.

Dudbridge, F. (2013). Power and predictive accuracy of polygenic risk scores. *PLoS Genet*, *9*(3), e1003348.

Duncan, L., et al. (2019). Analysis of polygenic risk score usage and performance in diverse human populations. *Nat Commun*, *10*(1), 3328.

Fusar-Poli, P. & Meyer-Lindenberg, A. (2016). Forty years of structural imaging in psychosis: promises and truth. *Acta Psychiatr Scand*, *134*(3), 207–224.

Fusar-Poli, P., et al. (2011). Neuroanatomy of vulnerability to psychosis: a voxel-based meta-analysis. *Neurosci Biobehav Rev*, *35*(5), 1175–1185.

Gaziano, J. M., et al. (2016). Million veteran program: a mega-biobank to study genetic influences on health and disease. *J Clin Epidemiol*, *70*, 214–223.

Green, E. K., et al. (2016). Copy number variation in bipolar disorder. *Mol Psychiatry*, *21*(1), 89–93.

Gong, Q., et al. (2015). A neuroanatomical signature for schizophrenia across different ethnic groups. *Schizophr Bull*, *41*(6), 1266–1275.

Goodkind, M., et al. (2015). Identification of a common neurobiological substrate for mental illness. *JAMA Psychiatry*, *72*(4), 305–315.

Gordovez, F. J. A. & **McMahon, F. J.** (2020). The genetics of bipolar disorder. *Mol Psychiatry*, *25*(3), 544–559.

Gulsuner, S., et al. (2020). Genetics of schizophrenia in the South African Xhosa. *Science*, *367*(6477), 569–573.

Guo, W., et al. (2015). Abnormal causal connectivity by structural deficits in first-episode, drug-naive schizophrenia at rest. *Schizophr Bull*, *41*(1), 57–65.

Harvey, P. D., et al. (2014). The genetics of functional disability in schizophrenia and bipolar illness: methods and initial results for VA cooperative study# 572. *Am J Med Genet B Neuropsychiatr Genet*, *165*(4), 381–389.

Hauberg, M. E., et al. (2016). Schizophrenia working group of the psychiatric genomics consortium analyzing the role of microRNAs in schizophrenia in the context of common genetic risk variants. *JAMA Psychiatry*, *73*(4), 369–377.

He, X., et al. (2020). The role of cytokines in predicting the efficacy of acute stage treatment in patients with schizophrenia. *Neuropsychiatr Dis Treat*, *16*, 191–199.

Huckins, L. M., et al. (2019). Gene expression imputation across multiple brain regions provides insights into schizophrenia risk. *Nat Genet*, *51*(4), 659–674.

International Schizophrenia Consortium, *et al.* (2009). Common polygenic variation contributes to risk of schizophrenia and bipolar disorder. *Nature*, *460*, 748–752.

Iwashiro, N., et al. (2012). Localized gray matter volume reductions in the pars triangularis of the inferior frontal gyrus in individuals at clinical high-risk for psychosis and first episode for schizophrenia. *Schizophr Res*, *137*(1–3), 124–131.

Katagiri, N., et al. (2015). A longitudinal study investigating sub-threshold symptoms and white matter changes in individuals with an 'at risk mental state' (ARMS). *Schizophr Res*, *162*(1–3), 7–13.

Kawano, M., et al. (2015). Hippocampal subfield volumes in first episode and chronic schizophrenia. *PLoS ONE*, *10*(2), e0117785.

Kim, J. Y., Jeon, H., Kwon, A., Jin, M. J., Lee, S. H., & **Chung, Y. C.** (2019). Self-awareness of psychopathology and brain volume in patients with first episode psychosis. *Front Psychiatry*, *10*, 839.

Kwak, Y. B., Kim, M., Cho, K. I. K., Lee, J., Lee, T. Y., & **Kwon, J. S.** (2019). Reduced cortical thickness in subjects at clinical high risk for psychosis and clinical attributes. *Aust N Z J Psychiatry*, *53*(3), 219–227.

Lancaster, T. M., et al. (2019). Structural and functional neuroimaging of polygenic risk for 537 schizophrenia: a recall-by-genotype-based approach. *Schizophr Bull*, *45*, 405–414, 538.

Lam, M., et al. (2019). Comparative genetic architectures of schizophrenia in East Asian and European populations. *Nat Genet*, *51*(12), 1670–1678.

Lee, S. H., Ripke, S., Neale, B. M., & **Cross-Disorder Group of the Psychiatric Genomics Consortium** (2013). International Inflammatory Bowel Disease Genetics Consortium (IIBDGC). Genetic relationship between five psychiatric disorders estimated from genome-wide SNPs. *Nat Genet*, *45*(9), 984–994.

Legge, S. E., et al. (2021). Genetic architecture of schizophrenia: a review of major advancements. *Psychol Med*, *51*(13), 2168–2177.

Luo, N., et al. (2019). Brain function, structure and genomic data are linked but show different sensitivity to duration of illness and disease stage in schizophrenia. *Neuroimage Clin*, *23*, 101887.

Maier, W., Hofgen, B., Zobel, A., & Rietschel, M. (2005). Genetic models of schizophrenia and bipolar disorder: overlapping inheritance or discrete genotypes? *Eur Arch Psychiatry Clin Neurosci, 255*, 159–166.

Malhotra, D., et al. (2011). High frequencies of de novo CNVs in bipolar disorder and schizophrenia. *Neuron, 72*(6), 951–963.

Malhotra, D. & Sebat, J. (2012). CNVs: harbingers of a rare variant revolution in psychiatric genetics. *Cell, 148*(6):1223–1241.

Mallas, E. J., et al. (2016). Genome-wide discovered psychosis-risk gene ZNF804A impacts on white matter microstructure in health, schizophrenia and bipolar disorder. *PeerJ, 4*, e1570.

Marconi, A., Di Forti, M., Lewis, C. M., Murray, R. M., & Vassos, E. (2016). Meta-analysis of the association between the level of cannabis use and risk of psychosis. *Schizophr Bull, 42*(5), 1262–1269.

Martin, A. R., et al. (2020). Erratum: human demographic history impacts genetic risk prediction across diverse populations (The American Journal of Human Genetics (2020) 107 (4)(583–588),(S000292972030286X),(10.1016/j. ajhg. 2020.08. 017)). *Am J Hum Genet, 107*(4), 788–789.

Martin, A. R., et al. (2017). Human demographic history impacts genetic risk prediction across diverse populations. *Am J Hum Genet, 100*(4), 635–649.

Mechelli, A., et al. (2011). Neuroanatomical abnormalities that predate the onset of psychosis a multicenter study. *Arch Gen Psychiatry, 68*(5), 489–495.

Miller, A. H., Haroon, E., Raison, C. L., & Felger, J. C. (2013). Cytokine targets in the brain: impact on neurotransmitters and neurocircuits. *Depress Anxiety, 30*(4), 297–306.

Mizrahi, R. (2010). Advances in PET analyses of stress and dopamine. *Neuropsychopharmacology, 35*, 472–476.

Mondelli, V., et al. (2015). Cortisol and inflammatory biomarkers predict poor treatment response in first episode psychosis. *Schizophr Bull, 41*(5), 1162–1170.

Mondelli, V., et al. (2010a). Abnormal cortisol levels during the day and cortisol awakening response in first-episode psychosis: the role of stress and of antipsychotic treatment. *Schizophr Res, 116*(2), 234–242.

Mondelli, V., et al. (2010b). Higher cortisol levels are associated with smaller left hippocampal volume in first-episode psychosis. *Schizophr Res, 119* (1), 75–78.

Morales, J., et al. (2018). A standardized framework for representation of ancestry data in genomics studies, with application to the NHGRI-EBI GWAS Catalog. *Genome Biol, 19*(1), 1–10.

Morgan, C., et al. (2014). Modelling the interplay between childhood and adult adversity in pathways to psychosis: initial evidence from the AESOP study. *Psychol Med, 44*, 407–419.

Mortensen, P. B., Pedersen, C. B., Melbye, M., Mors, O., & Ewald, H. (2003) Individual and familial risk factors for bipolar affective disorders in Denmark. *Arch Gen Psychiatry, 60*, 1209–1215.

Mostafavi, H., et al. (2020). Variable prediction accuracy of polygenic scores within an ancestry group. *eLife, 9*, e48376.

Myin-Germeys, I. & van Os, J. (2007). Stress-reactivity in psychosis: evidence for an affective pathway to psychosis. *Clin Psychol Rev, 27*(4), 409–424.

Murray RM & Vassos E. (2020). Nature, nurture, and the polygenic risk score for schizophrenia. *Schizophr Bull*, *46*(6), 1363–1365.

Nakamura, K., et al. (2013). Gray matter changes in subjects at high risk for developing psychosis and first-episode schizophrenia: a voxel-based structural MRI study. *Front Psychiatry*, *4*, 16.

Nakamura, M., et al. (2019). Surface morphology of the orbitofrontal cortex in individuals at risk of psychosis: a multicenter study. *Eur Arch Psychiatry Clin Neurosci*, *269*(4), 397–406.

Noto, C., et al. (2014). Effects of risperidone on cytokine profile in drug-naïve first-episode psychosis. *Int J Neuropsychopharmacol*, *18*(4), pyu042.

Noto, M. N., et al. (2019). Activation of the immune-inflammatory response system and the compensatory immune-regulatory system in antipsychotic naive first episode psychosis. *Eur Neuropsychopharmacol*, *29*(3), 416–431.

O'Donovan, M. C., Craddock, N. J., & Owen, M. J. (2009). Genetics of psychosis; insights from views across the genome. *Hum Genet*, *126* (1), 3–12.

Ota, M., Obu, S., Sato, N., & Asada, T. (2011). Neuroimaging study in subjects at high risk of psychosis revealed by the Rorschach test and first-episode schizophrenia. *Acta Neuropsychiatr*, *23*(3), 125–131.

Owen, S. M. (2016). Schizophrenia. *Lancet*, *388*(10039), 86–97.

Palaniyappan, L., Park, B., Balain, V., Dangi, R., & Liddle, P. (2015). Abnormalities in structural covariance of cortical gyrification in schizophrenia. *Brain Struct Funct*, *220*(4), 2059–2071.

Pardiñas, A. F., et al. (2018). Common schizophrenia alleles are enriched in mutation-intolerant genes and in regions under strong background selection. *Nat Genet*, *50*, 381–389.

Pariante, C. M. (2008). Pituitary volume in psychosis: the first review of the evidence. *J Psychopharmacol*, *22*(2), 76–81.

Pearlson, G. D. (2015). Etiologic, phenomenologic, and endophenotypic overlap of schizophrenia and bipolar disorder. *Ann Rev Clin Psychol*, *11*, 251–281.

Pereira, L., et al. (2021). African genetic diversity and adaptation inform a precision medicine agenda. *Nat Rev Genet*, *22*(5), 284–306.

Popejoy, A. B. & Fullerton, S. M. (2016). Genomics is failing on diversity. *Nature*, *538*(7624), 161.

Pinto, D., et al (2010). Functional impact of global rare copy number variation in autism spectrum disorders. *Nature*, *466*(7304), 368–372.

Psychiatric Genomics Consortium Schizophrenia Working Group (2014). Biological insights from 108 schizophrenia-associated genetic loci. *Nature*, *511*, 421–427.

Purcell, S. M., et al. (2009). Common polygenic variation contributes to risk of schizophrenia and bipolar disorder. *Nature*, *460*, 748–752.

Ratnayake, U., Quinn, T., Walker, D. W., & Dickinson, H. (2013). Cytokines and the neurodevelopmental basis of mental illness. *Front Neurosci*, *7*, 180.

Richards, A. L., et al. (2012). Schizophrenia susceptibility alleles are enriched for alleles that affect gene expression in adult human brain. *Mol Psychiatry*, *17*(2), 193–201.

Ripke, S., et al. (2014). Biological Insights From 108 Schizophrenia-Associated Genetic Loci. Nature, 511(7510), 421–427.

Roalf, D. R., et al. (2015). Heritability of subcortical and limbic brain volume and shape in multiplex-multigenerational families with schizophrenia. *Biol Psychiatry*, *77*(2), 137–146.

Roberts, T., et al. (2020). INTREPID II: protocol for a multistudy programme of research on untreated psychosis in India, Nigeria and Trinidad. *BMJ Open, 10*(6), e039004.

Ruderfer, D. M., et al. (2018). Genomic dissection of bipolar disorder and schizophrenia, including 28 subphenotypes. *Cell, 173*(7), 1705–1715.

Rujescu D, et al. (2009). Disruption of the neurexin 1 gene is associated with schizophrenia. *Hum Mol Genet, 18*, 988–996.

Saito, J., et al. (2017). Longitudinal study examining abnormal white matter integrity using a tract-specific analysis in individuals with a high risk for psychosis. *Psychiatry Clin Neurosci, 71*(8), 530–541.

Sakuma, A., et al. (2018). No regional gray matter volume reduction observed in young Japanese people at ultra-high risk for psychosis: a voxel-based morphometry study. *Asian J Psychiatr, 37*, 167–171.

Sanders, A. R., et al. (2008) No significant association of 14 candidate genes with schizophrenia in a large European ancestry sample: implications for psychiatric genetics. *Am J Psychiatry, 165*, 497–506.

Sasabayashi, D., et al. (2020). Subcortical brain volume abnormalities in individuals with an at-risk mental state. *Schizophr Bull, 46*(4), 834–845.

Schaufelberger, M. S., et al. (2007). Grey matter abnormalities in Brazilians with first-episode psychosis. *Br J Psychiatry Suppl, 51*, s117–122.

Schizophrenia Psychiatric Genome-Wide Association Study (GWAS) Consortium (2011). Genome-wide association study identifies five new schizophrenia loci. *Nat Genet, 43*(10), 969–976.

Schizophrenia Working Group of the Psychiatric Genomics Consortium (2014). Biological insights from 108 schizophrenia-associated genetic loci. *Nature, 511*(7510), 421–427.

Sekar, A., et al. (2016). Schizophrenia risk from complex variation of complement component 4. *Nature, 530*(7589), 177–183.

Selten, J. P., van der Ven, E., & Termorshuizen, F. (2020). Migration and psychosis: a meta-analysis of incidence studies. *Psychol Med, 50*(2), 303–313.

Serpa, M. H., et al. (2017). State-dependent microstructural white matter changes in drug-naïve patients with first-episode psychosis. *Psychol Med, 47*(15), 2613–2627.

Socrates, A., et al. (2021). Investigating the effects of genetic risk of schizophrenia on behavioural traits. *NPJ Schizophrenia, 7*(1), 1–9.

Smoller, J. W. (2013). Cross Disorder Group of the Psychiatric Genomics Consortium. Identification of risk loci with shared effects on five major psychiatric disorders: a genome-wide analysis. *Lancet, 381*(9875), 1360.

Song, X., et al. (2013). Elevated levels of adiponectin and other cytokines in drug naïve, first episode schizophrenia patients with normal weight. *Schizophr Res, 150*(1), 269–273.

Stahl, E. A., et al. (2019). Genome-wide association study identifies 30 loci associated with bipolar disorder. *Nat Genet, 51*(5), 793–803.

Stevenson, A., et al. (2019). Neuropsychiatric genetics of African populations-psychosis (neurogap-psychosis): a case-control study protocol and GWAS in Ethiopia, Kenya, South Africa and Uganda. *BMJ Open, 9*(2), e025469.

Sullivan, P. F. (2008). The dice are rolling for schizophrenia genetics. *Psychol Med, 38*, 1693–1696.

Sullivan, P. F. (2010). The psychiatric GWAS consortium: big science comes to psychiatry. *Neuron, 68*(2), 182–186.

Takahashi, T., et al. (2020). Gray matter changes in the insular cortex during the course of the schizophrenia spectrum. *Front Psychiatry, 11,* 659.

Takahashi, T., et al. (2020). Thalamic and striato-pallidal volumes in schizophrenia patients and individuals at risk for psychosis: a multi-atlas segmentation study. *Schizophr Res, 243,* 268–275.

Takahashi, T., et al. (2011). A follow-up MRI study of the fusiform gyrus and middle and inferior temporal gyri in schizophrenia spectrum. *Prog Neuropsychopharmacol Biol Psychiatry, 35*(8), 1957–1964.

Takayanagi, Y., et al. (2020). Structural MRI study of the planum temporale in individuals with an at-risk mental state using labeled cortical distance mapping. *Front Psychiatry, 11,* 593952.

Tang, Y., et al. (2019). Altered cellular white matter but not extracellular free water on diffusion MRI in individuals at clinical high risk for psychosis. *Am J Psychiatry, 176*(10), 820–828.

Tansey, K. E., et al. (2016). Common alleles contribute to schizophrenia in CNV carriers. *Mol Psychiatry, 21*(8), 1085–1089.

Torres, F., Barbosa, M., & Maciel, P. (2016). Recurrent copy number variations as risk factors for neurodevelopmental disorders: critical overview and analysis of clinical implications. *J Med Genet, 53*(2), 73–90.

Tosato, S., Dazzan, P., & Collier, D. (2005). Association between the neuregulin 1 gene and schizophrenia: a systematic review. *Schizophr Bull, 31,* 613–617.

Van, L., Boot, E., & Bassett, A. S. (2017). Update on the 22q11. 2 deletion syndrome and its relevance to schizophrenia. *Curr Opin Psychiatry, 30*(3), 191–196.

Van der Merwe, C., et al. (2018). Advancing neuropsychiatric genetics training and collaboration in Africa. *Lancet Glob Health, 6*(3), e246–e247.

Van Erp, T. G. M., et al. (2015). Subcortical brain volume abnormalities in 2028 individuals with schizophrenia and 2540 healthy controls via the ENIGMA consortium. *Mol Psychiatry, 21*(4), 547–553.

Van Os, J., Rutten, B. P., & Poulton, R. (2008). Gene-environment interactions in schizophrenia: review of epidemiological findings and future directions. *Schizophr Bull, 34*(6), 1066–1082.

Van Winkel, R., Stefanis, N. C., & Myin-Germeys, I. (2008). Psychosocial stress and psychosis. A review of the neurobiological mechanisms and the evidence for gene-stress interaction. *Schizophr Bull, 34*(6), 1095–1105.

Varese, F., et al. (2012). Childhood adversities increase the risk of psychosis: a meta-analysis of patient-control, prospective- and cross-sectional cohort studies. *Schizophr Bull, 38*(4), 661–671.

Vassos, E., Agerbo, E., Mors, O., & Pedersen, C. B. (2016). Urban-rural differences in incidence rates of psychiatric disorders in Denmark. *Br J Psychiatry, 208*(5), 435–440.

Velakoulis, D., et al. (2006). Hippocampal and amygdala volumes according to psychosis stage and diagnosis a magnetic resonance imaging study of chronic schizophrenia, first-episode psychosis, and ultra-high-risk individuals. *Arch Gen Psychiatry, 63*(2), 139–149.

Vieira, S., et al. (2021). Neuroanatomical abnormalities in first-episode psychosis across independent samples: a multi-centre mega-analysis. Psychol Med, *51*(2), 340–350.

Walker, E., Mittal, V., & Tessner, K. (2008). Stress and the hypothalamic pituitary adrenal axis in the developmental course of schizophrenia. *Annu Rev Clin Psychol, 4*, 189–216.

Walsh, K. M. & Bracken, M. B. (2011). Copy number variation in the dosage-sensitive 16p11.2 interval accounts for only a small proportion of autism incidence: a systematic review and meta-analysis. *Genet Med, 13*(5), 377–384.

Williams, H. J., et al. (2011). Most genome-wide significant susceptibility loci for schizophrenia and bipolar disorder reported to date cross-traditional diagnostic boundaries. *Hum Mol Genet, 20*(2), 387–391.

Witthaus, H., et al. (2009). Gray matter abnormalities in subjects at ultra-high risk for schizophrenia and first-episode schizophrenic patients compared to healthy controls. *Psychiatry Res, 173*(3), 163–169.

World Health Organization (1993). *The ICD-10 classification of mental and behavioural disorders: clinical descriptions and diagnostic guidelines.* Geneva: World Health Organization.

Wray, N. R., et al. (2014). Research review: polygenic methods and their application to psychiatric traits. *J Child Psychol Psychiatry, 55*(10), 1068–1087.

Wu, F., et al. (2018). Structural and functional brain abnormalities in drug-naive, first-episode, and chronic patients with schizophrenia: a multimodal MRI study. *Neuropsychiatr Dis Treat, 14*, 2889–2904.

Xiu, M. H., et al. (2014). Decreased interleukin-10 serum levels in first-episode drug-naïve schizophrenia: relationship to psychopathology. *Schizophr Res, 156*(1), 9–14.

Yao, X., et al. (2021). Integrative analysis of genome-wide association studies identifies novel loci associated with neuropsychiatric disorders. *Transl Psychiatry, 11*(1), 69.

Yue, Y., et al. (2016). Regional abnormality of grey matter in schizophrenia: effect from the illness or treatment? *PLoS One, 11*(1), e0147204.

Zajkowska, Z. & Mondelli, V. (2014). First-episode psychosis: an inflammatory state?' *Neuroimmunomodulation, 21*, 102–108.

Zaslavsky, K., et al. (2019). SHANK2 mutations associated with autism spectrum disorder cause hyperconnectivity of human neurons. *Nat Neurosci, 22*(4), 556–564.

Zeng, B., et al. (2016). Abnormal white matter microstructure in drug-naive first episode schizophrenia patients before and after eight weeks of antipsychotic treatment. *Schizophr Res, 172*(1–3), 1–8.

Zeni-Graiff, M., et al. (2016). Peripheral immuno-inflammatory abnormalities in ultra-high risk of developing psychosis Program for Recognition and Intervention in Individuals in At-Risk Mental States (PRISMA). *Schizophr Res, 176*(2), 191–195.

Zhang, R., et al. (2015). Disrupted brain anatomical connectivity in medication-naïve patients with first-episode schizophrenia. *Brain Struct Funct, 220*(2), 1145–1159.

Zhang, J. P., et al. (2019). Schizophrenia polygenic risk score as a predictor of antipsychotic efficacy in first-episode psychosis. *Am J Psychiatry, 176*(1), 21–28.

Zhao, C., et al. (2018). Structural and functional brain abnormalities in schizophrenia: a cross-sectional study at different stages of the disease. *Prog Neuropsychopharmacol Biol Psychiatry, 83*, 27–32.

Zhou, Y., et al. (2017). White matter integrity in genetic high-risk individuals and first-episode schizophrenia patients: similarities and disassociations. *Biomed Res Int, 2017*, 3107845.

Zhu, F., et al. (2018). Altered serum tumor necrosis factor and interleukin-1β in first-episode drug-naive and chronic schizophrenia. *Front Neurosci, 12,* 296.

Zugman, A., et al. (2015). Structural covariance in schizophrenia and first-episode psychosis: an approach based on graph analysis. *J Psychiatr Res, 71,* 89–96.

5

Psychosis across persons 4: Course and outcome

Jonathan K. Burns

Introduction

The question of course and outcome for people with psychotic illnesses, and with schizophrenia in particular, has preoccupied clinicians and researchers for more than a century and remains a controversial and often confused issue. Arguably, Kraepelin's classic construction of a category of illness he termed *dementia praecox* that included those individuals with a deteriorating pattern of illness, first placed an emphasis on course and outcome as epidemiologically and diagnostically key aspects of severe mental illness. And, in a sense, what has been called the 'Kraepelian dichotomy'—separating 'poor prognosis' non-affective psychoses from 'better prognosis' affective illness—has dominated both professional and public thinking well into the current era. More recently, however, it has become increasingly apparent that there is considerable heterogeneity in the course and outcome of psychosis related to many factors including gender, age of onset, exposure to treatment, and socioeconomic and geographic context, challenging old assumptions and demonstrating the need for more coordination in international research to improve our understanding of the long-term pattern and consequences of psychotic illness.

Adopting a global perspective on the course and outcome of psychosis is timely and, many would argue, key to better understanding psychotic disorders and developing appropriate and effective interventions that improve both the longevity and quality of patients' lives. In recent years, more and more evidence has emerged from research calling into question some of psychiatry's core articles of faith, including that psychosis, and schizophrenia in particular, has a chronic deteriorating course and pessimistic prognosis; and that in countries of the Global South, patients experience a better outcome than their counterparts living in the Global North. The 'better outcome' hypothesis (or 'axiom' as some authors, e.g. Cohen et al., 2008, have termed it) emerged from the three large, multi-country studies of the epidemiology, course, and outcome of schizophrenia and other psychoses conducted by the World Health Organization (WHO) between 1968 and 1999 (Hopper et al., 2007; Jablensky et al., 1992; WHO, 1973). More recent data, however, from later follow-up of some of the WHO cohorts and from newer cohorts studied in a wider range of countries, reveal a far more complex and variable picture. It may be that there is cause for some optimism as studies such as AESOP in the UK have reported much higher rates of symptom recovery than previously thought possible. At 10-year follow-up of this first-episode psychosis (FEP) cohort, almost half (46%) of the 303 participants for whom complete data was available had been free of psychotic symptoms for the preceding 2 years or more, demonstrating that 'sustained symptom remission is possible for many with a psychotic disorder' (Morgan et al., 2014). These authors point out that this finding is contrary to the widely held view that non-affective psychotic disorders such as schizophrenia are 'chronic and deteriorating' (Morgan et al., 2014). On the other hand, evidence from long-term follow-up (>8 years) of cohorts in Ethiopia (Shibre et al., 2015), China (Ran et al., 2006; Ran et al., 2007), and Indonesia (Kurihara et al., 2005), as well as from very long-term (25-year) follow-up of the Madras Longitudinal Study cohort in India (Thara, 2012), indicates that the long-term outcome of psychosis may not in fact be better in the Global South, and that rates of mortality and significant symptomatology appear to be high in these contexts. Perhaps what is most clear though from the growing evidence base of global psychosis research is that 'course' and 'outcome' are highly complex concepts that are difficult to measure reliably and are even more difficult to compare between persons across decades and across socioeconomic, cultural, and geographic contexts.

The multidimensional nature of course and outcome

Several reviews of the course and outcome of psychosis/schizophrenia have been published during the last 15 years (Bromet et al., 2005; Jaaskelainen et al., 2013; Lang et al., 2013; Menezes et al., 2006). What these reviews all have in common are their conclusions: (a) that researchers often conflate these concepts and it is important to remember that 'course' is a longitudinal measure of pattern, while 'outcome' is a cross-sectional measure of current status; (b) that both course and outcome vary considerably between populations and within populations in relation to multiple factors (see later in this chapter for discussion of these factors); and (c) that marked methodological differences characterize this field of research, making the comparison of and pooling of data from different studies very difficult. As McGrath (2008) states: 'Apart from the multidimensional nature of outcome measures, there are methodological concerns about how best to compare results from studies with different intake criteria, and different durations of follow-up.' In fact, most authors would probably agree that the following are the key areas of methodological difference hindering this research field and obstructing our ability to synthesize a reliable evidence base on the course and outcome of psychosis—both within discrete populations and across the global landscape.

Different definitions and measures of outcome

In their review of follow-up studies of FEP reported between 1980 and 2013, Morgan and colleagues (Morgan et al., 2014) observed that there was 'notable variation in how remission and recovery were operationalized'. In terms of *remission*, some researchers defined this as the total absence of symptoms, while others defined it as symptoms below a specific threshold as measured using rating scales such as the Positive and Negative Syndrome Scale (PANSS). Also, there was variation in terms of the duration required for participants to be either symptom-free or below a set threshold in order to be considered in remission. It is now widely accepted that simple measures of clinical remission of symptoms are insufficient in determining patient outcomes, and the more recent emphasis on achieving *recovery* requires consideration of *social functional* status also (Jaaskelainen et al., 2013; Menezes et al., 2006). This brings a further challenge as Jääskeläinen et al. (2013) note in their review of recovery in schizophrenia: 'In contrast to most clinical symptoms, outcomes related to recovery do not lend themselves to simple, reliable metrics.' Indeed, there are multiple ways of conceptualizing and measuring an individual's occupational, social, and relational functioning, not to mention his or her quality of life or sense of well-being, identity, and existential fulfilment. A quick scan of the outcome literature reveals a wide array of both symptom and functional measures that require a great deal of ingenuity (and a dose of subjectivity) in attempting comparisons across studies.

Heterogenous samples

Comparison of follow-up data is also frustrated by the fact that the research samples themselves often differ diagnostically and epidemiologically. It has been noted, for example, in reviews of outcome in schizophrenia that where broader or looser criteria have been used, outcome appears to be better; whereas studies with narrower or tighter diagnostic criteria (often based on Kraepelin's original criteria for dementia praecox) tend to report poorer outcomes (e.g. Hegarty et al., 1994; Lang et al., 2013). (Note, however, that the systematic review and meta-analysis by Jääskeläinen et al. (2013) did not support this conclusion.) The more positive outcome of psychosis reported from long-term follow-up of the AESOP study (Morgan et al., 2014) and from incidence cohorts in the International Study of Schizophrenia (ISoS) (Harrison et al., 2001) is notable since both cohorts comprised unselected FEP patients. Morgan et al. (2014) note that studies comprising unselected incident cases of all psychoses are rare and that they 'provide the optimum basis for investigating the variability and determinants of course and outcome over the long term'. This is because study designs focusing on schizophrenia or non-affective psychosis only and/or hospital admissions, bias samples towards those individuals with poorer outcome. Furthermore, the comparison of incidence versus prevalence samples is problematic as they differ in composition—as McGrath (2008) explains: 'Prevalent cases are enriched with those with chronic illness and depleted of those who have died'. Notably those with chronic illness are often treatment-refractory (Menezes et al., 2006). Thus, it is important to distinguish incidence from prevalence studies in considering course and outcome of psychoses across the globe.

Different follow-up periods

Outcome studies differ considerably in terms of duration of follow-up with some reporting at 1 year and some at 35+ years. In general, systematic reviews and meta-analyses have tended to compare and combine data irrespective of follow-up duration (Jaaskelainen et al., 2013; Lang et al., 2013; Menezes et al., 2006) leading McGrath (2008) to ask whether it is 'valid to compare 'proportions recovered' between studies with different durations of follow-up?' He goes on to critique the solution some have advocated for comparing outcome data from different follow-up periods—that is the derived annualized remission rate (where the rate is divided by the number of follow-up years)—arguing that 'this derived measure assumes that the chance of recovery is evenly distributed over time, which is an unlikely scenario for any disease' (McGrath, 2008). And while Hegarty et al. (1994) and Menezes et al. (2006) found that duration of follow-up was not a predictor of outcome, the latter authors noted that stratification by study duration did suggest some trends, with a tendency for longer duration studies to show reduced rates of good outcome and increased rates of intermediate and poor outcome. It is possible that this may reflect attrition from the cohort of 'better outcome' participants who have improved or recovered to the point they no longer need treatment and drop out of follow-up (Menezes et al., 2006). Conversely, it is possible that overall outcome may appear better with longer-term follow-up as individuals with a poorer course either die or drop out of the cohort due to non-adherence, homelessness, and/or becoming lost to contact. Finally, it is possible that both scenarios are true and this may depend on context; with different factors at play in high-resource versus low-resource settings.

Factors associated with better or worse outcome

A number of sociodemographic and clinical features of psychosis are robustly associated with either improved or poorer outcome. Most evidence has emanated from studies conducted in the Global North, but data from several longitudinal studies conducted in the Global South now provide us with a more global perspective that reveals some regional differences. Also, as cohorts are followed up for much longer periods, there is evidence that some of the apparent associations (such as gender) may change over time. In general, factors predictive of poorer clinical and social outcomes in relation to non-affective psychosis include: male gender; early age of illness onset; long duration of untreated psychosis (DUP); insidious onset of illness; more negative symptoms; cognitive deficits; a positive family history of schizophrenia or major psychoses; poor premorbid adjustment and functioning; poor social support; poor treatment adherence; and comorbid substance abuse (Jablensky et al., 1992; Lambert et al., 2010; Menezes et al., 2006). Conversely, factors associated with better outcomes include: female gender; acute illness onset; shorter DUP; predominant positive and affective symptoms; early treatment response; good adherence; and strong social support (Jablensky et al., 1992; Lambert et al., 2010; Menezes et al., 2006).

Of all the findings on factors associated with outcome of psychosis and schizophrenia, perhaps the most controversial is that suggesting 'better outcomes in developing countries'. This probably has something to do with the fact that engaging with this finding (either in support of it or in opposition to it) requires one to engage with the complex and often emotive issues of race, culture, tradition, language, social practices, and 'development'. Importantly, adopting a global perspective on outcome requires us to examine and reflect upon not just research data from geographically diverse locations, but also the extraordinary diversity of humanity and the manner in which this diversity manifests in the heterogeneous presentation and natural history of psychosis. As we move to a global perspective, however, we should not lose sight of two important epidemiological facts highlighted by McGrath in his 2008 editorial, 'Dissecting the heterogeneity of schizophrenia outcomes' (McGrath, 2008). Firstly, McGrath reminds us that modern population genetics shows that while there is considerable variation within spatially defined populations, there remains 'between-group differences that reflect ancient geographical origin' and that some of these variations have been linked to susceptibility to various diseases. The implication here of course is that we should not automatically attribute any differences we might find between populations or countries or world regions (in prevalence, incidence, course, and outcome of psychosis) to the 'black box' of culture (Edgerton & Cohen, 1994; Maguire et al., 2020). The other reminder from McGrath is that outcomes of schizophrenia are unlikely to map neatly according to national or regional borders and that differences within nations should be studied alongside differences between nations if we are to understand the epidemiology of psychosis.

So, for example, we know that urban birth and migrant status are associated with increased risk for schizophrenia, but do we understand the impact of these factors on course and outcome? In fact, there is very little data available and the only systematic review to date of psychosis outcomes in migrants identified only 14 studies and concluded that while clinical remission rates appear to be higher and suicide rates lower in migrants, they are more likely to experience involuntary hospitalization and disengage from services (Maguire et al., 2020). The AESOP study examined clinical, social, and service use outcomes by ethnicity, and found poorer outcomes across the board for the Black Caribbean people compared with the White British group, with the Black African group experiencing comparable clinical outcomes but worse social and service use outcomes (Lambo, 1960; Morgan et al., 2017). Few studies have yet examined physical health outcomes.

The WHO studies of schizophrenia

It is a fascinating but little-known historical footnote that the Nigerian psychiatrist Adeoye Lambo pre-empted the WHO multi-country studies by two decades in observing that people with chronic psychotic illness appeared to have a better course and outcome and increased rates of 'recovery' within an African context. Lambo is worth quoting: 'Permanent recovery . . . seems to occur much more readily in African patients . . . We feel that, other things being equal, the favourable social and environmental factors inherent in the community to which the mentally ill are exposed in Africa influence the threshold of incapacity' (Lambo, 1960). Lambo's observations were anecdotal; however, he hypothesized that the 'lack of chronicity' he observed could be attributed to 'primary cultural factors inherent in certain environments' and that there is a better therapeutic response in those treated 'within the framework of the community'. Interestingly, Lambo also suggested that it may be that 'institutionalisation tends to produce severe chronicity in patients of all races and in all cultures'.

The International Pilot Study of Schizophrenia (IPSS) was conducted in nine countries and included 1202 consecutive admissions to psychiatric facilities (WHO, 1973); arguably, then, it could not be considered a truly epidemiological sample. At 2-year follow-up, patients were grouped into five outcome categories and, surprisingly, while only 39% of patients in countries of the Global North fell into the two 'best outcome' groups combined, 59% fell into these groups in countries of the Global South. Conversely, in the Global North, 37% of patients fell into the two 'worst outcome' groups combined, while only 23% of patients in the Global South were categorized as such. This pattern persisted at 5-year follow-up with Agra (India) and Ibadan (Nigeria) reporting better clinical and social outcomes, and Cali (Colombia) reporting better social outcomes compared with Global North sites (Leff et al., 1992). Social outcomes here were operationalized as occupational adjustment, relationship with friends and degree of social interaction; and social outcome was dichotomized as 'severe social impairment' or 'moderate, mild, or no social impairment'. Later follow-up at 10–14 years confirmed these findings with 51% of patients in Cali (Leon, 1989) having good outcome and 59% in Agra reported to be clinically 'normal' (Dube et al., 1984) (although in Agra it is worth noting that 83% had 'behaviour symptoms' and 67% had 'thinking difficulties' and 'speech abnormality' during interview). In Washington DC, however, 11-year follow-up showed little improvement compared with the 2-year assessment of functioning (Carpenter & Strauss, 1991).

Because the IPSS cohort was not necessarily representative and there was concern that selection bias might have partly accounted for the unexpected findings, a second large multisite study was initiated in the early 1980s. The WHO Collaborative Study on the Determinants of Outcome of Severe Mental Disorders (DOSMeD)—also called the 'Ten Country Study'—included 12 sites in 10 countries (Jablensky et al., 1992). The DOSMeD study had a much-improved study design, used standardized instruments and methodology, and comprised 1,379 first-episode incident patients across all sites. At two-year follow-up, 37% of patients in Global South countries were assessed as being in complete remission compared with only 15% of Global North country patients. Patients in the former showed 'a more favourable evolution' than patients in the latter on five out of the six measures of outcome. The authors conclude their report by stating that: '(DOSMeD) replicated in a clear and, possibly, conclusive way the major finding of the IPSS, that of the existence of consistent and marked differences in the prognosis of schizophrenia between the centres in developed countries and the centres in developing countries' (Jablensky et al., 1992). This conclusion should perhaps be somewhat tempered by the important consideration regarding the validity of these outcome measures. For example, one might argue that within low-resourced settings the percentage of time on antipsychotic medication and the percentage time spent in hospital are more reflective of socioeconomic conditions and the nature of health systems than of illness course and outcome. For example, in South Africa an analysis of mental health burden and service use showed a 'treatment gap' of 80% for people with severe mental disorders; where actual admissions to hospital over 1 year represented only 19.8% of admissions predicted from the expected burden of disease per population (Burns, 2014).

The third major study of schizophrenia undertaken by the WHO was the International Study of Schizophrenia (ISoS) and it incorporated numerous cohorts including some of the original IPSS and DOSMeD cohorts (Edgerton & Cohen, 1994; Hopper et al., 2007). The final sample was 1,633 patients comprising 14 treated incidence cohorts and 4 prevalence cohorts from culturally diverse sites in 12 countries. Outcome was determined for all incidence cases (809) at 15 years. Hopper and Wanderling (2000) showed that the finding of a consistent outcome differential favouring the Global South remained robust. The finding remained when strict International Classification of Diseases (ICD) criteria were applied as well as when 'broad' versus 'narrow' definitions of schizophrenia were used. These authors argue that the ISoS analyses dealt adequately with various possible sources of bias in the previous studies and that such bias could not account for the differences in outcome.

Critiques of the WHO studies

From the outset, the findings of better outcome of schizophrenia in countries of the Global South have attracted scepticism and criticism (Cohen, 1992; Cohen et al., 2008; Edgerton & Cohen, 1994); and a sometimes-heated debate between critics and original authors has persisted to the present (e.g. Jablensky et al., 1994; Leff, 2008; Warner, 1992). Early criticisms concerned issues of methodology, arguing that some patients recruited in the Global South sites did not necessarily have schizophrenia (Luhrmann, 2007). For example, critics have noted that in the Global South there is a 10-times higher rate of 'non-affective remitting psychosis' (NARP), an acute psychotic illness with rapid complete remission and, thus, favourable outcome (Susser & Wanderling, 1994) and that within the WHO studies, cases of NARP were misdiagnosed as schizophrenia. Furthermore, the IPSS cohort utilized a broad definition of schizophrenia with the possibility that cases of affective psychoses may have been included, especially in Global South sites. It is well known that schizophrenia has been overdiagnosed in African-Americans in the past (Bell & Mehta, 1980) and the implication is that this may have impacted diagnostic practices in 'non-Western' samples. Burns (2009) has also questioned the true representativeness of samples from the Global South, arguing that it is well recognized by psychiatrists working in these regions 'that in contexts of scarce resource, it is very often only the acutely psychotic and socially disruptive patients that access the health services'. Conversely, those with an insidious onset, long duration of untreated illness, marked social and occupational decline, prominent negative symptoms, and a dependence on traditional sources of healthcare are less likely to access formal medical services. If this is the case, then one might wonder whether the WHO studies were able to reach many 'poorer outcome' individuals (either incident or prevalent) and whether in fact their Global South cohorts were, as early as recruitment, biased in terms of a better outcome sample.

In addition to criticisms of methodological and diagnostic inconsistencies between sites, concerns about selection bias, and the high attrition rates and loss to follow-up (especially in Global South sites), sceptics of the 'better outcome hypothesis' have expressed particular concern at whether the selected sites could be considered representative of the Global South. For example, in relation to the DOSMeD, Edgerton and Cohen (1994) state: 'But one thing is obvious. These five centres do not begin to represent the full range of social or cultural diversity in what might be called the developing world, nor can they be said to be typical of that world.' They also point out the significant social, economic, and cultural variability between sites in the Global North.

Defenders of the finding maintain that the ISoS dealt with all of the methodological concerns and eliminated six potential sources of bias, namely: differences in follow-up; arbitrary grouping of centres; diagnostic ambiguities; selective outcome measures; gender; and age. Hopper and Wanderling (2000) conclude that 'none of these potential confounders explains away the differential in course and outcome' and that the robustness of the differential 'is generally taken as prima facie evidence for the relevance of 'culture' in influencing course and outcome of schizophrenia'. The issue of 'culture' certainly came to the fore as a means of explaining the apparent better outcome in the Global South. Bresnahan and colleagues (2003) write: 'It appears, therefore, that some aspect of the economic or cultural circumstance in developing countries may provide a more therapeutic context for recovery.' These authors propose the following explanations with respect to the Global South context: that family relationships may be more conducive to recovery (Bresnahan et al., 2003; Leff et al., 1987; Susser et al., 1996); that informal subsistence economies may provide diverse opportunities for reintegration of patients into work roles (Warner, 1983); that individuals with mental illness are less likely to be segregated within institutions; and that there is better community cohesion (Bresnahan et al., 2003).

Thus, the cultural and social environment was cited as the likely explanation for the WHO findings of better outcomes in schizophrenia in the Global South.

Non-WHO findings from the last two decades

In terms of revisiting the 'better outcome' hypothesis and trying to reach a balanced view on how people across the world with psychosis and schizophrenia fair in the long term, this publication and the present review chapter come at a good time, because we now have much more data available from both ongoing and new longitudinal studies conducted in many countries over the last two decades. And, as mentioned earlier, these new data are not just shedding new light on course and outcome in the Global South, but are also giving us pause to reconsider some of the assumptions we have long held on course and outcome within the Global North.

Cohen et al. (2008) published a critical review of the better outcome hypothesis and assembled data from 23 longitudinal studies of schizophrenia in 11 countries in the Global South. This review improved significantly on the extent to which it could be considered representative of the Global South, including three in Africa, two in South America, two in the Caribbean, three in Asia, and one in Eastern Europe. From this review the authors reported marked variability in outcome with changing patterns over time, noting in particular that while those with chronic symptoms appeared to be a minority, the majority of participants experienced relapse over a period of time. In addition to regionally specific variations in disability and social outcome, including some cohorts with high marital failure and high unemployment, they also highlighted the generally high proportion of patients who had never received biomedical treatment and, in some areas, the very high mortality rates of people with schizophrenia—even higher standardized mortality rates than often cited in the Global North. Finally, they expressed their scepticism at the perceived positive role of family and relative lack of stigma reported in the WHO studies from the Global South. At Asian and African sites in particular they noted a breakdown of family support and high levels of stigma resulting in families abandoning mentally ill members (Gureje, 2007; Lauber & Rossler, 2007). However, the reviewed studies were methodologically highly heterogeneous, which—as discussed earlier and noted by several researchers—limits any general conclusions that can be drawn.

In the next section, an update of Cohen and colleagues' 2008 review will be presented primarily focused on outcome data published during the last two decades. Where sufficient available data allows it, this review is organized in terms of (a) different components of outcome; (b) different periods of follow-up;

and (c) different geographical regions; and (d) nature of samples (i.e. prevalence versus incidence samples). Notably, this review does not include issues of mortality and suicide, which are important components of outcome (Seeman, 2007), and where there is evidence for substantial variation across geographical regions (Saha et al., 2007), as these important issues are addressed in Chapter 6.

Clinical remission

Short-term follow-up (1–3 years)

Short-term follow-up from Asian studies (notably all except one were from India) show the majority of clinical remission rates lying between 50% and 60% (Chang et al., 2012; Chatterjee et al., 2014; Hassan & Taha, 2011; Saravanan et al., 2010; Thara et al., 2012; Verghese et al., 1985; Verghese et al., 1989; Verma et al., 2012). Kulhara and Chandiramani (1988) reported 37.4% in symptomatic remission in Chandigarh but notably this was a schizophrenia sample only; while the two other studies reporting low remission rates—22.1% (Ran et al., 2001) and 29% (Srinivasan et al., 2001; Tirupati et al., 2004)—comprised untreated individuals with schizophrenia. As noted previously, samples with more narrowly defined schizophrenia criteria tend to report poorer outcomes (Hegarty et al., 1994; Lang et al., 2013). The Worldwide Schizophrenia Outpatient Health Outcomes (SOHO) study detected clinical remission in 84.4% of the Asian sample at 3-year follow-up (Haro et al., 2011), but importantly nearly two-thirds of the sample were lost to follow-up and it is likely, therefore, that this removed a substantial proportion of poor prognosis individuals from the follow-up sample. African studies show a range of clinical remission rates including 60.0% from South Africa (Chiliza et al., 2014), 45.7% from Nigeria (Makanjuola & Adedapo, 1987), and 27.4% from Ethiopia (Alem et al., 2009). The SOHO study (Haro et al., 2011), reported 79.6% remission at 3 years but importantly only about half the sample were followed up and countries included were in North Africa and the Middle East, which is a region that is socially, culturally, and economically quite distinct from sub-Saharan Africa. In Latin America, Menezes and Mann (1996) in Sao Paolo found only 23.8% to be symptom-free at 2 years; while the SOHO study (Haro et al., 2011) reported a rate of 79.4% for the region at 3 years, but again only a little over half of the sample were followed up.

By comparison, short-term clinical remission rates from Europe are very similar, ranging from 53.7% at 1 year in Turkey (Ucok et al., 2011) to 65.1% at 3 years in the SOHO study sample from Central and Eastern European sample (Haro et al., 2011) where follow-up rates were much better (73.1%). Notably, in the Turkish study, remission rates dropped steadily to 47.1% at 2 years to 38% at 3 years (Ucok et al., 2011).

Medium-term follow-up (3.5–7 years)

Medium-term follow-up continues to show some relatively high clinical remission rates from Asia (and again these are predominantly from India) with Kulhara and Wig (1978) reporting a rate of 45% at 4.5–6 years from Chandigarh, and Johnson et al. (Johnson et al., 2012; Johnson et al., 2014a; 2014b) detecting 68.4% in remission at 5 years in Tamil Nadu. Notably, however, other studies from the region show much lower remission rates, including 25.4% at 5 years in Madras (Chennai) (Verghese et al., 1985) and 37% at 6 years in Bali (Kurihara et al., 2011). The only medium-term follow-up data from Africa comes from Teferra et al. (2011; 2012) in Ethiopia who found only 21.2% of their schizophrenia sample to be in clinical remission.

Medium-term clinical remission rates in Europe are generally lower than short-term rates, ranging from 29.5% at 4 years in Turkey (Ucok et al., 2011) to 52% at 7 years in the Czech Republic (Ceskova et al., 2011). Other studies report 43% at 4 years in Ireland (Crumlish et al., 2009), 42% at 5 years in Sweden (Wieselgren & Lindstrom, 1996), and 38.7% at 7 years in Greenland (Lynge & Jacobsen, 1995).

Long-term follow-up (8–14 years)

Apart from the high 10-year clinical remission rate of 72.3% reported by Thara et al. (1994) from the Madras Longitudinal Study, long-term rates in the Global South are very low. At 10-year follow-ups, Ran et al. (2006; 2007) detected a remission rate of only 25% in Sichuan, China, while Shibre et al. (2015) found only 18% of their Ethiopian sample met remission criteria. A low rate of 29% at 11 years was also reported from Bali (Kurihara et al., 2005; Kurihara et al., 2006). All of these studies reported low rates of attrition, but they did exclude those who died during the follow-up from the reported remission rates (see Chapter 6 for a discussion of mortality among individuals with psychosis and its implications for interpreting outcomes).

Contrary to the accepted wisdom of better outcome in the Global South, long-term remission rates appear to be highly variable across the world. Within the Global North these range from 41% in clinical remission at 10.5 years in the UK (White et al., 2009) to 61% in both the Danish OPUS cohort at 10 years (Wils et al., 2017) and the Nottingham (UK) IsoS sample at 13 years (Harrison & Mason, 2007). Other studies report 46% at 10 years in the UK AESOP study (Morgan et al., 2014), 47% and 49% at 8 years from Finland (Salokangas, 1983) and Ireland (Crumlish et al., 2009), respectively, 48% at 10 years from Norway

(Hegelstad et al., 2012), and 60% at 12 years from Ireland (Hill et al., 2012). Given the heterogeneity of studies in terms of their follow-up periods, outcome definitions, and sampling strategies, direct comparisons of course and outcome across settings are extremely challenging. To better understand the sources of the observed variation, and identify factors that might explain variation between contexts, coordination is required to apply comparable methods across multiple settings.

Very long-term follow-up (≥15 years)

While the clinical remission rates for the Madras Longitudinal Study (MLS) at very long follow-up at 20 years and 25 years were lower than the 10-year rate for the MLS—47.5% (Thara, 2004) and 45% (Thara, 2012), respectively, they are considerably higher than rates reported elsewhere. In their Balinese cohort, Kurihara et al. (2011) found only 32.2% to be in clinical remission at 17 years, while the only other very long-term follow-ups (both from the Global North) reported similarly low remission rates—27% at 15 years from the Netherlands (Wiersma et al., 1998) and 30% at 20 years from Iceland (Helgason, 1990).

Functional outcome

As alluded to earlier in this chapter, the comparison of functional outcome across studies is challenging, in part due to the heterogeneity of methods and measures adopted, but also because functional outcome is highly context-dependent and also defined variably in different social and cultural settings. Functional outcome is notoriously difficult to assess and compare across settings and contexts (Isaac et al., 2007; Srinivasan & Thara, 1999). Important components of functional outcome include: occupational status; social functioning; housing situation; socioeconomic status; relationship status and social supports and level of independent self-management. Evidence on some core components of functional outcome is summarized next.

The SOHO study provides recent and useful comparative data on short-term functional remission rates (Haro et al., 2011). Regional rates were highest for Northern Europe (35%) and lowest for North Africa and the Middle East (17.8%). Other rates included: 28.7% for Latin America; 24.6% for East Asia; 21.6% for Central and Eastern Europe; and 20.7% for Southern Europe. Surprisingly few other outcome studies report functional remission rates, but those that do show marked variability within regions. For example, in East Asia, short-term rates reported from two separate cohorts in Hong Kong are similar to the SOHO finding—24% (Hassan & Taha, 2011) and 20% (Thara, 2004); while a much higher remission rate of 58% was reported by Verma et al. (2012)

in their Singapore study. A high short-term rate of 51% was also reported from a German study (Kurihara et al., 2011). In terms of long-term functional remission, Jaracz et al. (2015) found that 36% of their Polish cohort met criteria for functional remission at 10-year follow-up.

Occupational function

The assessment of occupational function is complicated by the fact that 'employment' is a difficult concept to define in people with severe mental illness and across different social contexts (Hickling et al., 2001; Hopper, 1991). Two important trends have been noted in relation to employment rates in people with psychotic disorders including schizophrenia. The first is that rates appeared to be higher in earlier studies (especially in the UK) conducted between the 1950s and 1980s than in later studies; and the other is that most longitudinal studies of first-episode patients show a drop in employment rates from illness onset to later follow-up stages (Jaracz et al., 2015; Marwaha & Johnson, 2004; Spellmann et al., 2012). Importantly, in the UK, the drop over time does not reflect the pattern of employment rates over the same period in the general population where unemployment has generally fallen. Changes in mental health policy as well as labour market conditions in the UK over the last 50 years may partially explain the drop in employment rates in people with schizophrenia over this period. In the era of deinstutionalization there was a marked emphasis on getting patients into work as part of rehabilitation and community integration and the nature of this work was often 'manual, repetitive and monotonous and often on assembly lines' (Anonymous, 1969). The increasing emphasis in more modern times on productivity and the dominance of services industries and technology means the nature of most work has changed and within such a competitive market, job prospects for those with schizophrenia are likely to be lower (Marwaha & Johnson, 2004).

Thus, comparisons of employment rates in people with psychosis and schizophrenia across social, economic, and geographical contexts is complex and requires in-depth analyses of both the contemporary and historical conditions of all the contexts in which studies have been conducted. Such an analysis is far beyond the scope of this chapter and so the following comparison of employment rates from around the world needs to be regarded as simplistic and with significant limitations.

In the short-term (1–3 years), employment rates for people with psychosis in Asia (and to a lesser extent in Africa and Latin America) appear relatively high. In Asian studies, rates range between 30% in Hong Kong (Chang et al., 2016) and 56% in India (Kulhara & Chandiramani, 1988). Similarly, a rate of 43% was reported from Jamaica (Hickling et al., 2001), with a slightly lower rate of 36%

coming from a Nigerian study (Makanjuola & Adedapo, 1987). By contrast, all rates reported post-1990 from Global North contexts are lower, including 16% at 3 years (Singh et al., 2000) and 25% (Birchwood et al., 1992) and 13% (Barnes et al., 2000) from the UK at 1 year, as well as 23% at 1 year from Denmark (Byrne et al., 2002). The only higher employment rate—49% at 2 years—comes from an earlier UK study by Johnstone et al. (1986). However, the caveats about comparing across contexts needs to be held in mind.

This difference between the Asian settings studied and those from Europe appear to persist in longer-term assessments of employment outcome. Apart from one lower rate from India (Shrivastava et al., 2010), employment rates from Asian studies looking at long-term and very long-term outcome, range between 46% for men and 26% for women in the 25-year assessment of the Madras Longitudinal Study (MLS) (Thara, 2012) to 76% for men and 75% for women in the earlier 20-year follow-up of the same cohort (Thara, 2004). Given the earlier observation in Marwaha and Johnson's 2004 review (of mainly Global South studies) that employment rates seem to drop with persistence of the illness, the increased rate in the MLS is an interesting departure from this trend. Notably, in Singapore, a drop over time was reported in a cohort of 402 patients with first-admission schizophrenia, from 55% at 10 years to 48% at 15 years (Tsoi & Wong, 1991) to 47% at 20 years (Kua et al., 2003). The only longer-term African study to report on occupational functioning was from Nigeria, where Gureje and Bamidele (1999) found that at 13-year retrospective follow-up of 120 people with schizophrenia, 55% of men and 48% of women had good occupational outcome.

By contrast, most long-term studies in the Global North (with a couple of exceptions) report employment rates substantially lower, ranging from 11% in Norway and Denmark at 10 years (Hegelstad et al., 2012) to 38% in Ireland at 12 years (Hill et al., 2012). Others include 19% (White et al., 2009) and 22% in the AESOP study (Morgan et al., 2014) at 10 years from the UK, and 24% at 10-year follow-up of the Danish OPUS Trial cohort (Wils et al., 2017). Similar rates are reported from very long follow-up studies at 20 years or beyond (DeSisto et al., 1995; Helgason, 1990; Opjordsmoen & Opjordsmoen, 1989). Notably two long-term studies report higher employment rates, both at 11 years: 46% from Finland (Lauronen et al., 2007) and 42% from Poland (Jaracz et al., 2015).

Thus, in summary, there is marked variability and methodological differences cannot be conclusively ruled out as an explanation for the observed heterogeneity in outcomes. Given the vast diversity of countries within the Global South (even comparing settings within a subregion, such as Hong Kong and mainland China), it seems implausible to suggest that there is a single factor that these countries have in common that would contribute to differences in outcomes, and indeed the overall picture appears to be one of variation that requires explanation. As evidenced by higher employment rates in the UK and other Global North contexts in the 1950s to 1980s period, with a subsequent drop in more recent decades, it seems reasonable to suggest that the persistent higher employment rates in some Asian contexts may be attributed to persisting mental health policy and labour market conditions in that region that are perhaps more similar to the UK conditions of the 1950s–1980s. This hypothesis would need to be tested by careful analysis of those conditions in the countries in which the studies have been conducted. If correct, such a hypothesis would imply that differences in occupational outcome relate more to structural aspects of the social, political, and economic environment, rather than to differences in disease processes.

Social function and marriage

Comparing outcomes in social functioning across global contexts is particularly difficult due to the wide array of measures used across studies and over time, as well as the vast differences that exist between societies in terms of social norms, practices, and attitudes. As for the aforementioned review of occupational outcome, the following review of social outcome is simplistic, restricted to just a few conceptual measures, and is limited by the absence of a full analysis of the social context of each study discussed.

Social function

There are many measures of social impairment, based on specific scales such as the Social Functioning Assessment Scale (SOFAS) or on other criteria where authors categorize degrees of social impairment. There is insufficient data to compare across geographical regions according to period of follow-up and so for the purposes of this review, all results will be pooled. This strategy reveals some interesting differences across world regions. Indian studies report approximately a third of individuals showing no social impairment at outcome. For example, in the MLS, 34% showed no impairment at 2 years (Verghese et al., 1989), dropping to 26% at 5-year follow-up (Thara & Rajkumar, 1992); while in 75 never-treated schizophrenia patients also in Chennai, Tirupati et al. (2004) reported good social functioning in 35% at 1 year. Interestingly a lower rate of only 17% was reported from China (Ran et al., 2001). Similarly low rates are reported for the African region (14% at 4 years from Ethiopia (Teferra et al., 2011; Teferra et al., 2012) and 21% at 5 years from Tunisia (Rafrafi et al., 2009)). A review of longitudinal outcome studies from the Global North shows consistently low rates including 15% from Finland at 11 years (Lauronen et al., 2007) and 14% at 15-year follow-up from Germany (Bottlender et al., 2010) and from a 15-year follow-up of a multisite study in six European centres (Weirsma et al., 2000).

If one focuses on individuals having poor social outcome at follow-up, the lowest rates are reported from India, from the MLS (13% at 2 years (Verghese et al., 1989) rising to 22% at 5 years (Thara & Rajkumar, 1992). Intermediate rates of 35% and 33% come from long-term follow-ups of cohorts in Singapore (Tsoi & Wong, 1991) and Bali (Kurihara et al., 2000) respectively; while short-term follow-up of the Chinese cohort assessed over half of the patients (56%) as having poor social outcome (Ran et al., 2001). Studies outside of Asia report on average about 50–60% of patients as having poor social outcome at both short- and long-term assessments, e.g. 54% from Brazil (Menezes & Mann, 1996); 59% from the European multisite study (Wiersma et al., 2000); and 64% from both the Mannheim long-term study (an der Heiden et al., 1995) and a later German study from Munich (Bottlender et al., 2010). Interestingly, a wide variation in rates is reported from studies in Africa, with very poor social outcomes (86%) at 4 years in Ethiopia (Teferra et al., 2011; Teferra et al., 2012) and a relatively low rate of only 36% at 13 years from Nigeria (Gureje & Bamidele, 1999).

Marital outcome

In the discussion of functional and social outcome across global contexts, the task of comparing marriage and marriage outcomes is particularly obfuscated by sociocultural context and norms—as Cohen et al. put it: '(marriage) must be interpreted in the context of sociocultural norms and assessed, at least to some degree, qualitatively' (Cohen et al., 2008). Thus, in considering both rates of marriage and rates of separation or divorce (an indicator of sorts for marriage quality), it is essential to take into account general population rates as there are notable differences across national and cultural settings.

It has long been accepted that marital outcome for people with schizophrenia and other psychotic disorders is markedly better in the MLS and other Asian studies than in countries of the Global North (Hopper et al., 2007; Thara & Kamath, 2015). Findings from the MLS are mainly responsible for this assumption, with 54% of participants married at 5-year follow-up (Thara & Rajkumar, 1992), 70% at 10 years (Thara et al., 1994), 74% at 20 years (Thara, 2004), and 64% at 25 years (Thara, 2012). However, these rates are nonetheless lower than the general population locally. Table 5.1 builds on and updates a table in Cohen et al.'s (2008) seminal paper and comprises a review of longitudinal studies of schizophrenia and psychosis from around the world where marital rates have been reported at follow-ups of between 1 year and 25 years. Where rates are available for more than one study, a mean (unweighted) rate has been calculated for each country. Also, mean national general population marriage rates for the

Table 5.1 Marital and separation/divorce rates from longitudinal studies of schizophrenia and psychosis across the globe

Country	Marriage			Separation and divorce (SAD)		
	Mean % married: participants (P)	Mean % married: country (C)'	Ratio: C/P	Mean % SAD: participants (P)[s]	Mean % SAD: country (C)'[s]	Ratio: P/C
Asia	**50**	**76**	**1.5**	**19**	**3**	**6.2**
India (Iyer et al., 2010; Padmavathi et al., 1998; Srinivasa Murty et al., 2005; Suresh et al., 2012; Thara, 2004; Thara, 2012; Thara & Rajkumar, 1992; Thara et al., 1994)	58	84	1.4	40	2	20.0
China (Ran et al., 2001; Ran et al., 2015a; Ran et al., 2015b; Ran et al., 2017)	62	82	1.3	9	1	9.0
Hong Kong (Tang et al., 2014)	32	66	2.1	20	4	5.0
Indonesia (Bali) (Kurihara et al., 2000; Kurihara et al., 2005; Kurihara et al., 2006; Kurihara et al., 2011)	57	79	1.4			
South Korea (Jung et al., 2011)	37	68	1.8	5	5	1.0
Japan (Ogawa et al., 1987)	45	73	1.6	19	3	6.3
Africa	**30**	**72**	**2.4**	**35**	**5**	**7.0**
Ethiopia (Kebede et al., 2005; Teferra et al., 2011; Teferra et al., 2012)	41	79	1.9	39	6	6.5
Nigeria (Gureje & Bamidele, 1999; Jablensky et al., 1992; Makanjuola & Adedapo, 1987)	26	76	2.9	31	4	7.8
Tunisia (Rafrafi et al., 2009)	22	61	2.8			
Latin America	**20**	**55**	**2.8**	**29**	**5**	**5.8**

Brazil (Menezes & Mann, 1996; Rosa et al., 2005)	20	55	2.8	29	5	5.8
Middle East	**37**	**75**	**2.0**	**10**	**1**	**10.0**
Jordan (Rayan & Obiedate, 2017)	37	75	2.0	10	1	10.0
Europe	**26**	**56**	**2.2**	**39**	**21**	**1.9**
Finland (Moilanen et al., 2013; Salokangas et al., 2006)	33	47	1.4	61	24	2.5
Poland (Cechnicki et al., 2011; Jaracz et al., 2015; Szkultecka-Dębek et al., 2016)	20	68	3.4	28	7	4.0
Iceland (Helgason, 1990)	34	55	1.7	32	17	1.9
Norway (Friis et al., 2016; Melle et al., 2000)	29	47	1.4	45	20	2.3
Denmark (Friis et al., 2016; Gotfredsen et al., 2017; Secher et al., 2015; Simonsen et al., 2010)	28	44	1.6			
UK (Hutchinson et al., 1999; Morgan et al., 2014)	32	55	1.7	31	14	2.2
Spain (Usall et al., 2002)	39	58	1.5			
Italy (Marchesi et al., 2014)	19	62	3.3	31	3	10.3
Canada (Abdel-Baki et al., 2011; Iyer et al., 2010)	17	49	2.9			
Sweden (Olsson et al., 2016)	16	43	2.7	57	21	2.7
Japan (Ogawa et al., 1987)	45	73	1.6	19	3	6.3
Russia (Golovina, 1998)	30	61	2.0	51	16	3.2
Croatia (Szkultecka-Dębek et al., 2016)	18	67	3.7	40	6	6.7

(continued)

Table 5.1 Continued

Country	Marriage			Separation and divorce (SAD)		
	Mean % married: participants (P)	Mean % married: country (C)[*]	Ratio: C/P	Mean % SAD: participants (P)[s]	Mean % SAD: country (C)[*s]	Ratio: P/C
Estonia (Szkultecka-Dębek et al., 2016)	20	47	2.4	50	15	3.3
Hungary (Szkultecka-Dębek et al., 2016)	26	53	2.0	28	19	1.5
Slovakia (Szkultecka-Dębek et al., 2016)	23	62	2.7	48	12	4.0
Slovenia (Szkultecka-Dębek et al., 2016)	19	51	2.7	32	11	2.9
Serbia (Szkultecka-Dębek et al., 2016)	23	68	3.0	26	6	4.3

[*] Marriage and divorce statistics for countries are taken for the age range 20–65 years.

[s] Separated and divorced rates (SAD) are calculated as number of SAD/(married + SAD), i.e. this indicates what proportion of previously married people are now separated or divorced.

years corresponding to study dates have been extracted from the UNPD World Marriage Data 2012 online database (United Nations, 2012), so that comparisons can be made for each country. Thus, mean participant marital rates per country and world region can be expressed as a ratio of the expected mean general population rate to the actual mean participant rate, which can then be compared. Table 5.1 also shows rates of separation or divorce for participants and for national corresponding general populations so that the same ratios can be compared. Importantly, however, rates of separation or divorce increase with longer follow-up, but the general population data is cross-sectional for the entire population of marriageable age—this is a limitation of this analysis but cannot be avoided.

A simple comparison of mean marital rates in people with schizophrenia and psychosis across world regions shows that the highest rates at follow-up are in Asian studies (50%), followed by the Middle East (37%), Africa (30%), then studies from the Global North (26%), with the lowest rate coming from just one study in Latin America (20%). However, if these mean marital rates are expressed in relation to expected mean rates for the general population in each region, then a different picture emerges. While people with psychosis in Asia are most likely to be married with a rate only 1.5 times lower than the general population rate (followed by the Middle East with a rate of 2.0), we find that people with psychosis in Europe are only marginally more disadvantaged with a rate 2.2 times lower than the general population. By comparison, the gaps between patient and general population marital rates for Africa and Latin America are higher, with ratios of 2.4 and 2.8, respectively. This is because expected general population marital rates vary considerably between regions—based on this review, approximately three-quarters of adults in Africa are married, compared with half in countries of the Global North. Thus, in terms of marriage opportunities, it appears that individuals with psychosis in Africa and Latin America are more disadvantaged (relative to their neighbours) than similarly affected individuals in Europe.

An analysis of separation and divorce rates provides an insight into the quality of marriages and their outcome. In brief, while the rates of separation and divorce (SAD) in people with schizophrenia and psychosis are highest in the Global North (39%), with apparently better outcomes in Asia (19%) and the Middle East (10%), if one considers these rates relative to general adult population rates of SAD in the same regions, then as for marriage rates, a different picture emerges. While patients in the Global North are approximately twice as likely to be separated or divorced than the general population, patients in the Global South are between 5 and 10 times more likely to be separated or divorced than the general population in the same regions. It appears then that marriage outcomes for people with schizophrenia and psychosis in the Global South are substantially worse (relative to the general population) than those of similarly affected individuals in the Global North.

Summary of findings from the last two decades

Table 5.2 summarizes the findings on course and outcome from the last two decades of global research on schizophrenia and other psychoses.

Conclusions

The question of course and outcome in psychotic disorders is longstanding, highly complex, and often controversial. Both methodological variability and conceptual differences between researchers over time and across different centres and regions, have given rise to a huge volume of outcome data, which is highly heterogenous (McGrath, 2008) and, thus, very difficult to compare across diverse settings. Differences in diagnosis, sampling, case detection, and identification, definition and measurement of outcome, and periods of follow-up, characterize the literature on outcome. Against this background, it seems extraordinary that for so long, the academic and clinical community have accepted as fact certain early pronouncements that gained traction and secured a foothold in major textbooks of psychiatry, psychology, and epidemiology. For a century, a relatively pessimistic view on the outcome of non-affective psychoses and schizophrenia has held sway; while for over 40 years the 'better outcome in developing countries' hypothesis has been accepted as an 'axiom' (Cohen et al., 2008) of psychiatric epidemiology.

One of the main limitations of early comparative studies of outcome across geographical and sociocultural contexts was the relative paucity of data from which conclusions could be drawn. Now, well into the twenty-first century, we have made some progress in assembling and following-up cohorts of patients in many parts of the world—allowing us to adopt a much improved and more representative global perspective on course and outcome—but the methodological heterogeneity remains a barrier to making valid comparisons across contexts.

The first conclusion is that assessments of course and outcome (and recovery) cannot hinge on one-dimensional concepts such as clinical symptomatology or even functional impairment. The concept of 'outcome', and to an even greater extent the concept of 'recovery', cannot be easily operationalized (Jaaskelainen et al., 2013); and when one adds the problem of finding valid metrics that are relevant and appropriate across differing social, economic, and cultural contexts, it is clear that this is no easy task. It is likely that the balancing act of trying to maximize the consistency and comparability of outcome measures across

Table 5.2 Summary of outcome data from the last two decades

Topic	Summary points
Clinical remission	
Short term	% remission similar across settings (~50–60%)
Medium term	% remission similar across settings (~ 40–45%), except for a high % in Tamil Nadu, India
Long term	% remission variable (from ~30% to 72% in MLS study at 10 years)
Very long term	% remission low (~30%), except MLS, ~45% at 20–25 years
Functional outcome	
Functional remission	Very mixed % of functional remission across settings
Occupational function	Somewhat higher % employment in Asian countries than in Europe, in both short- and long-term follow-ups
Social function	Indian studies show a higher percentage of people with no social impairment (approx. 30%) at outcome than studies from other countries (approx. 15–20%) In Asian follow-up studies, around 30–35% experience poor social outcome, compared with approximately 50–60% from other regions (and a very high percentage from Ethiopia)
Marriage outcomes	% married are highest and % separated or divorced lowest in Asia and the Middle East Relative to the general population, people with psychosis in Africa and Latin America are more disadvantaged than those in Europe in terms of marriage opportunities Marriage outcomes highly variable, but relative to the general population, patients in Africa and Asia appear more likely to have poor marriage outcomes than those in Europe

contexts, against the imperative to make measures relevant to specific contexts, will continue to challenge this research field (and others!) for decades to come.

The second conclusion we can draw from this review is that the general pessimism of the twenty-first century regarding the outcome of psychosis, should definitely give way to a less certain, and possibly to a more positive, twenty-first century view on outcome. Long-term findings from studies such as AESOP are forcing us to reconsider 'the still common view that non-affective psychotic disorders, especially schizophrenia, are chronic and deteriorating' (Morgan et al., 2014).

The third conclusion emerging from this review pertains to the controversial 'better outcome in developing countries' hypothesis. A contemporary global perspective shows us that there is no evidence that course and outcome, multidimensionally defined, are better (or worse) in the Global South than in the Global North. There are some suggestions that there may be trends in variation of individual components of outcome across geographical regions—for example, a trend towards better employment rates in some Asian countries (note previous caveats on employment as a measure); a higher proportion of patients with better social functioning in Asian countries (and in particular in India); and higher marital rates and lower SAD rates in Asia and the Middle East. Also, and contrary to accepted wisdom, patients in the Global North appear to have on average higher long-term clinical remission rates and better marital outcomes (relative to the general population). But it is clear that the data supports McGrath's (2008) scepticism that 'schizophrenia outcomes will obediently map on to geopolitical boundaries'. Certainly, there can be no useful purpose in continuing to utilize the largely outdated economic constructs of 'developed' versus 'developing' countries in our discourse on psychosis outcomes. Rather, we should look to the obvious variability that exists within geographical regions and countries and even sites, in relation to social and economic factors such as gender, ethnic and minority status, migration, urban upbringing, income distribution, and poverty. McGrath (2008) articulates well this need for a change in our focus and attention: 'It is curious that the hypothesis related to economic status captured the attention of the research community at the expense of the more general finding to emerge from the WHO study, which was that clinical outcomes varied widely within and between sites, regardless of economic status.'

Finally, while science has in many ways moved on, and large funders are rapidly shifting the focus of their support and resources on much-needed interventional and translational research, there is a strong argument for continued efforts to better understand and unravel the complexities of course and outcome in psychosis. Necessarily these efforts require a global perspective if meaningful findings are to emerge that shed new light on the aetiology, drivers of course and outcome, as well as the lived experience of psychosis across the world.

References

Abdel-Baki, A., Lesage, A., Nicole, L., Cossette, M., Salvat, E., & Lalonde, P. (2011). Schizophrenia, an illness with bad outcome: myth or reality? *Can J Psychiatry, 56*(2), 92–101.

Alem, A., et al. (2009). Clinical course and outcome of schizophrenia in a predominantly treatment-naïve cohort in rural Ethiopia. *Schizophr Bull, 35*(30), 646–654.

an der Heiden, W., et al. (1995). [The Mannheim long-term study of schizophrenia. Initial results of follow-up of the illness over 14 years after initial inpatient treatment]. *Nervenarzt, 66*(11), 820–827.

Anonymous (1969). Industrial therapy in mental hospitals. *Br Med J*, 1(5638), 202–203.

Barnes, T. R., Hutton, S. B., Chapman, M. J., Mutsatsa, S., Puri, B. K., & Joyce, E. M. (2000). West London first-episode study of schizophrenia. Clinical correlates of duration of untreated psychosis. *Br J Psychiatry*, *177*, 207–211.

Bell, C. C. & Mehta, H. (1980). The misdiagnosis of black patients with manic depressive illness. *J Natl Med Assoc*, *72*(2), 141–145.

Birchwood, M., Cochrane, R., MacMillan, F. C. S., Kucharska, J., & Cariss, M. (1992). The influence of ethnicity and family structure on relapse in first-episode schizophrenia: a comparison of Asian, Afro-Caribbean, and White Patients. *Br J Psychiatry*, *161*, 783–790.

Bottlender, R., et al. (2010). Social disability in schizophrenic, schizoaffective and affective disorders 15 years after first admission. *Schizophr Res*, *116*(1), 9–15.

Bresnahan, M., Menezes, P., Varma, V., & Susser, E. (2003). Geographical variation in incidence, course and outcome of schizophrenia: a comparison of developing and developed countries. In **Murray, R., Jones, P., Susser, E., van Os, J., & Cannon, M.,** eds. *The epidemiology of schizophrenia.* Cambridge: Cambridge University Press, 5–17.

Bromet, E. J., Naz, B., Fochtmann, L. J., Carlson, G. A., & Tanenberg-Karant, M. (2005). Long-term diagnostic stability and outcome in recent first-episode cohort studies of schizophrenia. *Schizophr Bull*, *31*(3), 639–649.

Burns, J. (2009). Dispelling a myth: developing world poverty, inequality, violence and social fragmentation are not good for outcome in schizophrenia. *Afr J Psychiatry*, *12*(3), 200–205.

Burns, J. K. (2014). The burden of untreated mental disorders in KwaZulu-Natal Province—mapping the treatment gap. *S Afr J Psych*, *20*(1), 6–10.

Byrne, M., Agerbo, E., & Mortensen, P. B. (2002). Family history of psychiatric disorders and age at first contact in schizophrenia: an epidemiological study. *Br J Psychiatry Suppl*, *43*, s19–25.

Carpenter, W. T. & Strauss, J. S. (1991). The prediction of outcome in schizophrenia: IV. Eleven-year follow-up of the Washington IPSS cohort. *J Nerv Ment Dis*, *179*(9), 517–525.

Cechnicki, A., Angermeyer, M. C., & Bielańska, A. (2011). Anticipated and experienced stigma among people with schizophrenia: its nature and correlates. *Soc Psychiatry Psychiatr Epidemiol*, *46*(7), 643–650.

Ceskova, E., Prikryl, R., & Kasparek, T. (2011). Outcome in males with first-episode schizophrenia: 7-year follow-up. *World J Biol Psychiatry*, *12*(1), 66–72.

Chang, W. C., et al. (2016). Three-year clinical and functional outcome comparison between first-episode mania with psychotic features and first-episode schizophrenia. *J Affect Disord*, *200*, 1–5.

Chang, W. C., et al. (2012). Prediction of remission and recovery in young people presenting with first-episode psychosis in Hong Kong: a 3-year follow-up study. *Aust N Z J Psychiatry*, *46*(2), 100–108.

Chatterjee, S., et al. (2014). Effectiveness of a community-based intervention for people with schizophrenia and their caregivers in India (COPSI): a randomised controlled trial. *Lancet*, *383*(9926), 1385–1394.

Chiliza, B., et al. (2014). Combining depot antipsychotic with an assertive monitoring programme for treating first-episode schizophrenia in a resource-constrained setting. *Early Interv Psychiatry*, *10*(1), 54–62.

Cohen, A., Patel, V., Thara, R., & Gureje, O. (2008). Questioning an axiom: better prognosis for schizophrenia in the developing world? *Schizophr Bull, 34*(2), 229–244.

Cohen, A. (1992). Prognosis for schizophrenia in the Third World: a reevaluation of cross-cultural research. *Cult Med Psychiatry, 16*, 53–75.

Crumlish, N., et al. (2009). Beyond the critical period: longitudinal study of 8-year outcome in first-episode non-affective psychosis. *Br J Psychiatry, 194*(1), 18–24.

DeSisto, M. J., et al. (1995). The Maine and Vermont three-decade studies of serious mental illness. I. Matched comparison of cross-sectional outcome. *Br J Psychiatry, 167*(3), 331–338.

Dube, K. C., Kumar, N., & Dube, S. (1984). Long term course and outcome of the Agra cases in the International Pilot Study of Schizophrenia. *Acta Psychiatr Scand, 70*(2), 170–179.

Edgerton, R. B. & Cohen, A. (1994). Culture and schizophrenia: the DOSMD challenge. *Br J Psychiatry, 164*, 222–231.

Friis, S., et al. (2016). Early predictors of ten-year course in first-episode psychosis. *Psychiatr Serv, 67*(4), 438–443.

Golovina, A. G. (1998). Characteristics of family status of patients with schizophrenia. *Zh Nevrol Psikhiatr Im S S Korsakova, 98*(1), 16–21.

Gotfredsen, D. R., et al. (2017). Stability and development of psychotic symptoms and the use of antipsychotic medication—long-term follow-up. *Psychol Med, 47*(12), 2118–2129.

Gureje, O. & Bamidele, R. (1999). Thirteen-year social outcome among Nigerian outpatients with schizophrenia. *Soc Psychiatry Psychiatr Epidemiol, 34*, 147–151.

Gureje O. (2007). Psychiatry in Africa: the myths, the exotic, and the realities. *S Afr Psychiatry Rev, 10*(1), 11–14.

Haro, J. M., Novick, D., Bertsch, J., Karagianis, J., Dossenbach, M., & Jones, P. B. (2011). Cross-national clinical and functional remission rates: worldwide schizophrenia outpatient health outcomes (W-SOHO) study. *Br J Psychiatry, 199*(3), 194–201.

Harrison, G., et al. (2001). Recovery from psychotic illness: a 15- and 25-year international follow-up study. *Br J Psychiatry, 178*, 506–517.

Harrison, G. & Mason, P. (2007). Nottingham, UK. In Hopper, K., Harrison, G., Janca, A., & Sartorius, N. (eds) *Recovery from schizophrenia: an international perspective*. Oxford: Oxford University Press, 177–188.

Hassan, G. A. & Taha, G. R. (2011). Long term functioning in early onset psychosis: two years prospective follow-up study. *Behav Brain Func, 7*, 28.

Hegarty, J. D., Baldessarini, R. J., Tohen, M., Waternaux, C., & Oepen, G. (1994). One hundred years of schizophrenia: a meta-analysis of the outcome literature. *Am J Psychiatry, 151*(10), 1409–1416.

Hegelstad, W. T., et al. (2012). Long-term follow-up of the TIPS early detection in psychosis study: effects on 10-year outcome. *Am J Psychiatry, 169*(4), 374–380.

Helgason, L. (1990). Twenty years' follow-up of first psychiatric presentation for schizophrenia: what could have been prevented? *Acta Psychiatr Scand, 81*(3), 231–235.

Hickling, F. W., McCallum, M., Nooks, L., & Rodgers-Johnson, P. (2001). Outcome of first contact schizophrenia in Jamaica. *West Indian Med J, 50*(3), 194–197.

Hill, M., et al. (2012). Prospective relationship of duration of untreated psychosis to psychopathology and functional outcome over 12 years. *Schizophr Res, 141*(2–3), 215–221.

Hopper, K., Harrison, G., Janca, A., & Sartorius, N. (eds) (2007). *Recovery from schizophrenia: an international perspective.* Oxford: Oxford University Press.

Hopper, K., Wanderling, J., & Narayanan, P. (2007). To have and to hold: a cross-cultural inquiry into marital prospects after psychosis. *Glob Public Health, 2*(3), 257–280.

Hopper, K. & Wanderling, J. (2000). Revisiting the developed versus developing country distinction in course and outcome in schizophrenia: results from IsoS, the WHO collaborative followup project. *Schizophr Bull, 26*(4), 835–846.

Hopper, K. (1991). Some old questions for the new cross-cultural psychiatry. *Med Anthropol Q, 5*, 299–330.

Hutchinson, G., Bhugra, D., Mallett, R., Burnett, R., Corridan, B., & Leff, J. (1999). Fertility and marital rates in first-onset schizophrenia. *Soc Psychiatry Psychiatr Epidemiol, 34*, 617–621.

Isaac, M., Chand, P., & Murthy, P. (2007). Schizophrenia outcome measures in the wider international community. *Br J Psychiatry, 191*(suppl. 50), s71–s77.

Iyer, S., Mangala, R., Thara, R., & Malla, A. (2010). Preliminary findings from a study of first-episode psychosis in Montreal, Canada and Chennai, India: comparison of outcomes. *Schizophr Res, 121*(1–3), 227–233.

Jaaskelainen, E., et al. (2013). A systematic review and meta-analysis of recovery in schizophrenia. *Schizophr Bull, 39*(6), 1296–1306.

Jablensky, A., Sartorius, N., Cooper, J. E., Anker, M., Korten, A., & Bertelsen, A. (1994). Culture and schizophrenia: criticisms of WHO studies are answered. *Br J Psychiatry, 165*, 434–436.

Jablensky, A., et al. (1992). Schizophrenia: manifestations, incidence and course in different cultures: a World Health Organization ten-country study. *Psychol Med, 20*(Supplement 20), 1–97.

Jaracz, K., et al. (2015). Psychosocial functioning in relation to symptomatic remission: a longitudinal study of first episode schizophrenia. *Eur Psychiatry, 30*(8), 907–913.

Johnson, S., Sathyaseelan, M., Charles, H., & Jacob, K. S. (2014a). Predictors of disability: a 5-year cohort study of first-episode schizophrenia. *Asian J Psychiatr, 9*, 45–50.

Johnson, S., Sathyaseelan, M., Charles, H., Jeyaseelan, V., & Jacob, K. (2012). Insight, psychopathology, explanatory models and outcome of schizophrenia in India: a prospective 5-year cohort study. *BMC Psychiatry, 12*(1), 159.

Johnson, S., Sathyaseelan, M., Charles, H., Jeyaseelan, V., & Jacob, K. S. (2014b). Predictors of insight in first-episode schizophrenia: a 5-year cohort study from India. *Int J Soc Psychiatry, 60*(6), 566–574.

Johnstone, E. C., Crow, T. J., Johnson, A. L., & MacMillan, J. F. (1986). The Northwick Park Study of first episodes of schizophrenia. I. Presentation of the illness and problems relating to admission. *Br J Psychiatry, 148*, 115–120.

Jung, S. H., et al. (2011). Factors affecting treatment discontinuation and treatment outcome in patients with schizophrenia in Korea: 10-year follow-up study. *Psychiatry Investig, 8*(1), 22–29.

Kebede, D., Alem, A., Shibre, T., Negash, A., Deyassa, N., Beyero, T., & Medhin, G. (2005). Short-term symptomatic and functional outcomes of schizophrenia in Butajira, Ethiopia. *Schizophr Res, 78*(2–3), 171–185.

Kua, J., Wong, K. E., Kua, E. H., & Tsoi, W. F. (2003). A 20-year follow-up study on schizophrenia in Singapore. *Acta Psychiatr Scand, 108*(2), 118–125.

Kulhara, P. & Chandiramani, K. (1988). Outcome of schizophrenia in India using various diagnostic systems. *Schizophr Res*, *1*(5), 339–349.

Kulhara, P. & Wig, N. N. (1978). The chronicity of schizophrenia in North West India: results of a follow-up study. *Br J Psychiatry*, *132*, 186–190.

Kurihara, T., Kato, M., Kashima, H., Takebayashi, T., Reverger, R., & Tirta, I. G. R. (2006). Excess mortality of schizophrenia in the developing country of Bali. *Schizophr Res*, *83*(1), 103–105.

Kurihara, T., Kato, M., Reverger, R., & Tirta, I. G. (2005). Eleven-year clinical outcome of schizophrenia in Bali. *Acta Psychiatr Scand*, *112*(6), 456–462.

Kurihara, T., Kato, M., Reverger, R., & Tirta, I. (2011). Remission in schizophrenia: a community-based 6-year follow-up study in Bali. *Psychiatry Clin Neurosci*, *65*(5), 476–482.

Kurihara, T., Kato, M., Reverger, R., & Tirta, I. (2011). Seventeen-year clinical outcome of schizophrenia in Bali. *Eur Psychiatry*, *26*(5), 333–338.

Kurihara, T., Kato, M., Reverger, R., & Yagi, G. (2000). Outcome of schizophrenia in a non-industrialized society: comparative study between Bali and Tokyo. *Acta Psychiatr Scand*, *101*(2), 148–152.

Lambert, M., Karow, A., Leucht, S., Schimmelmann, B. G., & Naber, D. (2010). Remission in schizophrenia: validity, frequency, predictors, and patients' perspective 5 years later. *Dialogues Clin Neurosci*, *12*(3), 393–407.

Lambo, T. A. (1960). Further neuropsychiatric observations in Nigeria with comment on the need for further epidemiological study in Africa. *BMJ*, *2*, 1696–704.

Lang, F. U., Kösters, M., Lang, S., Becker, T., & Jäger, M. (2013). Psychopathological long-term outcome of schizophrenia—a review. *Acta Psychiatr Scand*, *127*(3), 173–182.

Lauber, C. & Rossler, W. (2007). Stigma towards people with mental illness in developing countries in Asia. *Int Rev Psychiatry*, *19*(2), 157–178.

Lauronen, E., et al. (2007). Outcome and its predictors in schizophrenia within the Northern Finland 1966 birth cohort. *Eur Psychiatry*, *22*(2), 129–136.

Leff, J., Sartorius, N., Jablensky, A., Korten, A., & Ernberg, G. (1992). The international pilot study of schizophrenia: five-year follow-up findings. *Psychol Med*, *22*(1), 131–145.

Leff, J., et al. (1987). Expressed emotion and schizophrenia in north India. III. Influence of relatives' expressed emotion on the course of schizophrenia in Chandigarh. *Br J Psychiatry*, *151*, 166–173.

Leff, J. (2008). Comment on paper by Cohen, Patel, Thara, and Gureje. *Schizophr Bull*, *34*(2), 251–252.

Leon, C. A. (1989). Clinical course and outcome of schizophrenia in Cali, Colombia: a 10-year follow-up study. *J Nerv Ment Dis*, *177*(10), 593–606.

Luhrmann, T. M. (2007). Social defeat and the culture of chronicity: or, why schizophrenia does so well over there and so badly here. *Cult Med Psychiatry*, *31*(2), 135–172.

Lynge, I. & Jacobsen, J. (1995). Schizophrenia in Greenland: a follow-up study. *Acta Psychiatr Scand*, *91*(6), 414–422.

Maguire, J., Sizer, H., Mifsud, N., & O'Donoghue, B. (2020). Outcomes for migrants with a first episode of psychosis: a systematic review. *Schizophr Res*, *222*, 42–48.

Makanjuola, R. O. A. & Adedapo, S. A. (1987). The DSM-III concepts of schizophrenic disorder and schizophreniform disorder: a clinical and prognostic evaluation. *Br J Psychiatry*, *151*, 611–618.

Marchesi, C., Affaticati, A., Monici, A., De Panfilis, C., Ossola, P., & Tonna, M. (2014). Predictors of symptomatic remission in patients with first-episode schizophrenia: a 16years follow-up study. *Compr Psychiatry*, *55*(4), 778–784.

Marwaha, S. & Johnson, S. (2004). Schizophrenia and employment—a review. *Soc Psychiatry Psychiatr Epidemiol*, *39*(5), 337–349.

McGrath, J. (2008). Dissecting the heterogeneity of schizophrenia outcomes. *Schizophr Bull*, *34*(2), 247–248.

Melle, I., Friis, S., Hauff, E., & Vaglum, P. (2000). Social functioning of patients with schizophrenia in high-income welfare societies. *Psychiatr Serv*, *51*(2), 223–228.

Menezes, N. M., Arenovich, T., & Zipursky, R. B. (2006). A systematic review of longitudinal outcome studies of first-episode psychosis. *Psychol Med*, *36*(10), 1349–1362.

Menezes, P. R. & Mann, A. H. (1996). Mortality among patients with non-affective functional psychoses in a metropolitan area of south-eastern Brazil. *Rev Saude Publica*, *30*(4), 304–309.

Moilanen, J., et al. (2013). Characteristics of subjects with schizophrenia spectrum disorder with and without antipsychotic medication—a 10-year follow-up of the Northern Finland 1966 Birth Cohort study. *Eur Psychiatry*, *28*(1), 53–58.

Morgan, C., et al. (2014). Reappraising the long-term course and outcome of psychotic disorders: the AESOP-10 study. *Psychol Med*, *44*(13), 2713–2726.

Morgan, C., et al. (2017). Ethnicity and long-term course and outcome of psychotic disorders in a UK sample: the ÆSOP-10 study. *BJPsych*, *211*(2), 88–94.

Ogawa, K., Miya, M., Watarai, A., Nakazawa, M., Yuasa, S., & Utena, H. (1987). A long-term follow-up study of schizophrenia in Japan—with special reference to the course of social adjustment. *Br J Psychiatry*, *151*, 758–765.

Olsson, A. K., Hjärthag, F., & Helldin, L. (2016). Predicting real-world functional milestones in schizophrenia. *Psychiatry Res*, *242*, 1–6.

Opjordsmoen, S. & Opjordsmoen, S. (1989). Long-term course and outcome in unipolar affective and schizoaffective psychoses. *Acta Psychiatr Scand*, *79*(4), 317–326.

Padmavathi, R., Rajkumar, S., & Srinivasan, T. N. (1998). Schizophrenic patients who were never treated—a study in an Indian urban community. *Psychol Med*, *28*, 1113–1117.

Rafrafi, R., Zaghdoudi, L., Mahbouli, M., Bouzid, R., Labbane, R., & El Hechmi, Z. (2009). Social outcome of schizophrenics in Tunisia: a transversal study of 60 patients. *L'Encephale*, *35*(3), 234–240.

Ran, M., Xiang, M., Huang, M., Shan, Y., & Cooper, J. (2001). Natural course of schizophrenia: 2-year follow-up study in a rural Chinese community. *Br J Psychiatry*, *178*, 154–158.

Ran, M. S., Chan, C. L., Chen, E. Y., Xiang, M. Z., Caine, E. D., & Conwell, Y. (2006). Homelessness among patients with schizophrenia in rural China: a 10-year cohort study. *Acta Psychiatr Scand*, *114*(2), 118–123.

Ran, M. S., et al. (2007). Mortality in people with schizophrenia in rural China: 10-year cohort study. *Br J Psychiatry*, *190*(3), 237–242.

Ran, M. S., Mao, W. J., Chan, C. L., Chen, E. Y., & Conwell, Y. (2015a). Gender differences in outcomes in people with schizophrenia in rural China: 14-year follow-up study. *Br J Psychiatry*, *206*(4), 283–288.

Ran, M. S., et al. (2015b). Different outcomes of never-treated and treated patients with schizophrenia: 14-year follow-up study in rural China. *Br J Psychiatry*, *207*(6), 495–500.

Ran, M. S., et al. (2017). Marriage and outcomes of people with schizophrenia in rural China: 14-year follow-up study. *Schizophr Res, 182*, 49–54.

Rayan, A. & Obiedate, K. (2017). The correlates of quality of life among Jordanian patients with schizophrenia. *J Am Psychiatr Nurses Assoc, 23*(6), 404–413.

Rosa, M. A., Marcolin, M. A., & Elkis, H. (2005). Evaluation of the factors interfering with drug treatment compliance among Brazilian patients with schizophrenia. *Rev Bras Psiquiatr, 27*(3), 178–184.

Saha, S., Chant, D., & McGrath, J. (2007). A systematic review of mortality in schizophrenia: is the differential mortality gap worsening over time? *Arch Gen Psychiatry, 64*(10), 1123–1131.

Salokangas, R. K., Honkonen, T., Stengård, E., & Koivisto, A. M. (2006). Subjective life satisfaction and living situations of persons in Finland with long-term schizophrenia. *Psychiatr Serv, 57*(3), 373–381.

Salokangas, R. K. (1983). Prognostic implications of the sex of schizophrenic patients. *Br J Psychiatry, 142*, 145–151.

Saravanan, B., Jacob, K. S., Johnson, S., Prince, M., Bhugra, D., & David, A. S. (2010). Outcome of first-episode schizophrenia in India: longitudinal study of effect of insight and psychopathology. *Br J Psychiatry, 196*(6), 454–459.

Secher, R. G., et al. (2015). Ten-year follow-up of the OPUS specialized early intervention trial for patients with a first episode of psychosis. *Schizophr Bull, 41*(3), 617–626.

Seeman, M. V. (2007). An outcome measure in schizophrenia: mortality. *Can J Psychiatry, 52*(1), 55–60.

Shibre, T., et al. (2015). Long-term clinical course and outcome of schizophrenia in rural Ethiopia: 10-year follow-up of a population-based cohort. *Schizophr Res, 161*(2–3), 414–420.

Shrivastava, A., Shah, N., Johnston, M., Stitt, L., & Thakar, M. (2010). Predictors of long-term outcome of first-episode schizophrenia: a ten-year follow-up study. *Indian J Psychiatry, 52*(4), 320–326.

Simonsen, E., et al. (2010). Early identification of non-remission in first-episode psychosis in a two-year outcome study. *Acta Psychiatr Scand, 122*(5), 375–383.

Singh, S. P., et al. (2000). Three-year outcome of first-episode psychoses in an established community psychiatric service. *Br J Psychiatry, 176*, 210–216.

Spellmann, I., et al. (2012). One-year functional outcomes of naturalistically treated patients with schizophrenia. *Psychiatry Res, 198*(3), 378–385.

Srinivasa Murty, R., Kishore Kumar, K. V., Chisholm, D., Thomas, T., Sekar, K., & Chandrashekar, C. R. (2005). Community outreach for untreated schizophrenia in rural India: a follow-up study of symptoms, disability, family burden and costs. *Psychol Med, 35*(3), 341–351.

Srinivasan, T. N., Rajkumar, S., & Padmavathi, R. (2001). Initiating care for untreated schizophrenia patients and results of one year follow-up. *Int J Soc Psychiatry, 47*(2), 73–80.

Srinivasan, T. N. & Thara, R. (1999). The long-term home-making functioning of women with schizophrenia. *Schizophr Res, 35*(1), 97–98.

Suresh, K., et al. (2012). Work functioning of schizophrenia patients in a rural south Indian community: status at 4-year follow-up. *Soc Psychiatry Psychiatr Epidemiol, 47*(11), 1865–1871.

Susser, E., Collins, P., Schanzer, B., Varma, V. K., & Gittelman, M. (1996). Topics for our times: can we learn from the care of persons with mental illness in developing countries? *Am J Public Health, 86*(7), 926–928.

Susser, E. & Wanderling, J. (1994). Epidemiology of nonaffective acute remitting psychosis vs schizophrenia: sex and sociocultural setting. *Arch Gen Psychiatry, 51*, 294–301.

Szkultecka-Dębek, M., et al. (2016). Schizophrenia causes significant burden to patients' and caregivers' lives. *Psychiatr Danub, 28*(2), 104–110.

Tang, J. Y.-M., et al. (2014). Prospective relationship between duration of untreated psychosis and 13-year clinical outcome: a first-episode psychosis study. *Schizophr Res, 153*(1), 1–8.

Teferra, S., et al. (2012). Five-year clinical course and outcome of schizophrenia in Ethiopia. *Schizophr Res, 136*(1–3), 137–142.

Teferra, S., et al. (2011). Five-year mortality in a cohort of people with schizophrenia in Ethiopia. *BMC Psychiatry, 11*(1), 165.

Thara, R. (2012). Twenty-five years of schizophrenia: the Madras longitudinal study. *Indian J54*(2), 134.

Thara, R., Henrietta, M., Joseph, A., Rajkumar, S., & Eaton, W. W. (1994). Ten-year course of schizophrenia—the Madras longitudinal study. *Acta Psychiatr Scand, 90*, 329–336.

Thara, R. & Kamath, S. (2015). Women and schizophrenia. *Indian J Psychiatry, 57*(Suppl 2), S246–S251.

Thara, R., Mangala, R., Mohan, G., Joseph, J., & John, S. (2012). Early intervention for first-episode psychosis in India. *East Asian Arch Psychiatry, 22*(3), 94–99.

Thara, R. & Rajkumar, S. (1992). Gender differences in schizophrenia. Results of a follow-up study from India. *Schizophr Res, 7*(1), 65–70.

Thara, R. (2004). Twenty-year course of schizophrenia: the Madras Longitudinal Study. *Can J Psychiatry, 49*, 564–569.

Tirupati, N. S., Thara, R., & Padmavati, R. (2004). Duration of untreated psychosis and treatment outcome in schizophrenia patients untreated for many years. *Aust N Z J Psychiatry, 38*(5), 339–343.

Tsoi, W. F. & Wong, K. E. (1991). A 15-year follow-up study of Chinese schizophrenic patients. *Acta Psychiatr Scand, 84*, 217–220.

Ucok, A., Serbest, S., & Kandemir, P. E. (2011). Remission after first-episode schizophrenia: results of a long-term follow-up. *Psychiatry Res, 189*(1), 33–37.

United Nations (2012). Department of Economic and Social Affairs, Population Division. *World Population Prospects [2012], archive.* Retrieved from https://population.un.org/wpp/Download/Archive/Standard/

Usall, J., Haro, J. M., Ochoa, S., Marquez, M., & Araya, S. (2002). Influence of gender on social outcome in schizophrenia. *Acta Psychiatr Scand, 106*(5), 337–342.

Verghese, A., et al. (1985). Factors associated with the course and outcome of schizophrenia: a multicentred follow-up study. *Indian J Psychiatry, 27*, 201–206.

Verghese, A., John, J. K., Rajkumar, S., Richard, J., Sethi, B. B., & Trivedi, J. K. (1989). Factors associated with the course and outcome of schizophrenia in India: results of a two-year multicentre follow-up study. *Br J Psychiatry, 154*, 499–503.

Verma, S., Subramaniam, M., Abdin, E., Poon, L. Y., & Chong, S. A. (2012). Symptomatic and functional remission in patients with first-episode psychosis. *Acta Psychiatr Scand, 126*(4), 282–289.

Warner, R. (1992). Commentary on Cohen, 'Prognosis for schizophrenia in the Third World'. *Cult Med Psychiatry, 16*, 85–88.

Warner, R. (1983). Recovery from schizophrenia in the third world. *Psychiatry, 46*(3), 197–212.

White, C., et al. (2009). Predictors of 10-year outcome of first-episode psychosis. *Psychol Med, 39*(9), 1447–1456.

Wiersma, D., et al. (2000). Social disability in schizophrenia: its development and prediction over 15 years in incidence cohorts in six European centres. *Psychol Med, 30*(5), 1155–1167.

Wiersma, D., Nienhuis, F. J., Slooff, C. J., & Giel, R. (1998). Natural course of schizophrenic disorders: a 15-year follow-up of a Dutch incidence cohort. *Schizophr Bull, 24*(1), 75–85.

Wieselgren, I. M. & Lindstrom, L. H. (1996). A prospective 1–5 year outcome study in first-admitted and readmitted schizophrenic patients; relationship to heredity, premorbid adjustment, duration of disease and education level at index admission and neuroleptic treatment. *Acta Psychiatr Scand, 93*(1), 9–19.

Wils, R. S., et al. (2017). Antipsychotic medication and remission of psychotic symptoms 10 years after a first-episode psychosis. *Schizophr Res, 182*, 42–48.

World Health Organization (**WHO**) (1973). *Report of the international pilot study of schizophrenia*. Geneva: World Health Organization.

6

Mortality and psychosis

Alex Cohen

Introduction

Interest in mortality rates among individuals with severe mental illness began about 200 years ago, with a focus on those in asylums (Burrows, 1820), and continued as a prominent topic in English language medical journals throughout the nineteenth century (Crookshank, 1899; Farr, 1841; Francis, 1840; Gardiner Hill, 1842). This topic continued to garner attention through the first half of the twentieth century (Alstrom, 1942; Malzberg, 1934; Malzberg, 1949). However, with the advent of deinstitutionalization in the mid-1950s, research on mortality among individuals with severe mental illness expanded its focus and began to consider mortality rates among individuals with psychosis who were living in the community. To our knowledge, the earliest population-based study of the association between mortality and severe mental illness was conducted by Babigian and Odorous (1969) who calculated the ratio between the observed number of deaths in a population of persons with a mental illness and the expected number of deaths in the general population. They found that persons with schizophrenia or affective disorders had elevated rates of mortality, up to twice the rate of the general population in which they lived. Three decades later, Brown (1997) conducted a meta-analysis of 12 studies that linked psychiatric case and death registers and confirmed that the risk of all-cause mortality among persons with schizophrenia was about 1.5 times higher than the general population. (Brown expressed this risk as the standardized mortality ratio (SMR), which is a ratio of the observed number of deaths in a study population to the number of deaths that would be expected.) Furthermore, compared with the general populations in which they lived, persons with schizophrenia were twice as likely to die in accidents, seven times as likely to be the victims of homicide, and eight times as likely to die from suicide. It is necessary to also note that natural causes accounted for 80% of mortality among people with schizophrenia.

In the decades after the publication of the meta-analysis by Brown (1997), many other studies have examined the association between mortality and psychosis (e.g. Doyle et al., 2019; Hallgren et al., 2019; Taipale et al., 2020) and many of the results have been aggregated and summarized in meta-analyses (Gondek et al., 2015; Hjorthoj et al., 2017; Lee et al., 2018; Piotrowski et al., 2017). To the best of our knowledge, the most comprehensive systematic review of SMRs among individuals with schizophrenia was conducted by Saha et al. (2007) who used data derived from 37 studies in 25 countries. This review estimated that the median all-cause SMR for individuals with schizophrenia was 2.58. In other words, individuals with schizophrenia, world-wide, had all-cause mortality rates that were elevated a little more than two and a half times above that found in the general population. Median all-cause SMRs for men and women were 3.02 and 2.37, respectively. The median SMRs for natural (2.41) and unnatural causes (7.50) were elevated, and the SMR for suicide was 12.86. Perhaps the most disturbing finding was that the median all-cause SMR had increased from 1.84 in the 1970s to 3.20 in the 1990s, suggesting 'that people with schizophrenia [had] not fully benefited from the improvements in health outcomes available to the general population'.

Research on mortality and psychosis has increased in recent years (Firth et al., 2019; Seeman, 2007; Seeman, 2019; Thornicroft, 2011; Thornicroft, 2013) and this has prompted the organization of a World Psychiatric Association (WPA)/ World Health Organization (WHO) forum to develop 'a comprehensive approach to excess mortality in persons with severe mental disorders' (Liu et al., 2017). This is commendable but has at least one serious limitation: these efforts were based on research conducted almost exclusively in Northern Europe and North America. Thus, although the reviews cited here are informative, the evidence may not be directly relevant to the health systems and burden of disease profiles of countries in other settings. This biased evidence base becomes especially limiting when attempts to develop 'clinical practice, policy and research agendas to decrease excess mortality in persons with severe mental disorders' all but ignore evidence from diverse socioeconomic and sociocultural settings (Liu et al., 2017). As a corrective, this chapter will offer a narrative review of research on mortality and psychosis by providing evidence from a diversity of settings.

Approach

PubMed was searched for research on the epidemiology of mortality among individuals with psychosis.* After eliminating duplicates, reading through titles

---

* Search terms were: *((Psychotic Disorders/epidemiology/mortality) OR (Schizophrenia / epidemiology/mortality))* in titles or abstracts.

and abstracts, and conducting manual searches of PubMed, Google Scholar, and bibliographies of literature already identified, the following evidence was located: 46 peer-reviewed journal articles and book chapters that reported on 37 research projects in 17 countries.[†] Table 6.1 summarises the findings of these research projects. Rather than grouping the projects by the countries in which they were conducted, projects are grouped in the following categories: population-based, community-based, first-episode, and clinical/hospital samples. Whenever possible, the number of cases lost to follow-up is indicated and the number of located cases in the final cohort is used as the denominator when calculating the percentage of deaths in each cohort. The final cohort numbers are used because it cannot be assumed that mortality rates among those lost to follow-up are the same as among those not lost; and because lack of data on cases lost to follow-up might have resulted in underestimates of SMRs. When available, SMRs are listed for each cohort and by gender and/or cause of death.

Population-based studies

Hassall et al. (1988) suggest that psychiatric case registers linked with death registers provide what can be considered the best 'opportunities to carry out mortality studies of large [samples] of unselected psychiatric patients from defined geographical areas'. Such studies have been conducted in Taiwan (Chen et al., 2010; Pan et al., 2017; Pan et al., 2020; Tsai et al., 2014), South Korea (Kim et al., 2017), Israel (Gur et al., 2018; Kodesh et al., 2012), Hungary (Bitter et al., 2017), and Czech Republic (Krupchanka et al., 2018). Although it did not use a register of any kind, the research in China (Liu et al., 2014) is included in this category because it was based on a national, random sample of individuals with schizophrenia.

Several mortality studies in Taiwan used the National Health Insurance database to identify cohorts of individuals with schizophrenia (Chen et al., 2010; Pan et al., 2017; Pan et al., 2020; Tsai et al., 2014). These studies span the period 1998–2013 and include similar cohorts, although Chen et al. (2010) only included individuals under the age of 45 years. The mortality rates in the studies by Tsai et al. (2014) and Chen et al. (2010) differed (15.1% vs. 6.8%, respectively); however, the follow-up period in the latter was shorter (10 vs. 6 years) and the cohort was younger (<45 years). Tsai et al. (2014) did not report mortality rates for specific conditions. The studies by Pan et al. (2017; 2020) examined mortality rates in several consecutive cohorts (2003–2013) identified through the

---

[†] Eleven projects in seven countries were components of the WHO International Study of Schizophrenia (Hopper et al., 2007).

Table 6.1 Studies of mortality and psychosis in the global south

Country	Type of study Diagnosis	Original cohort n (%) Lost to follow-up n (%) Final cohort n (% original)	Mortality rates final cohort n (%) all-cause SMR [95%CI]	Leading causes n (% final cohort; *deaths*)
Population-based studies				
China (Liu et al., 2014)	4-year prospective National prevalence sample schizophrenia [ICD-10 Symptom Checklist for Mental Disorders]	922 (45.5) (m) 1149 (55.5) (f) 2071 (100) **lost** 52 (2.5) **final** 898 (97.4) (m) 1121 (97.6) (f) 2019 (97.4)	69 (7.7) (m) 77 (6.9) (f) 146 (7.2) (T) **SMR** 10.17 [n/a] (m) 12.42 [n/a] (f)	disease: 123 (6.1; *84.2*) other: 5 (0.2; *3.4*) accident: 11 (0.4; *7.5*) suicide: 7 (0.3; *4.8*)
Taiwan (Tsai et al., 2014)	10-year follow-up 1999–2008 National Health Insurance database schizophrenia [ICD-9-CM: 295]	33,069 (54.7) (m) 27,333 (45.3) (f) 60,402 (100) (T) **lost** n/a	n/a (m) n/a) (f) 9150 (15.1) (T) **SMR** n/a	n/a

Country (Study)	Design / Database / Diagnosis	Sample size (%)	Mortality / Risk	Cause-specific
Taiwan (Chen et al., 2010)	6-year follow-up 1998–2004 National Health Insurance database‡ schizophrenia [ICD-9-CM: 295* except 295.7 (schizoaffective disorder)]	3256 (59.0) (m) 2259 (41.0) (f) 5515 (100) (T) **lost** n/a **final** n/a	n/a (m) n/a (f) 377 (6.8) **HR§** 4.61 [3.87–5.50] natural: 3.46 [2.78–4.34] unnat'l: 7.95 [6.01–10.51]	cancer 26 (0.5; 6.9) circulatory, respiratory & digestive diseases 71 (1.3; 18.8) symptoms, signs & ill-defined conditions 33 (0.6; 8.8) other natural 77 (1.4; 20.4) injury & poisoning 69 (1.3; 18.3) suicide 101 (1.8; 26.8)
Taiwan (Pan et al., 2017)	3-year retrospective National Health Insurance database 2003 cohort schizophrenia [ICD-9 CM codes: 295*]	49,718 (53.9) (m) 42,509 (46.1) (f) 92,227 (T) **lost** n/a	2649 (5.3) (m) 1689 (4.0) (f) 4338 (4.7) (T) **SMR** 3.40 [3.30–3.50] natural: 2.78 [2.68–2.88] unnat'l: 6.99 [6.57–7.44]	natural: 3149 (3.4; 72.6)** unnatural: 1006 (1.1; 23.2)†† unknown: 183 (0.2; 4.2)
Taiwan (Pan et al., 2020)	3-year retrospective National Health Insurance database 2010 cohort schizophrenia [ICD-9 CM codes: 295*]	54,953 (52.2) (m) 49,608 (47.8) (f) 104,561 (100) (T) **lost** n/a	3014 (5.5) (m) 2036 (4.1) (f) 5050 (4.8) (T) **SMR** 3.27 [3.18–3.36] natural: 3.23 [3.13–3.33] unnat'l: 5.79 [5.41–6.18] cancer: 1.37 [1.27–1.47] CVD: 3.02 [2.80–3.24] diabetes: 3.23 [2.86–3.64] suicide: 9.57 [8.80–10.38]	natural: 3934 (3.8; 77.9) unnatural: 876 (0.8; 17.3) unknown: 240 (0.2; 4.8) cancer: 697 (0.7; 13.8) CVD: 876 (0.7; 14.9) diabetes: 250 (0.3; 5.4) suicide: 250 (0.5; 11.3)

(continued)

Table 6.1 Continued

Country	Type of study Diagnosis	Original cohort n (%) Lost to follow-up n (%) Final cohort n (% original)	Mortality rates final cohort n (%) all-cause SMR [95%CI]	Leading causes n (% final cohort; *deaths*)
South Korea (Kim et al., 2017)	9-year retrospective random sample National Health Insurance database schizophrenia [ICD-10: F20, F25]	4532 (48.3) (m) 4855 (51.7) (f) 9387 (100) **lost** none **final** see above	520 (11.5) (m) 460 (9.5) (f) 980 (10.4) (T) **SMR** 2.4 [2.2–2.5] suicide: 8.4 [7.2–9.6]	suicide: 183 (1.9; 18.7)
Israel (Kodesh et al., 2012)	6-year retrospective national sample large healthcare provider schizophrenia [ICD-9 codes 295.*–298.*][‡‡]	n/a (m) n/a (f) 8848 (100) (T)	n/a **SMR** 2.43 [1.96–2.96] (T) 2.78 [1.98–3.78] (m) 2.21 [1.64–2.92] (f)	n/a
Israel (Gur et al., 2018)	9-year retrospective case control large healthcare provider schizophrenia [ICD-10: F 20]	893 (64.3) (m) 496 (35.7) (f) 1389 (100) **lost** n/a **final** n/a	n/a (m) n/a (f) 97 (7.0) (T) **HR**[§§] 1.89 [1.46–2.44]	n/a

Study	Design			
Hungary (Bitter et al., 2017)	National register-based prospective matched-cohort study Nat'l Health Insurance Fund schizophrenia*** [ICD-10 F20.0–F20.9]	27,221 (41.8) (m) 37,948 (58.2) (f) 65,169 (100) **lost** n/a	5843 (21.5) (m) 8638 (22.8) (f) 14,481 (22.2) **RR**[†††] 2.4 [n/a]	n/a
Czech Republic (Krupchanka et al., 2018)	20-years National register-based retrospective discharged inpatients psychotic disorders [ICD-10: F20-29]	n/a (m) n/a (f) 49,822 (100) **lost** n/a	n/a (m) 724 (1.5) **SMR** 2.3 [2.1–2.5]	cancer: 130 (0.3; *18.0*) circulatory diseases: 273 (0.5; *37.7*) other natural: 190 (0.4; 26.2) external causes: 67 (0.1; *9.3*)[‡‡] self-harm: 64 (0.1; 8.8)
Community-based studies				
China RA-invited centres/ ISoS 8 urban centres (Chen & Shen, 2007; Hopper et al., 2007)	12-year retrospective random urban sample schizophrenia [ICD-9 criteria]	45 (50.6) (m) 44 (49.4) (f) 89 (100) **lost** 11 (12.4) **final** 39 (86.7) (m) 39 (88.6) (f) 78 (87.6)	10 (25.6) (m) 10 (25.6) (f) 20 (25.6) (T) **SMR** 2.97 [n/a] (T) 3.37 [n/a] (m) 2.59 [n/a] (f)	natural: 17 (21.8; *85.0*) suicide: 2 (2.6; *10.0*) unknown: 1 (1.3; *5.0*)

(continued)

Table 6.1 Continued

Country	Type of study Diagnosis	Original cohort n (%) Lost to follow-up n (%) Final cohort n (% original)	Mortality rates final cohort n (%) all-cause SMR [95%CI]	Leading causes n (% final cohort; *deaths*)
China Rural (Ran et al., 2007; Ran et al., 2015; Ran et al., 2020)	21-year prospective community sample schizophrenia [ICD-10 criteria]	237 (46.5) (m) 273 (53.5) (f) 510 (100)§§§ **lost** 69 (13.5) **final** n/a (m) n/a (f) 441 (86.5)	n/a (m) n/a (f) 196 (44.4) (T) **SMR** n/a	suicide: 27 (6.1; *13.8*) other:**** 169 (38.3; *86.2*)
India (Bagewadi et al., 2016)	3-year community sample schizophrenia [MINI-International Neuropsychiatric Interview]	n/a (m) n/a (f) 325 (100) **lost** n/a **final** n/a	n/a (m) n/a (f) 12 (3.7) (T) **SMR** 1.79 [n/a]	Medical: 6 (1.8; *50.0*) unknown: 1 (0.3; *8.3*) accident: 1 (0.3; *8.3*) suicide: 4 (1.2; *33.3*)

Study	Design/sample	Cohort n (%)	Lost / Final	Deaths n (%)	SMR	Cause of death
Ethiopia (Fekadu et al., 2015)	10-year prospective follow-up community prevalence schizophrenia [Schedules for Clinical Assessment in Neuropsychiatry]	296 (82.7) (m) 62 (17.3) (f) 358 (100)[†††]	**lost** none **final** see above	57 (15.9) (m) 8 (2.2) (f) 65 (18.2) (T)	**SMR** 3.03 [2.34–3.86]	suicide: 9 (2.5; 13.8) n/a: 56 (15.6; 86.2)[‡‡‡]

First episode studies

Study	Design/sample	Cohort n (%)	Lost / Final	Deaths n (%)	SMR	Cause of death
Hong Kong (Lo & Lo, 1977)	10-year retrospective 1st episode clinical sample schizophrenia (Mayer-Gross et al., 1960)	88 (66.2) (m) 41 (30.8) (f) 133 (100)	**lost** 47 (35.3) 57 (64.8) (m) 25 (61.0) (f) 82 (61.7)[§§§§]	n/a (m) n/a (f) 4 (4.9) (T)[*****]	**SMR** n/a	traffic accident: 1 (1.1; 25.0) suicide: 3 (3.4; 75.0)
Hong Kong RA-invited/ISoS (Hopper et al., 2007; Lee et al., 2007)[†††††]	15-year retrospective 1st episode clinical sample schizophrenia (ICD-9 criteria)	51 (51.0) (m) 41 (49.0) (f) 100 (100)[‡‡‡‡]	**lost** 19 (19.0) **final** 41 (80.4) (m) 40 (97.6) (f) 81 (81.0)	8 (19.5) (m) 3 (7.5) (f) 11 (13.6) (T)	**SMR** 5.76 [n/a] (T) 7.16 [n/a] (m) 3.78 [n/a] (f)	natural: 2 (2.5; 18.2) suicide: 9 (11.1; 81.8)

(continued)

Table 6.1 Continued

Country	Type of study Diagnosis	Original cohort n (%) Lost to follow-up n (%) Final cohort n (% original)	Mortality rates final cohort n (%) all-cause SMR [95%CI]	Leading causes n (% final cohort; *deaths*)
Hong Kong (Chan et al., 2015)	10-year outcomes early intervention clinical sample psychotic disorders Structured Clinical Interview for DSM-IV, Axis I	74 (50.7) (m) 71 (49.3) (f) 145 (100) (T) **lost** n/a	n/a (m) n/a (f) 7 (4.8) (T) **SMR** n/a	unnatural: 1 (0.7; 14.3) suicide: 6 (4.1; 85.7)
Japan DOSMeD/ISoS Nagasaki (Hopper et al., 2007; Nakane et al., 2007)	15-year follow-up treated incidence psychotic disorders ICD-9 / ICD-10§§§§§	61 (57.0) (m) 46 (43.0) (f) 107 (100) **lost** 43 (41.7) **final** 33 (54.1) (m) 31 (67.4) (f) 64 (59.8)	4 (12.1) (m) 3 (9.7) (f) 7 (10.9) **SMR** 5.71 [n/a] (T) 5.06 [n/a] (m) 6.90 [n/a] (f)	natural: 2 (3.1; 28.6) accident: 1 (1.6; 14.3) suicide: 4 (6.3; 57.1)

Country (Study)	Design	Sample	Deaths	SMR	Cause of death
Singapore (Kua et al., 2003)	20-year follow-up first admissions schizophrenia ICD-9 criteria[††††††]	244 (60.7) (m) 158 (39.3) (f) 402 (100) (T) **lost** 127 (31.6) **final** n/a (m) n/a (f) 275 (68.4)	n/a (m) n/a (f) 59 (21.5) **SMR** n/a		natural: 20 (7.3; 33.9) suicide: 39 (14.2; 66.1)[‡‡‡‡‡]
India DOSMeD/ISoS Chandigarh Rural (Hopper et al., 2007; Varma & Malhotra, 2007)	15-year follow-up first-episode community psychotic disorders[§§§§§§]	27 (49.1) (m) 28 (50.9) (f) 55 (100) **lost** 7 (12.7) **final** 23 (41.8) (m) 25 (45.5) (f) 48 (87.3)	7 (30.4) (m) 3 (12.0) (f) 10 (20.8) (T) **SMR** 3.02 [n/a] (T) 4.71 [n/a] (m) 1.76 [n/a] (f)		natural: 6 (12.5; 60.0) other/unknown: 3 (6.3; 30.0) suicide: 1 (2.1; 10.0)
India DOSMeD/ISoS Chandigarh Urban (Hopper et al., 2007; Varma & Malhotra, 2007)	15-year follow-up first-episode community psychotic disorders[*******]	91 (58.7) (m) 64 41.3 (f) 155 (100) **lost** 61 (39.4) **final** 51 (64.8) (m) 43 (67.2) (f) 94 (60.6)	8 (15.7) (m) 6 (14.0) (f) 14 (14.9) (T) **SMR** 1.88 [n/a] (T) 2.05 [n/a] (m) 1.70 [n/a] (f)		natural: 4 (4.3; 28.6) unknown: 5 (5.3; 35.7) accident: 1 (1.1; 7.1) suicide: 4 (4.3; 28.6)

(continued)

Table 6.1 Continued

Country	Type of study Diagnosis	Original cohort n (%) Lost to follow-up n (%) Final cohort n (% original)	Mortality rates final cohort n (%) all-cause SMR [95%CI]	Leading causes n (% final cohort; *deaths*)
India (Rangaswamy & Cohen, 2020)	35-year follow-up first-episode clinic patients schizophrenia ICD-9 & Feighner criteria[††††††]	45 (50.0) (m) 45 (50.0) (f) 90 (100) **lost** 28 (31.1) **final** 36 (80.0) (m) 26 (57.8) (f) 62 (68.9)	20 (55.6) (m) 12 (46.2) (f) 32 (51.6) (T) **SMR** n/a	CVD 8 (12.9; *25.0*) infections 5 (8.1; *15.3*) TB: 3 (4.8; *9.4*) other natural 5 (8.0; *15.6*) injury: 1 (1.6; *3.1*) suicide 7 (11.3; *21.9*) unknown: 3 (4.8; *9.4*)
Russia DOSMeD/ISoS (Hopper et al., 2007; Tsirkin, 2007)	15-year follow-up treated incidence schizophrenia [ICD-9 / ICD-10][‡‡‡‡‡‡]	29 (40.3) (m) 43 (59.7) (f) 72 (100) **lost** 7 (9.7) **final** n/a (m) n/a (f) 65 (92.3)	4 (n/a) (m) 6 (n/a) (f) 10 (15.4) **SMR** 1.41 [n/a] (T) 0.99 [n/a] (m) 1.98 [n/a] (f)	natural: 2 (3.1; *20.0*) suicide: 1 (1.5; *10.0*) possible suicide: 3 (4.6; *30.0*) unknown: 4 (6.2; *40.0*)

Study	Design/diagnosis	Baseline/follow-up N (%)	Deaths N (%)	SMR	Cause of death
Bulgaria RAPyD/ISoS Sofia (Ganev et al., 2007; Hopper et al., 2007)	16-year follow-up treated incidence non-affective psychosis [ICD-9: 295, 297, 298.3, 298.4, 298.8, 298.9]	21 (35.0) (m) 39 (65.0) (f) 60 (100) **lost** 3 (5.0) **final** 19 (31.7) (m) 38 (63.3) (f) 57 (95.0)	n/a (m) n/a (f) 2 (3.5)	**SMR** 1.04 [n/a] (T) 1.12 [n/a] (m) 0.96 [n/a] (f)	suicide: 2 (3.5; 3.5)
Czech Republic DOSMeD /ISoS Prague (Hopper et al., 2007; Skoda et al., 2007)	15-year follow-up treated incidence psychotic disorders [ICD-9/ICD-10§§§§§§]	43 (36.4) (m) 75 (63.6) (f) 118 (100) **lost** 28 (23.7) **final** 30 (25.4) (m) 60 (50.8) (f) 90 (76.3)	3 (10.0) (m) 8 (13.3) (f) 11 (12.2) (T)	**SMR** 2.53 [n/a] (T) 1.44 [n/a] (m) 3.55 [n/a] (f)	natural: 5 (5.6; 45.5) suicide: 6 (6.7; 54.5)

Clinical/hospital samples

Study	Design/diagnosis	Baseline/follow-up N (%)	Deaths N (%)	SMR	Cause of death
Taiwan (Ko et al., 2018)	13-year retrospective hospital sample schizophrenia [ICD-9 CM at baseline; ICD-10 CM at follow-up]	2297 (53.4) (m) 2001 (46.6) (f) 4298 (T) **lost** n/a	201 (8.8) (m) 166 (8.3) (f) 367 (8.5) (T)	**SMR** 8.8 [7.8–9.6]****** suicide: 31.3 [23.3–38.0] accidents/injury: 7.7 [5.1–10.2]	cancers: 60 (1.4; 16.3) CVD:30 (0.7; 8.2) cerebro dis: 16 (0.4; 4.4) diabetes: 20 (0.5; 5.4) pneumonia: 11 (0.3; 3.0) other natural: 20 (0.5; 5.4) accidents/injury: 37 (0.9; 10.1) suicide: 74 (1.7; 20.2) homicide: 2 (0.05; 0.5)

(continued)

Table 6.1 Continued

Country	Type of study Diagnosis	Original cohort n (%) Lost to follow-up n (%) Final cohort n (% original)	Mortality rates final cohort n (%) all-cause SMR [95%CI]	Leading causes n (% final cohort; *deaths*)
Taiwan (Cheng et al., 2014)	10-year retrospective long-stay inpatients schizophrenia [ICD-9: 295]	n/a (m) n/a (f) 2737 (100)[††††††] **lost** 280 (10.2)[†††††††] **final** 1998 (n/a) (m) 459 (n/a) (f) 2457 (89.8)	934 (46.7) (m) 59 (12.9) (f) 993 (40.4) (T) **SMR** 2.17 [2.04–2.31][$$$$$$$$] suicide: 0.70 [0.19–1.80] accidents: 2.28 [1.65–3.07]	respiratory dis: 232 (9.4; *23.4*) circulatory dis: 151 (6.1; *15.2*) digestive dis: 108 (4.4; *10.9*) genitourinary dis: 89 (3.6; *9.0*) other natural: 362 (14.7; *36.5*) suicide: 4 (0.2; *0.4*) accident: 43 (1.8; *4.3*) other external: 4 (0.2; *0.4*)
Japan (Ogawa et al., 1987)	21–27 years follow-up inpatients schizophrenia [ICD-9: 295.1-3]	67 (47.9) (m) 73 (52.1) (f) 140 (100) **lost** 10 (7.1) **final** 62 (44.3) (m) 68 (48.6) (f) 130 (92.9)	14 (22.6) (m) 11 (16.2) (f) 25 (19.2) (T) SMR n/a	suicide: 14 (10.8; *56.0*) unknown: 8 (6.2; *32.0*)[·········] other: 3 (2.3; *12.0*)

Country (Study)	Design / Diagnosis	Sample (lost/final)	Mortality / SMR	Causes of death
Japan (Saku et al., 1995)	3–37 years retrospective inpatients schizophrenia [diagnosis at discharge][††††††††]	n/a[†††††††] **lost** n/a **final** 1433 (63.2) (m) 835 (36.8) (f) 2268 (100)	323 (22.5) (m) 146 (17.5) (f) 469 (20.7) (T) **SMR**[§§§§§§§§§] 2.55 [2.28–2.85] (m) 3.02 [2.55–3.55 (f)[**********] **suicide:** 9.94 [7.74-12.71] (m) 10.53 [6.53–16.13] (f) **TB:** 4.14 [2.90–5.74] (m) 4.35 [2.32–7.43] (f)	cancer: 41 (1.8; 8.7) TB: 49 (2.2; 10.4) heart disease: 40 (1.8; 8.5) CVD: 32 (1.4; 6.8) respiratory: 24 (1.1; 5.1) other: 25 (1.1; 5.3) accidents: 33 (1.5; 7.0) suicide: 84 (3.7; 17.9) missing: 141 (6.2; 30.1)
South Korea (Park et al., 2015)	3 to 14 years retrospective inpatients/outpatients general hospital schizophrenia schizoaffective disorder [ICD-10: F20]	n/a	112: inpatients[††††††††††] 99: outpatients **SMR** inpatients: 4.56 [3.75–5.48] outpatients: 3.59 [2.91-4.37] suicide: 15.08 [12.05–18.65] accident: 5.49 [3.73–7.79]	n/a
Indonesia (Kurihara et al., 2011)	17-year prospective follow-up consecutive admissions schizophrenia [PPDGJ-II criteria][†††††††††]	37 (62.7) (m) 22 (37.3) (f) 59 (100) **lost** none **final** see above	11 (29.7) (m) 4 (18.2) (f) 15 (25.4) (T) **SMR** 4.85 [2.4–7.3 (T) 5.98 [2.4–9.5] (m) 3.11 [0.1–6.2] (f)	natural: 13 (22.0; 86.7)[§§§§§§§§§§] accident: 1 (1.7; 6.7) suicide: 1 (1.7; 6.7)

(continued)

Table 6.1 Continued

Country	Type of study Diagnosis	Original cohort n (%) Lost to follow-up n (%) Final cohort n (% original)	Mortality rates final cohort n (%) all-cause SMR [95%CI]	Leading causes n (% final cohort; *deaths*)
India (Ponnudurai et al., 2006)	13-year follow-up outpatients schizophrenia	n/a (m) n/a (f) 121 (100) **lost** 61 (50.4) **final** 28 n/a (m) 32 n/a (f) 60 (49.6)	n/a (m) n/a (f) 7 (11.7) (T) SMR 5.42 [1.40–9.44]	natural: 5 (8.3; 71.4) accident: 1 (1.7; 14.3) suicide: 1 (1.7; 14.3)
India **IPSS/ISoS** **Agra** (Dube & Kumar, 2007; Hopper et al., 2007)	25-year follow-up outpatients********** psychotic disorders††††††††††	85 (60.7) (m) 55 (39.3) (f) 140 (100) **lost** 36 (25.7) **final** n/a (m) n/a (f) 104 (74.3)	n/a (m) n/a (f) 43 (41.3) (T) **SMR** 1.86 [n/a] (T) 1.34 [n/a] (m) 2.88 [n/a] (f)	natural: 26 (25.0; 60.4) homicide: 2 (1.9; 4.7) accident: 1 (1.0; 2.3) unknown: 10 (9.6; 26.5) suicide: 4 (3.8; 9.3)

Country (reference)	Study description	lost / final	SMR	Cause of death
Nigeria (Makanjuola & Adedapo 1987)	25–38 month follow-up consecutive new patients psychotic disorders[††††††††] [DSM-III criteria]	65 (56.0) (m) 51 (44.0) (f) 116 (100) **lost** 22 (19.0) **final** n/a (m) n/a (f) 94 (100)	n/a (m) n/a (f) 9 (9.6) (T) **SMR** n/a	unknown: 6 (6.4; 66.7)[§§§§§§§§§§] suicide: 1 (1.1; 11.1) killed: 2 (2.1; 22.2)[**********]
Brazil (Menezes & Mann, 1996)	2-year follow-up consecutive hospital admissions psychotic disorders [ICD-9: 295; 297; 298][††††††††††††]	n/a (m) n/a (f) 120 (100) **lost** 4 (3.3) **final** n/a n/a 116 (96.7)	3 (n/a) (m) 4 (n/a) (f) 7 (6.0) (T) **SMR** 8.4 [4.0–15.9] (T) 4.5 [1.2–11.5] (m) 25.5 [8.7–58.5] (f) suicide: 3.18 [1.25–6.68]	stomach haemorrhage: 1 (0.9; 14.3) sudden death: 1 (0.9; 14.3) suicide: 5 (4.3; 71.4)[††††††††††††]
Colombia **IPSS/ISoS** (Hopper et al., 2007; Leon & Leon, 2007)	26-year follow-up clinical sample schizophrenia	56 (44.1) (m) 71 (55.9) (f) 127 (100) **lost** 43 (33.9) **final** 46 (36.2) (m) 38 (30.0) (f) 84 (66.1)	9 (19.6) (m) 3 (7.9) (f) 12 (14.3) (T) SMR 1.31 [n/a] (T) 1.68 [n/a] (m) 0.79 [n/a] (f)	natural: 8 (9.5; 66.7) suicide: 1 (1.2; 8.3) homicide: 1 (1.2; 8.3) unknown: 2 (2.4; 16.7)

(continued)

Table 6.1 Continued

Country	Type of study Diagnosis	Original cohort n (%) Lost to follow-up n (%) Final cohort n (% original)	Mortality rates final cohort n (%) all-cause SMR [95%CI]	Leading causes n (% final cohort; *deaths*)
Czech Republic IPSS /ISoS **Prague** (Hopper et al., 2007; Skoda et al., 2007)	26-year follow-up inpatients psychotic disorders[§§§§§§§§§§§§]	43 (34.4) (m) 82 (65.6) (f) 125 (100)	10 (35.7) (m) 36 (59.0) (f) 46 (51.7)	natural: 25 (28.1; *54.3*) suicide: 19 (21.3; *41.3*) accident: 1 (1.1; *2.2*) unknown: 1 (1.1; *2.2*)
		lost 36 (28.8)	**SMR**	
		final 28 (22.4) (m) 61 (48.8) (f) 89 (71.2)	3.84 [n/a] (T) 1.59 [n/a] (m) 6.30 [n/a] (f)	

[‡] Inclusion criteria: history of psychiatric hospitalization, <45 years old.

[§] Control group was patients receiving appendectomies. Cases and controls <45 years. Adjusted for age, gender, medical comorbidity, urbanization, and geographical location.

[**] About one-third of cases had the following medical conditions at baseline: CVD (10.5%), diabetes (7.5%), COPD (9.3%), renal disease (2.6%), and cancer (1.3%).

[††] Accidents and adverse effects (ICD-10 codes: E800–E949), homicide and injury inflicted by other persons' (E960–E969) and suicide and self-inflicted injury (E950–E959).

[‡‡] Excluding depression with or without a psychotic component.

[§§] Controls from same community cohort; matched on age, gender, and socioeconomic status.

[***] Individuals with 'at least two records of schizophrenia diagnosis' during a period of 9 years (1 January 2005 and 31 December 2013).

[†††] Compared with national cohort of controls alive during inclusion period.

‡‡‡ ICD-10: V01–Y98.

§§§ Includes 10 individuals lost to follow-up but not included in two earlier studies.

**** Accidents and medical conditions combined.

†††† A leakage study identified an additional 40 individuals with schizophrenia (31 men & 9 females).

‡‡‡‡ Data about other causes of death are not provided. However, infectious and parasitic diseases were the leading causes for individuals with severe mental illness, in general, while accidents and homicide were also prominent.

§§§§ Four individuals who died were not included in the final research analyses.

***** Four individuals who died were not included in the final research analyses, but are included here.

††††† Updated version of Lee et al. (1998)

‡‡‡‡‡ Randomly selected from 797 individuals seen in 1977–1978.

§§§§§ ICD-9 criteria baseline; ICD-10 criteria at follow-up.

****** A continuation of previous studies in Singapore, but sample limited to those ≤39 years at baseline.

†††††† To confirm diagnosis following Slater and Roth guidelines (1970).

‡‡‡‡‡‡ 34 suicides in first 10 years.

§§§§§§ 'At least one major psychotic symptom (i.e. hallucinations or delusions, qualitative thought or speech disorder, qualitative psychomotor disorder, or gross behavioural abnormalities), failing which at least two of a list of six lesser disturbances'.

******* The same as above.

††††††† ICD-11 used to reconfirm.

‡‡‡‡‡‡‡ ICD-9 criteria baseline; ICD-10 criteria at follow-up.

§§§§§§§ ICD-9 criteria baseline; ICD-10 criteria at follow-up.

******** SMR for suicide higher among women (46.1) than men (23.9).

†††††††† Gender information n/a.

‡‡‡‡‡‡‡‡ Gender information n/a.

§§§§§§§§ SMRs elevated for all causes except cancers and suicide.

********* Six cases experienced 'sudden' deaths.

††††††††† Converted to DSM-IIIR: 295.

(continued)

Table 6.1 Continued

######## Full sample included all psychiatric patients (n=4980); many were missing follow-up data (n=1,232, 24.7%) and, of these, an indeterminant number were individuals with schizophrenia.

§§§§§§§§§ Highest SMRs for men and women were suicide, pneumonia, and bronchitis, and tuberculosis; kidney disease and accidents and adverse events were especially high for women, but less so for men.

********** SMRs for accidents and renal disease particularly elevated for women: 7.92 [3.95–14.16] and 6.42 [2.58–13.23], respectively.

†††††††††† No information on distribution of genders.

########## *Pedoman Penggolongan dan Diagnosis Gangguan Jiwa di Indonesia Edisi II* (in Indonesian), which is based on the DSM-III and ICD-9.

§§§§§§§§§§ Only three had received treatment at time of death.

*********** 'Typical patients', i.e. 'very young, very old [or] chronic patients' were excluded.

††††††††††† '... presence of delusions, inappropriate or unusual behaviour, hallucinations, gross psychomotor disorder, social withdrawal, thinking disorder, overwhelming fear, depersonalization, or self-neglect'.

########### Schizophreniform disorder, schizophrenia, and residual schizophrenia.

§§§§§§§§§§§ Five died in establishments of traditional healers.

************ Two beaten to death.

†††††††††††† 295-schizophrenic disorders; 297-delusional disorder; 298-other non-organic psychoses.

############ Four died by suicide during first year after discharge; three women died by suicide.

§§§§§§§§§§§§ affective and non-affective psychoses.

National Health Insurance database. Table 6.1 summarises the findings concerning the 3-year follow-up of the 2010–2013 cohort and the 2003–2005 cohort to provide evidence of changes over time. Over the course of this period, all-cause SMRs remained similar (3.40 [95%CI: 3.30–3.50] vs. 3.27 [95%CI: 3.18–3.36]). However, while mortality rates due to natural causes increased (2.78 [95%CI: [2.68–2.88] vs. 3.23 [95%CI: 3.13–3.33]), rates due to unnatural causes decreased (6.99 [95%CI: 6.57–7.44] vs. 5.79 [95%CI: 5.41–6.18]), the result of decreased rates of suicide (Pan et al., 2020).

The Taiwan studies did not always report specific causes of death (Pan et al., 2017; Tsai et al., 2014), and even when causes were reported (Chen et al., 2010; Pan et al., 2020), the results are not exactly comparable given the differences in length of follow-up, and that Chen et al. (2010) only considered persons with schizophrenia under the age of 45 years and compared their rates of mortality with a control group of appendectomy patients rather than the general population of Taiwan. Nevertheless, at least two general findings were evident. First, rates of all-cause mortality among individuals with schizophrenia were more than three times greater than the general population of Taiwan. Second, SMRs for suicide were 13.79 [95%CI: 12.81–14.82] (Pan et al., 2017) and 9.57 [95%CI: 8.80–10.38] (Pan et al., 2020) in the 2005–2008 and 2010–2013 cohorts, respectively.

The studies from South Korea (Kim et al., 2017), Israel (Gur et al., 2018; Kodesh et al., 2012), Hungary (Bitter et al., 2017), and Czech Republic (Krupchanka et al., 2018) all suggest that the rates of mortality among individuals with psychotic disorders were lower than those found in Taiwan. Of these studies, only the one from South Korea (Kim et al., 2017) reported an SMR for suicide (8.4 [95% CI 7.2–9.6]), which was slightly lower than the SMR for suicide in the 2010-2013 cohort in Taiwan (Pan et al., 2020).

Another perspective would be to consider, when available, the percentage of deaths attributed to suicide and 'unnatural' deaths, which may include suicide, homicide, injury, poisoning, and accidents. For suicide, this ranges from 8.8% in the Czech Republic (Krupchanka et al., 2018), to 26.8% in one study in Taiwan (Chen et al., 2010). For 'unnatural' deaths, the range is from 17.3% in Taiwan (Pan et al., 2020) and 18.1% in the Czech Republic (Krupchanka et al., 2018) to 45.1% in another study in Taiwan (Chen et al., 2010). 'Natural' deaths generally comprise 75% or more of mortality (Chen et al., 2010; Krupchanka et al., 2018; Pan et al., 2017; Pan et al., 2020).

The research by Liu et al. (2014) is in contrast to the findings of research in the other population-based studies. For example, the all-cause SMRs for men and women in China, 10.17 [95%CI: n/a] and 12.42 [95%CI: n/a], respectively, are much higher than equivalent SMRs in the other countries. Only one of the studies in Israel (Kodesh et al., 2012) presents separate all-cause SMRs for men (2.78 [1.98–3.78]) and women (2.21 [1.64–2.92]); the other population-based studies found men and women, in the aggregate, to have risks of mortality that are about 2.0 to 4.5 times greater than the general populations in which they live. Thus, the large all-cause SMRs in China are outliers. Given that the research by Liu et al. (2014) is the only study that was conducted in a middle-income country, speculation about the differences across high- and middle-income countries should be avoided until further evidence is produced.

Community-based studies

The following community-based studies were identified: urban China (Chen & Shen, 2007), rural China (Ran et al., 2007; Ran et al., 2015; Ran et al., 2020), India (Bagewadi et al., 2016), and Ethiopia (Fekadu et al., 201; Kebede et al., 2004; Teferra et al., 2011). Such studies have the potential to provide detailed information about specific populations but, at the same time, are prone to bias due to case-finding strategies that miss specific subpopulations of individuals with psychosis, e.g. those who are homeless, do not seek care, or seek care in settings that do not provide access or are unknown to researchers.

Of the two studies in China, only one (Chen & Shen, 2007) reported an all-cause SMR (2.97). Neither study reported an SMR for suicide but did report that 2.6% and 6.1% of the urban and rural cohorts, respectively, had died by suicide. These rates are lower than urban (17.0%) and rural (9.1%) estimates of suicide rates among individuals with schizophrenia in the period 1995–1999 (Phillips et al., 2004). Suicide rates in the general population of China decreased 58% between the late 1990s and 2011, a decline that has been attributed to rapid socioeconomic development, urbanization, improvements in healthcare, and restrictions on the use of pesticides (Wang et al., 2014). However, whether these social changes resulted in substantial improvements in the lives of persons with schizophrenia is a question that awaits future research. Ran et al. (2020) report that older participants had suicide rates that were lower than their younger counterparts. This is in contrast to the findings of Wang et al. (2014) who reported that older adults (≥50 years) living in rural China account for almost 60% of all suicide deaths in the country.

The Ethiopian study of mortality was one aspect of research on the 10-year functional outcomes among a community cohort of 358 individuals with schizophrenia residing in the rural district of Butajira (Kebede et al., 2019). All-cause SMR was 3.03 [95%CI: 2.34–3.86], with infectious disease being the leading cause of death (Fekadu et al., 2015). Nearly 14% of deaths were the result of suicide.

First-episode studies

The 10 research projects (Chan et al., 2015; Ganev et al., 2007; Kua et al., 2003; Lee et al., 2007; Lo & Lo, 1977; Nakane et al., 2007; Rangaswamy & Cohen, 2020; Skoda et al., 2007; Tsirkin, 2007; Varma & Malhotra, 2007) included as first-episode studies appear to mostly meet Bromet's (2008) criteria for 'a clinical cohort [that has] a uniform starting point (the closer to the actual onset, the better for minimizing lead-time bias), a transparent and systematic method of case ascertainment, and a reliable method of assessment and assignment of diagnosis'. However, differences in case ascertainment in each of the sites (i.e. first admission to hospital vs. first episode identified in the community) and differences in diagnostic criteria may have introduced bias into and limit comparability between the samples. Rates of attrition in the first-episode studies are also problematic. Five (Kua et al., 2003; Lo & Lo, 1977; Nakane et al., 2007; Rangaswamy & Cohen, 2020; Varma & Malhotra, 2007) of the 10 first-episode studies had attrition rates over 30%, and it cannot be assumed that those lost to follow-up had the same mortality rates as the rest of their cohorts (Rangaswamy & Cohen, 2020).

The only estimates of all-cause SMRs come from six of the first-episode studies (Ganev et al., 2007; Lee et al., 2007; Nakane et al., 2007; Skoda et al., 2007; Tsirkin, 2007; Varma & Malhotra 2007) conducted under the aegis of the International Study of Schizophrenia (ISoS) (Hopper et al., 2007). Relatively high all-cause SMRs were found in Hong Kong (5.76 [95%CI:not reported) (Lee et al., 2007) and Japan (5.71 [95%CI: not reported]) (Nakane et al., 2007); much lower rates were found in Russia (1.41 [95%CI: not reported]) (Tsirkin, 2007) and Bulgaria (1.04 [95%CI: not reported]) (Ganev et al., 2007) and the urban site in India (1.88 [95%CI: not reported); slightly higher rates were found in the Czech Republic (2.53 [95%CI:not reported]) (Skoda et al., 2007) and the rural site in India (3.02 [95%CI: not reported]). A comparison of the all-cause SMR estimate from the ISoS study was in accord with the all-cause SMR estimate from population-based research in the Czech Republic (2.3 [95%CI: 2.1–2.5]) (Krupchanka et al., 2018). However, when considering the all-cause SMR estimates from the ISoS research, it is important to consider that four of these studies had samples with fewer than or equal to 100, all SMR estimates were based on between 2 and 14 deaths in each cohort, and two of the studies had attrition rates of about 40% (Hopper et al., 2007; Nakane et al., 2007; Varma & Malhotra, 2007).

SMRs for suicide were not reported in either the ISoS studies or the others. However, the proportion of deaths attributed to suicide is reported in most. This proportion is above 80% in two studies (Chan et al., 2015; Lee et al., 2007) and above 50% in four (Kua et al., 2003; Lo & Lo, 1977; Nakane et al., 2007; Skoda et al., 2007). However, because the risk for suicide is heightened in the 10 years following a first episode of psychosis there may be an over-representation of individuals who died by suicide (Sher & Kahn, 2019). This might account for the outsize proportion of deaths attributed to suicide in several of the studies under review (Chan et al., 2015; Kua et al., 2003; Lee et al., 2007; Lo & Lo, 1977; Nakane et al., 2007; Skoda et al., 2007; Tsirkin, 2007). The relative youth of these samples may also account for rates of 'natural' deaths that are lower than in the population-based samples. And, as noted previously, many of these studies had samples in which the number of deaths was small.

A further challenge is posed to the interpretation of findings about mortality rates in first-episode samples because, other than suicide, few specific causes are reported. 'Natural causes' are often grouped together, and when compared with those population and community-based studies that report causes of death, medical conditions appear to account for relatively fewer deaths among the first-episode studies. Thus, generalisations about causes or comparisons across the first-episode studies must remain either speculative or be avoided entirely.

Clinic and hospital studies

Research based on clinic or hospital samples or on some combination of out-patients and inpatients are prone to sample bias because individuals who are able and willing to access such services may not be representative. It is also true that characteristics of institutional care, e.g. expense, location, or reputation, will also determine who and how individuals access services. Therefore, it is difficult to interpret the findings of this group of studies. For example, samples may be relatively small (Kurihara et al., 2011; Makanjuola & Adedapo, 1987; Skoda et al., 2007), subject to large amounts of attrition (Leon & Leon, 2007; Ponnudurai et al., 2006), or from a specialised hospital for long-term patients (Cheng et al., 2014). A further limitation is that several of these studies are based on samples in which the number of deaths was no more than 25 and often much fewer (Kurihara et al., 2011; Leon & Leon, 2007; Makanjuola & Adedapo, 1987; Menezes & Mann, 1996; Ogawa et al., 1987; Ponnudurai et al., 2006).

Despite these limitations, the research suggests that individuals in these studies consistently have mortality rates that are elevated, as indicated by all-cause SMRs that range from 1.31 [95%CI:n/a] in specialist services in Cali, Colombia (Craig et al., 2007; Leon & Leon, 2007) to 8.8 [95%CI: 7.8–9.6] in a general hospital in southern Taiwan (Ko et al., 2018). Individuals with psychosis also appear to be at elevated risk of suicide in all the clinic and hospital studies. Four of the studies that report suicide SMRs found highly elevated rates: from 3.18 [1.25–6.68] in Brazil (Menezes & Mann, 1996) to 31.3 [23.3–38.0] in Taiwan (Ko et al., 2018), with rates in Japan of 9.94 [95%CI:7.74–12.71] and 10.53 [95%CI:6.53–16.13] for men and women, respectively (Saku et al., 1995), and 15.08 [12.05–18.65] in South Korea (Park et al., 2015). A fifth study reported suicide rates that were about the same as the general population, but this was among a cohort of long-term inpatients in a hospital in Taiwan (Cheng et al., 2014).

Life expectancy

Three population-based studies reported life expectancy estimates. In Taiwan, Pan et al. (2020) found that, as of 2013, average life expectancies at birth were 59.53 [95%CI:57.83–61.22] and 65.65 [63.90–67.39] years for men and women, respectively, or about 15 years less than for the general population.

In Hungary, Bitter et al. (2017) determined that the mean ages at death for men and women with schizophrenia were 61.37 (SD = 14.51) and 69.69 (SD = 13.92) years, respectively, whereas men and women in the control group had mean ages at death of 65.21 (SD = 13.12) and 74.42 (SD = 12.64) years, respectively. Thus, men and women with schizophrenia had life expectancies about 4 and 5 years lower, respectively, than men and women in the general population. Another perspective on life expectancy is, having reached a certain age, the number of additional years on average an individual can expect to live. At the age of 20 years, men and women with schizophrenia could expect to live an additional 36.5 and 43.2 years, respectively, whereas in the control group men and women at that age could expect to live an additional 48.0 and 56.9 years. Thus, men and women with schizophrenia had life expectancies that were 11.5 and 13.7 years, respectively, shorter than the general population. At the age of 45 years, men and women with schizophrenia could expect to live an additional 17.9 and 23.2 years, respectively—8.1 and 9.6 years shorter than men and women in the general population.

In Israel, Kodesh et al. (2012) computed life expectancies at the age of 20 years for individuals with schizophrenia and the general population. Men and women with schizophrenia could expect to live to the ages of 71 and 72 years, respectively, whereas men and women in the general population could expect to live to 82 and 85 years. Thus, at the age of 20 years, men and women with schizophrenia could expect to live 11 and 13 fewer years than the general population of Israel.

There are several other studies of life expectancy. Two studies in China reported estimates of life expectancy. In a 21-year follow-up of a rural cohort,

Ran et al. (2020) found, 'The life expectancy of our participants was 58.5 years for women and 50.6 years for men, which was 13.4 and 17.1 years shorter than that for women and men in the general population in China during the same time period'. Chen and Shen (2007), in a 12-year follow-up study in eight urban centres, found, '... the mean age of death [was] 56.6 years for men and 59 years for women' in the cohort, which meant that men and women with schizophrenia died about 15 and 12 years earlier than men and women in the general population of China (The World Bank, 2020). The 10-year follow-up study in Ethiopia found that individuals with schizophrenia had a life expectancy at birth of about 46 years, almost 10 years shorter than the general population of Southern Ethiopia (Fekadu et al., 2015). The ISoS study in Cali, Colombia (Leon & Leon, 2007) reported no differences in life expectancies—about 70 years—between individuals with schizophrenia and the general population. If this is accurate, it is likely to be an outlier, given the evidence to the contrary.

Other studies have compared average age of deaths. Thara and Cohen (2020) reported that the average age at death was 40 years in their 35-year follow-up of a first-episode cohort in Chennai, India. This 'is in stark contrast to the average life expectancy' (about 58 years) in Tamil Nadu in 1981 at the initiation of the Madras Longitudinal Study (Kumar, 1991) or at the time of follow-up (about 71 years) (Indian Council of Medical Research et al., 2017). The Kurihara et al. (2011) 17-year follow-up of a cohort in Indonesia calculated that the average age at death of individuals with schizophrenia was 35.7 years, which was 40% shorter than the average life expectancy of the general population at the beginning of the study and almost 50% shorter than at the time of follow-up. Of the 13 individuals who died from medical conditions, 'only three had received medical treatment for the illness at the time of death'.

Ko et al. (2018) estimated the years of potential life lost (YPLL) among persons with schizophrenia to be almost 14 years greater than the general population of Taiwan, a finding in accord with other research in Taiwan (Leng et al., 2016) and with a meta-analysis of global research (Hjorthoj et al., 2017). Regarding specific causes of mortality, Ko et al. (2018) found that individuals with schizophrenia experienced more YPLL for cancer, cardiovascular disease, diabetes, pneumonia, renal disease, and suicide than the general population of Taiwan.

In sum, the estimates reviewed here are generally in agreement with the substantial evidence that individuals with schizophrenia have life expectancies that are as much as 20 years shorter than the general populations in which they live (Thornicroft, 2013).

Conclusions

Despite the relative lack of research from settings outside Western and Northern Europe and North America, it is apparent that individuals with psychosis residing in the rest of the world are at increased risk of premature mortality. For example, compared with the general populations in which they reside, individuals with psychosis in Taiwan (Pan et al., 2020) have a risk of suicide that is about 10 times higher than the general population. In Ethiopia (Fekadu et al., 2015) and China (Ran et al., 2020), suicide comprised almost 14% of all deaths in cohorts of individuals with schizophrenia. Despite the high prevalence of suicide, medical conditions accounted for a majority of deaths. However, only 7 of the 37 studies provide information about the specific medical conditions that were the leading causes of death. All the other studies aggregated medical conditions into the category 'natural' deaths. Similarly, few studies delineate the specific causes of 'unnatural' deaths, which includes suicide as well as deaths due to accidents, poisonings, and homicide. As a result, it is not possible to derive rates of suicide from statistics about 'unnatural' mortality.

In sum, the evidence provided by this review is broadly consistent with the findings of the Saha et al. (2007) review: (i) mortality risk for individuals with psychosis is high throughout the world; (ii) suicides comprise a substantial portion of this mortality, although our review does not suggest the risk is as much as 12 times greater than in general populations; and (iii) individuals with psychosis have elevated risk of mortality for 'natural' causes of death.

At the same time, methodological challenges are evident in the studies under review. First, diagnostic criteria were not consistent across the studies. For example, although several studies relied on ICD-9 criteria for psychosis, the inclusion codes varied: ICD-9 designates codes 295 to 299 for psychoses and code 296 specifically for 'episodic mood disorders'. Pan et al. (2017) included individuals who were diagnosed with most, but not all, of the 296 subheadings, while Kodesh et al. (2012) apparently included individuals diagnosed with all of the 296 subheadings, which include bipolar disorders without psychotic features. At the same time, research in Brazil (Menezes & Mann, 1996) and Bulgaria (Ganev et al., 2007) did not include individuals who were diagnosed as experiencing any of the 296 codes. Similar inconsistencies are also evident in the studies that used ICD-10 codes (Kim et al., 2017; Krupchanka et al., 2018; Liu et al., 2014). Second, the nature of samples varies, i.e. inpatient, outpatient, treated incidence, first-episode, recent cohorts, and population-based samples. This variation, and the potential biases in the samples, makes it imperative to be cautious when attempting to generalize from the available evidence (Bromet, 2008). Finally, the percentage of cohort members who were lost to follow-up varied from around 3% (Liu et al., 2014) to around 40% (Nakane et al., 2007; Varma & Malhotra, 2007), and many studies did not provide any information about the extent of attrition. Thus, the cohorts with high or unknown rates of attrition may not be representative (Brown, 1997), making it difficult, again, to make generalizations about the studies.

The need for more research on mortality among individuals residing in settings other than Western and Northern Europe and North America may be the primary finding of this review, a need also expressed by ISoS investigators (Craig et al., 2007). But more research is not a complete solution. Methodological issues must be addressed:

- Diagnostic categories must be clearly specified, and research should consider a range of psychotic disorders, both affective and non-affective.
- Sample inclusion and exclusion criteria must be reported in greater detail so that ascertainment bias might be assessed.
- Average ages of death in the cohorts are needed.
- Analyses must consider the proportion of cohort members who were lost to follow-up because it is difficult to be confident about the reliability of research in which a high percentage of the cohort could not be traced.

In addition, specific causes of death (organized by ICD categories) are necessary if we are to achieve a broad understanding of mortality and psychosis in diverse settings. Of course, this is easier said than done because death registers may not exist everywhere and, thus, investigations of mortality often must rely on broad and uninformative categories, e.g. 'natural' and 'unnatural' causes. Taking on the task of the documenting causes of death among individuals with psychosis may be beyond the capability of epidemiologists and psychiatric researchers, but at times it might be possible to initiate verbal autopsies (Fottrell & Byass, 2010) of representative samples. An alternative approach might be to conduct health assessments among representative samples of individuals with psychosis (Blomqvist et al., 2018; Nishanth et al., 2017) and use those data to estimate the extent to which specific comorbidities may contribute to overall mortality. That detail of health data would be invaluable in focusing the medical care of individuals with psychosis (Leucht et al., 2007).

In conclusion, excess mortality among individuals with psychosis has garnered increased attention in recent years (Thornicroft, 2011; Thornicroft, 2013; Seeman, 2007; Seeman, 2019). All too often, however, discussions about addressing the challenge of the so-called mortality gap are based on research conducted in a small fraction of the global population (Liu et al., 2017). A broader focus, one that encompasses a greater diversity of populations, is necessary.

References

Alstrom, C. H. (1942). Mortality in mental hospitals with special regard to tuberculosis. *Acta Psychiat Neurol Scand, 24*, 416–422.

Babigian, H. M., & Odoroff, C. L. (1969). The mortality experience of a population with psychiatric illness. *Am J Psychiatry, 126*, 470–480.

Bagewadi, V. I., et al. (2016). Standardized mortality ratio in patients with schizophrenia—findings from Thirthahalli, a rural south indian community. *Indian J Psychol Med, 38*(3), 202–206.

Bitter, I., et al. (2017). Mortality and the relationship of somatic comorbidities to mortality in schizophrenia. A nationwide matched-cohort study. *Eur Psychiatry, 45*, 97–103.

Blomqvist, M., et al. (2018). Health risks among people with severe mental illness in psychiatric outpatient settings. *Issues Ment Health Nurs, 39*(7), 585–591.

Bromet, E. J. (2008). Cross-national comparisons: problems in interpretation when studies are based on prevalent cases. *Schizophr Bull, 34*(2), 256–257.

Brown, S. (1997). Excess mortality of schizophrenia. A meta-analysis. *Br J Psychiatry, 171*, 502–508.

Burrows, G. M. (1820). *An inquiry into certain errors relative to insanity: and their consequences: physical, moral, and civil.* London: Underwood.

Chan, S. K., et al. (2015). 10-year outcome study of an early intervention program for psychosis compared with standard care service. *Psychol Med, 45*(6), 1181–1193.

Chen, C. & Shen, Y. (2007). RA: Beijing, China. In Hopper, K., Harrison, G., Janca, A., & Sartorius, N. (eds) *Recovery from schizophrenia: an international perspective.* Oxford: Oxford University Press, 243–254.

Chen, Y. H., et al. (2010). Mortality among psychiatric patients in Taiwan--results from a universal National Health Insurance programme. *Psychiatry Res, 178*(1), 160–165.

Cheng, K.-Y., et al. (2014). Mortality among long-stay patients with schizophrenia during the setting-up of community facilities under the Yuli model. *Health Psychol Behav Med, 2*(1), 602–612.

Craig, T. J., et al. (2007). Long-term mortality experience of international cohorts of persons with schizophrenia and related psychoses. In Hopper, K., Harrison, G., Janca, A., & Sartorius, N. (eds) *Recovery from schizophrenia: an international perspective.* Oxford: Oxford University Press, 61–68.

Crookshank, F. G. (1899). The frequency, causation, prevention, and treatment of phthisis pulmonalis in asylums for the insane. *Br J Psychiatry, 45*(191), 657–683.

Doyle, R., et al. (2019). The iHOPE-20 study: mortality in first episode psychosis-a 20-year follow-up of the Dublin first episode cohort. *Soc Psychiatry Psychiatr Epidemiol, 54*(11), 1337–1342.

Dube, K. C. & Kumar, N. (2007). IPSS: Agra, India. In Hopper, K., Harrison, G., Janca, A., & Sartorius, N. (eds) *Recovery from schizophrenia: an international perspective.* Oxford: Oxford University Press, 77–84.

Farr, W. (1841). Report upon the mortality of lunatics. *J Stat Soc Lond, 4*(1), 17–33.

Fekadu, A., et al. (2015). Excess mortality in severe mental illness: 10-year population-based cohort study in rural Ethiopia. *Br J Psychiatry, 206*(4), 289–296.

Firth, J., et al. (2019). The Lancet Psychiatry Commission: a blueprint for protecting physical health in people with mental illness. *Lancet Psychiatry, 6*(8), 675–712.

Fottrell, E. & Byass, P. (2010). Verbal autopsy: methods in transition. *Epidemiol Rev*, *32*(1), 38–55.

Francis, C. (1840). Mortality in lunatic asylums. *Lancet*, *35*(894), 129.

Ganev, K., et al. (2007). RAPyD: Sofia, Bulgaria. In **Hopper, K., Harrison, G., Janca, A., & Sartorius, N.** (eds) *Recovery from schizophrenia: an international perspective*. Oxford: Oxford University Press, 227–239.

Gardiner Hill, R. (1842). Statistics of lunacy. Mortality at the Wakefield Asylum. *Lancet*, *38*(972), 88–89.

Gondek, T. M., et al. (2015). The European studies on mortality in schizophrenia. *Psychiatr Pol*, *49*(6), 1139–1148.

Gur, S., et al. (2018). Mortality, morbidity and medical resources utilization of patients with schizophrenia: a case-control community-based study. *Psychiatry Res*, *260*, 177–181.

Hallgren, J., et al. (2019). Mortality trends in external causes of death in people with mental health disorders in Sweden, 1987–2010. *Scand J Public Health*, *47*(2), 121–126.

Hassall, C., et al. (1988). A preliminary study of excess mortality using a psychiatric case register. *J Epidemiol Community Health*, *42*(3), 286–289.

Hjorthoj, C., et al. (2017). Years of potential life lost and life expectancy in schizophrenia: a systematic review and meta-analysis. *Lancet Psychiatry*, *4*(4), 295–301.

Hopper, K., et al. (eds) (2007). *Recovery from schizophrenia: an international perspective*. Oxford: Oxford University Press.

Indian Council of Medical Research, et al. (2017). *India: health of the nation's states—the India state-level disease burden initiative*. New Dehli: ICMR, PHFI & IHME.

Kebede, D., et al. (2019). The 10-year functional outcome of schizophrenia in Butajira, Ethiopia. *Heliyon*, *5*(3), e01272.

Kebede, D., et al. (2004). The sociodemographic correlates of schizophrenia in Butajira, rural Ethiopia. *Schizophr Res*, *69*(2–3), 133–141.

Kim, W., et al. (2017). Mortality in schizophrenia and other psychoses: data from the South Korea national health insurance cohort, 2002–2013. *J Korean Med Sci*, *32*(5), 835–842.

Ko, Y. S., et al. (2018). Higher mortality and years of potential life lost of suicide in patients with schizophrenia. *Psychiatry Res*, *270*, 531–537.

Kodesh, A., et al. (2012). Epidemiology and comorbidity of severe mental illnesses in the community: findings from a computerized mental health registry in a large Israeli health organization. *Soc Psychiatry Psychiatr Epidemiol*, *47*(11), 1775–1782.

Krupchanka, D., et al. (2018). Mortality in people with mental disorders in the Czech Republic, a nationwide, register-based cohort study. *Lancet Public Health*, *3*(6), e289–e295.

Kua, J., et al. (2003). A 20-year follow-up study on schizophrenia in Singapore. *Acta Psychiatr Scand*, *108*(2), 118–125.

Kumar, A. K. S. (1991). UNDP's human development index: a computation for Indian states. *Econ Polit Wkly*, *26*(41), 2343–2345.

Kurihara, T., et al. (2011). Seventeen-year clinical outcome of schizophrenia in Bali. *Eur Psychiatry*, *26*(5), 333–338.

Lee, E. E., et al. (2018). A widening longevity gap between people with schizophrenia and general population, a literature review and call for action. *Schizophr Res*, *196*, 9–13.

Lee, P. W., et al. (1998). The 15-year outcome of Chinese patients with schizophrenia in Hong Kong. *Can J Psychiatry, 43*(7), 706–713.

Lee, P. W. H., et al. (2007). RA: Hong Kong. In **Hopper, K., Harrison, G., Janca, A., & Sartorius, N.** (eds) *Recovery from schizophrenia: an international perspective*. Oxford: Oxford University Press, 255–265.

Leng, C. H., et al. (2016). Estimation of life expectancy, loss-of-life expectancy, and lifetime healthcare expenditures for schizophrenia in Taiwan. *Schizophr Res, 171*(1–3), 97–102.

Leon, C. A. & Leon, A. (2007). IPSS: Cali, Colombia. In **Hopper, K., Harrison, G., Janca, A., & Sartorius, N.** (eds) *Recovery from schizophrenia: an international perspective*. Oxford: Oxford University Press, 85–99.

Leucht, S., et al. (2007). Physical illness and schizophrenia: a review of the literature. *Acta Psychiatr Scand, 116*(5), 317–333.

Liu, N. H., et al. (2017). Excess mortality in persons with severe mental disorders: a multilevel intervention framework and priorities for clinical practice, policy and research agendas. *World Psychiatry, 16*(1), 30–40.

Liu, T., et al. (2014). Prevalence of schizophrenia disability and associated mortality among Chinese men and women. *Psychiatry Res, 220*, 181–187.

Lo, W. H. & Lo, T. (1977). A ten-year follow-up study of Chinese schizophrenics in Hong Kong. *Br J Psychiatry, 131*, 63–66.

Makanjuola, R. O. & Adedapo, S. A. (1987). The DSM-III concepts of schizophrenic disorder and schizophreniform disorder. A clinical and prognostic evaluation. *Br J Psychiatry, 151*, 611–618.

Malzberg, B. (1949). Mortality among patients with mental disease in the New York civil state hospitals. *J Insur Med, 5*, 5–13.

Malzberg, B. (1934). *Mortality among patients with mental diseases*. New York: State Hospitals Press.

Mayer-Gross, W., et al. (1960). *Clinical psychiatry*. London: Cassell.

Menezes, P. R. & Mann, A. H. (1996). Mortality among patients with non-affective functional psychoses in a metropolitan area of south-eastern Brazil. *Rev Saude Publica, 30*(4), 304–309.

Nakane, Y., et al. (2007). DOSMeD: Nagasaki, Japan. In **Hopper, K., Harrison, G., Janca, A., & Sartorius, N.**, eds. *Recovery from schizophrenia: an international perspective*. Oxford: Oxford University Press, 164–176.

Nishanth, K., et al. (2017). Physical comorbidity in schizophrenia and its correlates. *The Indian J Med Res, 146*(2), 281.

Ogawa, K., et al. (1987). A long-term follow-up study of schizophrenia in Japan—with special reference to the course of social adjustment. *Br J Psychiatry, 151*, 758–765.

Pan, Y. J., et al. (2020). Excess mortality and shortened life expectancy in people with major mental illnesses in Taiwan. *Epidemiol Psychiatr Sci, 29*, e156.

Pan, Y. J., et al. (2017). Transformation of excess mortality in people with schizophrenia and bipolar disorder in Taiwan. *Psychol Med, 47*(14), 2483–2493.

Park, S., et al. (2015). Cause-specific mortality of psychiatric inpatients and outpatients in a general hospital in Korea. *Asia Pac J Public Health, 27*(2), 164–175.

Phillips, M. R., et al. (2004). Suicide and the unique prevalence pattern of schizophrenia in mainland China, a retrospective observational study. *Lancet, 364*(9439), 1062–1068.

Piotrowski, P., et al. (2017). Causes of mortality in schizophrenia: an updated review of European studies. *Psychiatr Danub, 29*(2), 108–120.

Ponnudurai, R., et al. (2006). Assessment of mortality and marital status of schizophrenic patients over a period of 13 years. *Indian J Psychiatry, 48*(2), 84–87.

Ran, M.-S., et al. (2020). Mortality and suicide in schizophrenia: 21-year follow-up in rural China. *BJPsych Open, 6*(6), e121.

Ran, M. S., et al. (2015). Gender differences in outcomes in people with schizophrenia in rural China: 14-year follow-up study. *Br J Psychiatry, 206*(4), 283–288.

Ran, M. S., et al. (2007). Mortality in people with schizophrenia in rural China: 10-year cohort study. *Br J Psychiatry, 190*(3), 237–242.

Rangaswamy, T. & Cohen, A. (2020). Invited commentary from a LAMIC country: thirty-five years of schizophrenia—the Madras Longitudinal study. *Schizophr Res, 220*, 27–28.

Saha, S., et al. (2007). A systematic review of mortality in schizophrenia: is the differential mortality gap worsening over time? *Arch Gen Psychiatry, 64*(10), 1123–1131.

Saku, M., et al. (1995). Mortality in psychiatric patients, with a specific focus on cancer mortality associated with schizophrenia. *Int J Epidemiol, 24*(2), 366–372.

Seeman, M. V. (2007). An outcome measure in schizophrenia: mortality. *Can J Psychiatry, 52*(1), 55–60.

Seeman, M. V. (2019). Schizophrenia mortality: barriers to progress. *Psychiatr Q, 90*(3), 553–563.

Sher, L. & Kahn, R. S. (2019). Suicide in schizophrenia: an educational overview. *Medicina (Kaunas), 55*(7), 361.

Skoda, C., et al. (2007). IPSS: Prague, Czech Republic. In **Hopper, K., Harrison, G., Janca, A., & Sartorius, N.**, eds. *Recovery from schizophrenia: an international perspective.* Oxford: Oxford University Press, 100–112.

Slater, E. & Roth, M. (1970). *Clinical psychiatry.* London: Bailliere Tindall and Cassell.

Taipale, H., et al. (2020). 20-year follow-up study of physical morbidity and mortality in relationship to antipsychotic treatment in a nationwide cohort of 62,250 patients with schizophrenia (FIN20). *World Psychiatry, 19*(1), 61–8.

Teferra, S., et al. (2011). Five-year mortality in a cohort of people with schizophrenia in Ethiopia. *BMC Psychiatry, 11*(1), 165.

The World Bank (2020). Life expectancy at birth, total (years)—China. Retrieved from https://data.worldbank.org/indicator/SP.DYN.LE00.IN?locations=CN

Thornicroft, G. (2011). Physical health disparities and mental illness: the scandal of premature mortality. *Br J Psychiatry, 199*(6), 441–442.

Thornicroft, G. (2013). Premature death among people with mental illness. *BMJ, 346*, f2969.

Tsai, K. Y., et al. (2014). Is low individual socioeconomic status (SES) in high-SES areas the same as low individual SES in low-SES areas: a 10-year follow-up schizophrenia study. *Soc Psychiatry Psychiatr Epidemiol, 49*(1), 89–96.

Tsirkin, S. (2007). DOSMeD: Moscow, Russia. In **Hopper, K., Harrison, G., Janca, A., & Sartorius, N.** (eds) *Recovery from schizophrenia: an international perspective.* Oxford: Oxford University Press, 152–163.

Varma, V. K. & Malhotra, S. (2007). DOSMeD: Chandigarh, India. In **Hopper, K., Harrison, G., Janca, A., & Sartorius, N.** (eds) *Recovery from schizophrenia: an international perspective.* Oxford: Oxford University Press, 115–128.

Wang, C. W., et al. (2014). Suicide rates in China from 2002 to 2011: an update. *Soc Psychiatry Psychiatr Epidemiol, 49*(6), 929–941.

7

Psychosis, phenomenology, and culture: Welcoming the 'black box'

Neely Anne Laurenzo Myers

Introduction

This chapter builds on an earlier critical review of literature (through 2011) concerning the relationships between culture and schizophrenia (Myers, 2011). It updates that review with new literature on the influences of culture on all aspects of psychosis (i.e. onset, manifestations, course, and outcome, and so on) and literature invoking culture as an explanation for variations in psychosis (i.e. in phenomenology, incidence, course, and outcome) across countries and populations. As an addition to the original review, this chapter also comments on the paucity of literature on the phenomenology of psychosis across cultures and the importance of taking a global perspective to build a complete view of psychotic phenomena and their relation to the cultures in which people live and grow. It also argues that there is an urgent need for further attention to phenom-enology, as well as a plea for re-theorizing the role of culture, at least in part, as a source of 'moral agency' that people can use to seek out mental health re-covery in locally meaningful ways (Mattingly, 2014; Myers, 2015; Myers, 2016; Myers, 2019).

It is clear in the psychiatric and epidemiological literature that social con-text makes a difference for people with schizophrenia—a feature frequently attributed to 'culture'. In this literature, 'culture' is often shorthand for com-plex assemblages of ways of life that account for social orderings (e.g. insti-tutional hierarchies) and environments while also capturing the ways that individuals and their families use culturally available meanings like explana-tory models to make sense of their illness experience and find relief (Myers, 2011). Anthropologists have long argued that the term culture often operates as a 'black box' explanation to account for otherwise 'unexplained variance' (Edgerton & Cohen, 1994; Jenkins & Barrett, 2004; Jenkins & Karno, 1992;

Lende & Downey, 2012; Luhrmann, 2007). They argue that the public health and epidemiological literature uses the term 'culture' without really engaging with the implications that a real role for culture might suggest.

This chapter adds a focus on the moral dimensions of 'culture' and so highlights local pathways that can lead to a person becoming misunderstood and not trusted as a 'good' person worthy of intimate relationships with others, including everyday social intimacies like employment opportunities, community group membership (e.g. book club, volunteer positions), and satisfying friendships. Culture, in this reading, can be thought of as a set of instructions about how to perform the tasks of everyday life that make it possible to become seen as a 'good' person in one's 'local moral world' (Kleinman, 1999; Luhrmann, 2001; Myers, 2015). By using the term 'local moral world', anthropologist-psychiatrist Kleinman tries to account for the ways one's culture defines what it means to be a 'good' person, not according to some broader sense of a human ethical code, but rather, according to 'local' history, politics, economics, religious practices, pathways to care, and experiences of care, common ways of expressing one's self, and styles of familial involvement and assistance (Biehl et al., 2007; DelVecchio Good et al., 2008). In this usage, 'local' means less of a geographic orientation and more of an orientation to others with whom one hopes to have social connections.

This approach makes plain that culture cannot be limited to population-level categories of nationality or ethnicity or reduced to national or ethnic differences as there are complex variations within 'cultures' and beyond geographic boundaries (Kirmayer & Ban, 2013). Thus, while there is no doubt that social context plays a role in the population-level differences we can identify in primarily statistical global health research (many of which will be presented next), these approaches lack nuanced analyses (Kleinman, 1999). Nonetheless, extending our view beyond the places where most research on psychoses is conducted— namely, North America, Western Europe, and Australia—is essential to understand the diversity of psychosis understandings, experiences, and treatments across settings.

This review, following the lead of others, suggests that the future investigation of the role of 'culture' includes attention to the often-demoralizing experience of the biomedical approach to psychosis, as well as the ways often-stigmatizing local cultural responses to the need for mental health treatment can cause a person to become disheartened or lose hope. Social scientists working on these issues note how Western biomedical approaches to mental illness can be disabling (Estroff, 1981; Luhrmann, 2008; Luhrmann & Marrow, 2016; Myers & Ziv, 2016; Spandler et al., 2015), and typically overlook nonclinical efforts to return to mental health in settings of creative work, religious practice, mutual support, education, and political action (Mattingly, 2014; Mead & Hilton, 2003; Myers, 2019; Ware et al., 2007; Wexler et al., 2013). Anthropologists and first-person perspectives have shown that psychotic behaviour and the societal response to psychosis often breaks down one's own sense and the sense of other people that one is a 'good' person capable of acting in ways that make possible intimate connections with others, which I call moral agency (Barrett, 1998; Jenkins & Carpenter-Song, 2008; Myers, 2015; Myers, 2016). In the United States, people who want to have moral agency are often asked to prove they can become a hardworking, independent, taxpaying adult (Myers, 2015). In India, someone may need to alternatively prove that they can be a dutiful son or obedient wife (Thara et al., 2003). Among Maasai women in northern Tanzania, my own preliminary work suggests that 'having heart', which locally means offering a calm and nurturing relationship to one's family and children and animals so that all are healthy and happy, is what makes one a 'good' woman. What it takes to be seen as a 'good person' and act as a moral agent varies across social contexts.

Moreover, the Western biomedical response to psychosis, I have argued, breaks down one's existing moral agency while offering few opportunities for a person to replenish their sense of moral agency in the aftermath of a psychotic episode (Myers, 2015; Myers & Ziv, 2016; Myers, 2019). In my published work, based on fieldwork, interviews, and the literature about people in mental health recovery, I have shown how protecting and carefully replenishing moral agency is an essential driver of well-being after a psychotic episode (Myers, 2016). Thus, the moral dimensions of the culture of mental healthcare, as well as local notions of what makes a person 'good' and how those intersect with the experience and treatment of psychosis, deserves further attention despite its messiness and the difficulties of operationalizing and measuring its effects.

If this sounds like the old plea for taking explanatory models into account, it is, but it is also much more. The complexities of understanding culture and the importance of moral negotiations of serious illness demand careful ethnographic work. We know that the experience of psychosis is intimately related to culture and morality in terms of boundaries of acceptable behaviour, explanations, and experiences of unusual states, response, and outcome. Building on the work of others, I would add that moral agency, or one's capacity to act in a way that enables them to be recognized as a 'good' person and so makes possible intimate connections with desired others, is an essential driver of mental health recovery (Hopper, 2007; Lewis et al., 2012; Myers, 2015; Myers, 2016; 2007; Ware et al., 2008). Understanding how moral agency is cultivated, protected, and replenished is an important future direction for work on psychosis and culture.

Culture and the psychosis continuum

Some argue that psychotic symptoms are part of a common spectrum of mental experiences that only become pathological when a person with a certain neurodevelopmental and genetic profile (e.g. working memory deficits, family history of psychosis) experiences repeated social adversities (Van Os et al., 2009). For example, a person who experienced childhood trauma and adolescent discrimination, and who also has a neurodevelopmental 'proneness', may develop an overactive response to stress over time ('sensitization') that leaves them more likely to have psychotic experiences and ultimately, a full psychotic break (Harrison et al., 2001; Howes & Kapur, 2009). This literature positions schizophrenia and other psychotic disorders as the endpoint of a 'psychosis-proneness-persistence continuum' across which susceptibility to and low-level expression of psychoses varies (Van Os et al., 2009). The psychosis continuum concept builds on a survey of high income countries showing that 5–8% of the general population reported psychotic experiences (PE), of which 75–90% were typically transient and did not disrupt social functioning (Van Os et al., 2009), but still met criteria for inclusion within a 'non-clinical psychosis' phenotype (Kelleher & Cannon, 2011). Van Os and colleagues (2009) argue that genetic vulnerabilities and adverse experiences likely push a person along the spectrum via transient psychotic experiences towards a psychotic disorder.

More research will help clarify this proposed notion of a psychosis continuum and the ways local configurations of culture (in tandem with vulnerability factors) may complicate, arrest, or accelerate one's progress along that continuum for people who have symptoms of a psychotic disorder or PEs (Myers, 2012). Based on findings about moral agency being important for mental health recovery in the Global North, it is likely that cultures that do not cultivate or protect one's sense of moral agency alongside the experience of psychotic symptoms—or that actually diminish one's moral agency through the process of care—may be more likely to push people along the continuum into psychosis. When a person finds it difficult to be seen as a 'good' person by people with whom they desire to have intimate connections, they suffer the stress of rejection, which can move them towards worsening symptoms according to this model.

Culture and positive symptoms

The experience of positive symptoms—the delusions and hallucinations of psychosis—seems to be inconsistent across 'cultures'. Larøi and colleagues (2014) argue that culture shapes hallucinations in both their pathological and non-pathological forms. For example, in one study of 1,080 patients who met DSM-IV criteria for schizophrenia in seven countries (Austria, Poland, Lithuania, Georgia, Pakistan, Nigeria, and Ghana), the highest one-year prevalence of auditory or visual hallucinations was observed in West African participants (e.g. 90.8% in Ghana, 85.4% in Nigeria; and 53.9% in Ghana, 50.8% in Nigeria, respectively) (Bauer et al., 2010). The lowest prevalence for auditory hallucinations in this sample was found in Austria (66.9%), and for visual hallucinations in Pakistan (3.9%) (Bauer et al., 2010). One Turkish study found that hallucinations and delusions varied regionally within the same country, suggesting (as anthropologists have long warned (e.g. Appadurai, 1990; Bhabha, 1994)) that 'cultural effects' may not necessarily map onto geopolitical boundaries (Gecici et al., 2010). Luhrmann's work makes a notable effort as she compares the experience of voice-hearing between patients with schizophrenia in Ghana, India, and northern California noting the variation in how patients experience their voices, how these experiences seem to be culturally shaped via a kind of 'social kindling', and arguing that in particular American experiences of voices as violent command hallucinations made them more distressing (Luhrmann et al., 2015; Luhrmann et al., 2015). As in many studies of culture and psychosis, however, the extent to which the individuals in these studies are representative of all those with psychosis in the population is open to question. It is possible that the different healthcare systems from which the patients in these studies were sampled included people that were seeking help for different reasons (e.g. differing levels of severity, more overt or flagrant symptoms), or who differed in other ways from people with equivalent symptoms in the community (e.g. those who could afford care were more likely to be identified through services in settings where there are financial barriers to psychiatric treatment), making it necessary to consider how much we are able to compare them across cultures.

In addition, different social contexts may be more or less likely to make people feel more or less comfortable reporting that they hear voices as some cultures do not immediately pathologize and stigmatize hearing voices (Al-Issa, 1995). For example, an interesting recent piece out of South Africa suggested that people experiencing early psychosis in KwaZulu-Natal were first offered the opportunity to undergo culturally accepted training, *ukuthwasa*, to become a traditional health practitioner (van der Zeijst et al., 2021). In this local moral world, symptoms of mental illness, including unusual perceptual experiences, were interpreted as an ancestral calling for which *ukuthwasa* was the locally accepted 'cure'. In the case of *uthukwasa*, the training process may be seen as a therapeutic intervention for psychosis, which includes therapy, traditional medication, and integration ceremonies, van der Jeist and colleagues (2020) argued. If they are amenable to training, and many are, a young person experiencing early psychotic symptoms used *uthukwasa* to enhance their sense of moral agency and secure a source of gainful employment as a healer. Social contexts that offer valued social roles to people experiencing psychosis—as 'traditional healers'— or even as peer providers (Myers, 2015b)—may be helpful in protecting one's sense that they are a moral agent and point to the importance of the moral dimensions of care for people experiencing psychosis. Preserving one's sense that they are a 'good' person in their local context capable of doing good things for others is likely a crucial part of the healing process for psychosis.

Culture and negative symptoms

Cultural elements also seem to interact with the negative symptoms of schizophrenia. Critiques of the ways cognitive assessments are shaped by and reinforce Western cultural values about the right way to think are important (Bromley, 2012). One study claims to have validated five factors that all future studies of negative symptoms of schizophrenia cross-culturally should aim to use, but notably these domains were validated in high-income countries only (Italy, Spain, China, Switzerland, and the USA) (Ahmed et al., 2019). This kind of assumption—researchers from the Global North assuming what they do applies automatically to the Global South—has led to calls to 'decolonize' global mental health.

Even though the way we measure cognition requires attention to cultural factors, there are some studies that suggest culture shapes the social impact of cognitive deficits or strengths for people diagnosed with schizophrenia. One 20-year follow-up study in the US followed participants who met the criteria for 'deficit schizophrenia,' or who met criteria for schizophrenia along with multiple, enduring negative symptoms for over one year, such as poverty of speech, restricted affect, diminished sense of purpose, and social drive even during times of stability (Kirkpatrick and Galderisi, 2008). In this study, only 13% showed one or more one-year periods of global recovery compared with 63% of their non-deficit schizophrenia counterparts (Strauss et al., 2010). This is important because Americans with schizophrenia who receive disability incomes live well below the poverty line, and unless they want to take on low-paying, high-stress jobs to supplement their income—such as working as a cashier or in fast food restaurants, which are especially challenging for people with cognitive deficits—they have limited access to affordable housing (Myers, 2015). Many then live a refugee-like existence on an 'institutional circuit' of makeshift housing, which includes the streets, shelters, nursing homes, and jails (Hopper et al., 1997; Luhrmann, 2008; Myers, 2015). Another study found that Swedish participants (versus their cognitive and functional counterparts in New York

City) lived independently more often and for longer periods because the process of obtaining and keeping housing was less cognitively demanding (Harvey et al., 2009). While this kind of comparison may seem like a stretch given the massive differences in the social welfare state between the US and Sweden, the authors argue for 'divergent real-world outcomes among individuals who show evidence of the same levels of ability and potential' based on social context. This should surprise no one who takes economic context, the stress of modern life, and the potential role of the state in exacerbating that stress seriously (Cooper & Sartorius, 1977).

These findings raise interesting questions. Does one's ability to recover from the effects of deficit schizophrenia symptoms depend in part on the massive efforts required to meet basic needs if state or familial assistance is unavailable? Further research on the interplay of cognitive capabilities and social context is needed (Koelkebeck & Wilhelm, 2014). It may be especially fruitful to collect data on this topic in non-Western contexts where cognitive demands, employment opportunities, and sources of social support (such as affordable housing) may be radically different (as proposed years ago by the late Richard Warner (2004)). Clearly, more work is needed.

Culture as risk

From a critical anthropological perspective, 'cultural features' such as diagnostic bias and error, or other epidemiological 'factors' like urbanicity, migration status, racial/ethnic discrimination, socioeconomic status, adverse life events, and cumulative social disadvantage (all described in detail in Chapters 2 through 5), each contribute to the ways that cultural context imposes 'risk' on individuals over time. However, anthropologists focused on phenomenology look specifically at how these factors—often taken together—play out in people's everyday lives. The epidemiological literature surveyed in this book makes it clear that something about 'seeming different' from the majority culture in various social contexts appears to increase one's risk for developing psychosis (Myers, 2011). People who 'seem different' may be more vulnerable to experiences of structural violence and structural racism, which diminish moral agency and can be deleterious to health outcomes (Farmer, 1999; Kelly, 2005; Luhrmann, 2007; Luhrmann & Marrow, 2016; Myers & Ziv, 2016; Anglin et al., 2021).

However, phenomenological anthropologists also describe ways that people find agency despite these top-down impositions of culture. People resist and push back and make intimate connections in ways that are comfortable for them so that they can move forward. We can see this in the work of Corin and Lauzon, for example, in their description of 'positive withdrawal'—a social strategy people diagnosed with schizophrenia in Montreal used to engage socially while protecting themselves from becoming overwhelmed by symptoms triggered by the stress of social interaction (Corin & Lauzon, 1992).

This is also evident in my own ethnographic engagement with young Black men experiencing early psychosis who welcomed the opportunity to tell their own stories in their own ways because, as they explained, 'no one has ever even asked me that before' despite years of engagement with American public mental health services for a serious psychotic disorder (Myers & Ziv, 2016). When people are not allowed to tell their own story, it can diminish their moral agency. When people find a social context where people understand or empathize with their experience and can see them as a good person, they may be less vulnerable to the lived experience of discrimination and stigma.

Diagnostic bias

As an example, let us consider the case of diagnostic bias. High rates of psychotic disorders in minoritized populations may be explained by cultural norms that promote the erroneous reporting or diagnosis of psychotic experiences in minoritized groups. Zandi and colleagues, for example, critiqued the role of clinician bias in the reportedly increased rates of psychosis among Moroccan immigrants to the Netherlands (Zandi et al., 2008). For first-generation Moroccan immigrants, the authors argued, these symptoms reflected a 'dissociative possession state' common in Moroccan culture that had been misinterpreted by Western psychiatrists. With a 'more sensitive' and 'culturally adapted' tool being used with the Moroccan groups,[1] the statistical differences in the risk of developing schizophrenia between Moroccan immigrants and Dutch natives disappeared (Zandi et al., 2010). However, other studies showed the opposite, and studies that have attempted to rigorously control for clinician bias still demonstrate elevated rates of psychosis among racially and ethnically minoritized populations (Morgan & Hutchinson, 2010).

In another relevant study, Latino patients displayed psychotic symptoms that were associated with distress, disability, and mental health service utilization but did not meet diagnostic criteria for a psychotic disorder. The authors concluded that these were best understood as culturally acceptable ways to signal 'interpersonal vulnerability' rather than serious disorder in people who were unmarried

---

[1] Zandi and colleagues (2010) rated symptoms of Western 'psychotic disorder' such as hearing voices and seeing things or dead persons as 'not significantly present' if these experiences did not negatively impact the patient's functioning.

and had experienced trauma exposure (Lewis-Fernandez et al., 2009). It is possible that PEs are, in some social contexts, culturally acceptable ways of signalling distress that may even facilitate the healing process by summoning social support (Jenkins, 1988; Lewis-Fernandez et al., 2009). Psychotic symptoms, while clinically significant, may be manifestations of culturally acceptable reactions to war, displacement, trauma exposure, dissociation, and anxiety (Desjarlais et al., 1995; Good, 1997). On the other hand, as Morgan and Hutchinson (2010) argue, we must be careful not to dismiss all psychotic symptoms in socially disadvantaged populations as merely a product of diagnostic bias because the social adversity experienced across the life course by such populations leads to an increased risk for psychosis, and we do not want to deny people treatment who may benefit. While diagnostic bias cannot be ignored, lived experiences of adversity, discrimination, and structural violence endured by many over the lifecourse are also key for fully understanding these phenomena.

Stigma

Studies of stigma can also be linked to phenomenological experiences of moral agency and social disadvantage. Rates of both anticipated and experienced stigma are consistently high across cultures with regard to mental illness (Thornicroft et al., 2009). Cross-cultural 'expressed emotion' (EE) research in European American and Mexican American families suggests that when families are hostile and critical (high EE), the symptoms of their family member with schizophrenia increase and they experience higher rates of rehospitalization (Aguilera et al., 2010; Jenkins & Karno, 1992; Leff et al., 1987). Anglo-American families in the United States seem to typically be more hostile and critical of their family member with a psychotic disorder (high EE) and recovery outcomes from schizophrenia are less frequent (Lopez et al., 2009). Stigma is also prevalent in sub-Saharan Africa, including Nigeria, where Gureje and colleagues found high levels of negative views of mental illness and stigma against people perceived as mentally ill even when no specific mental illness was named (Gureje et al., 2005). Even primary care providers in East Africa (who have no training in specialty mental health) often have stigmatizing attitudes towards people with mental health concerns as can traditional healers who are also frontline providers of mental healthcare there (Gureje et al., 2006, 2015; Ndetei et al., 2011). In India, recent work by Koschorke and colleagues (2017), suggests that many family caregivers of persons living with schizophrenia said they were too uncomfortable to disclose a family member's condition and 'high caregiver stigma' was independently associated with higher levels of positive symptoms among those receiving care.

Culture as protective

However, caregiver stigma can also be protective as families around the world may also protect their ill relatives' sense of moral agency and belonging via exertions prompted by their own stigma against schizophrenia (Goffman, 1963). Where a whole family may be seen as less worthy of intimate relationships with others if one member is 'not good', there may be more of an effort to protect moral agency. For example, Yang and colleagues (Yang et al., 2009) described families' use of the term *xiang tai duo* or 'excessive thinking' as an alternative explanation for unsettling behaviour that mimicked schizophrenia symptoms in Beijing or Mainland China. Jenkins (1988) argued that Mexican Americans used the more neutral term *nervios* for disturbing behaviours, thereby offering flexible 'cultural protection' and inclusiveness than provided by a diagnostic label. Similarly, Sousa (2016) wrote about the 'diagnostic neutrality' of families in India who knew their child had a diagnosis of a psychotic disorder, but never used that diagnostic term. Such linguistic devices, these authors argue, had a 'normalizing power' that allowed families to recognize behaviours as socially unusual, but not too abnormal (e.g. 'sometimes we all think excessively'), to prevent further stigma. In southern India, where recovery outcomes are consistently high, families also used 'excessive thinking' as an alternative explanation for schizophrenia (Saravanan et al., 2008). Here, family members, the general public, and patients comfortably seemed to hold multiple, contradictory models of serious emotional distress (Halliburton, 2004). For example, they might agree that there was something 'abnormal in the brain' without calling it the result of a 'disease;' or patients might refuse to accept the illness as something wrong with them and attribute it to external spiritual factors instead (Saravanan et al., 2008). Such strategies may contribute to the increased recovery outcomes observed in some cultural contexts as families work behind the scenes to offset stigma and preserve an ill family member's social standing and local 'moral worth' (Hopper et al., 2007; Saravanan et al., 2008; Yang et al., 2009). Of course, families also provide much-needed financial and moral support, especially if they focus on minimizing the social repercussions of psychosis rather than the diagnostic category and its implications (Luhrmann & Marrow, 2016).

There is also a growing body of research suggesting that culturally specific, faith-based interventions can be helpful for people experiencing psychosis, including in areas with limited access to mental health professionals (Burns & Tomita, 2015; Griffith et al., 2016; Luhrmann & Marrow, 2016) and perhaps especially if they help people manage stress (Myers, 2010). Many people perceive psychosis as a spiritual problem and half of individuals seeking formal mental healthcare for mental disorders choose traditional and religious healers as their frontline provider in sub-Saharan Africa (Burns & Tomita, 2015). In low- and middle-income countries, religious healers are often the primary providers of care—admittedly, sometimes perhaps with deleterious effects (Arias et al., 2016). Negative outcomes can likely be overcome with training, though, perhaps especially if public health workers and faith healers can learn to collaborate (Gureje et al., 2020; Read, 2019), although more in-depth qualitative research is needed (van der Watt et al., 2018).

Experts by experience across cultures

Another underdeveloped area globally are first-person accounts of the phenomenology of psychosis, including the experience of treatments for psychosis, particularly in non-Western countries. This approach asks what experiences of psychotic symptoms and the societal response to them are like for people who experience them in everyday life. Such an understanding requires a first-person perspective, or at least some attempt to elicit and understand that perspective, which is often the aim of anthropology and ethnographic fieldwork (see, e.g. Corin et al. 2004).

From the anthropological fieldwork on record, as well as the growing availability of autobiographical first-person narratives,[2] we are beginning to understand that the level of impairment one experiences from psychotic symptoms likely depends on both the social response *and* how one learns to live with these extreme states in local contexts with varying resources and possibilities (Jenkins, 2015; Luhrmann & Marrow, 2016; Myers, 2015). The best literature we have on a phenomenological perspective on psychosis is from anthropological research and scholarship from those with lived experience, which gives us a preliminary sense that the ways people experience the onset and treatment of symptoms of psychosis can vary radically (Jones & Luhrmann, 2016; Jones et al., 2016; Luhrmann et al., 2015). User-survivor researchers are 'experts by experience', or people with lived experience of psychosis who are writing and conducting research on that experience (Beresford, 2016; Rose, 2009; Rose, 2017), as well as challenging the links between psychosis and disability and the ways they ignore race, class, and gender (Jones & Kelly, 2015). Some of these works, at times self-identified as 'mad studies', offer not only personal, autobiographical accounts, but ideas for research development, analysis, and interpretation 'produced by people

---

[2] Gail Hornstein maintains a list of first-person publications here as a Bibliography of First-Person Narratives of Madness in English, 5th edition, 2011 (PDF): gailhornstein.com/works.htm

who have been there (and back) and who absolutely resist medical explanations of their experiences' (Russo & Sweeney, 2016; Spandler et al., 2015). Interesting work from user-survivors has come out about issues ranging from the sense that Americans diagnosed with schizophrenia have somehow brought on the onset of psychosis wilfully (Jones et al., 2016), to reflections on the role of spiritual explanations in cultural contexts as also being relevant for lifelong recovery (Bidois, 2012; Chadwick, 2010; Jones et al., 2016). While there are a couple of excellent volumes offering (at least some) first-person perspectives (e.g. Geekie et al., 2012; Nudel, 2009), more first-person phenomenological accounts, especially from less Western social contexts would be helpful when trying to understand the cross-cultural experience of psychosis and treatment.

We also need more user-survivor perspectives on treatment cross-culturally. There are few first-person narratives and little user-survivor scholarship available from outside of mainstream Western culture, although both would contribute to the development of person-centred cross-cultural psychiatry (Jain, 2016). In my own work in Tanzania, when I try to tell people about recovery from psychosis, they want me to introduce them to someone or hear a personal account, accounts that I have not personally been able to collect in that social context. Letting people know that recovery is possible in ways that are meaningful to them may be especially helpful in reducing stigma and may be an important new avenue for research (Koschorke et al., 2017).

In addition, user-survivor perspectives from non-Western settings may or may not align with Western activists' experiences. For example, while many user-survivors in the west advocate for freedom from the oppression of biomedical psychiatry, user-survivors I have met from Liberia were campaigning for more access to biomedical psychiatry in a place with few resources. All of these perspectives are needed.

Conclusions

For too long the 'black box' of culture has served as a placeholder for reminding us to attend to local culture—in all its multifarious, indeterminate, inconsistent, and increasingly hybrid splendour—when attempting to plot the prospects of recovery. More recent work in the social sciences has suggested that important factors have emerged from the 'black box', such as structural violence, structural racism, social adversity, and moral agency, which can all shape psychosis risk, stigma, and people's abilities to recover across cultural contexts (Luhrmann, 2007; Myers & Ziv, 2016; Selten & Cantor-Graae, 2005; Wright, 2012).

Cultural analyses raise our awareness of the host of value-laden commitments that people must learn to meet in order to thrive in sometimes highly specified local moral worlds; for example, the Bedouin with a psychiatric disability who is more valued if she is experiencing spiritual attacks than if she has a biological illness (Sartorius, 2010); or the Indian son or daughter whose psychiatric disability is tolerated once they are married, and especially if they have children (Hopper et al., 2007; Myers, 2011). The point is that when people become ill and the ways they perceive themselves and others shifts—and that shift can be negative, positive, or neutral for one's moral agency. As the work reviewed here attests, substantial progress has been made in understanding how culture may exacerbate or assuage symptom trajectories and manifestations and the ways 'local moral worlds' can work to protect and replenish moral agency and the social intimacies it secures to counterbalance some of the stress of social adversities. This recent work excepted, the reach and yield of research into culture as an improvised playbook—a toolkit that moral agents and those invested in supporting them may draw upon as they grapple with psychosis-associated experiences—has only just begun, and deserves much more attention on a global scale. We need to engage further in the hard work of understanding what is at stake morally for people experiencing psychosis and their intimate others as they struggle to find a 'good life' and recover from a serious psychotic disorder on their own terms. This demands the hard work of observation, getting to know people over the long term, trying to understand people's life projects in context and what it means to be a moral agent in any given place where we seek to create clinical supports—work that anthropologists, working in partnership with patients, clinicians, and families, are well poised to do. One cannot operationalize cultural criteria or create checklists from this endeavour, but one may better be able to promote recovery for each person more effectively by taking stock of their life projects and local moral resources. In the process, we must accept and continue to peer into the ever-present 'black box' as a tool for understanding and promoting recovery.

References

Aguilera, A., et al. (2010). Expressed emotion and sociocultural moderation in the course of schizophrenia. *J Abnorm Psychol*, *119*(4), 875–885.

Ahmed, A. O., et al. (2019). Cross-cultural validation of the 5-factor structure of negative symptoms in schizophrenia. *Schizophr Bull*, *45*(2), 305–314.

Al-Issa, I. (1995). The illusion of reality or the reality of illusion. Hallucinations and culture. *Br J Psychiatry*, *166*, 368–373.

Anglin, D. M., et al. (2021). From womb to neighborhood: a racial analysis of social determinants of psychosis in the United States. *Am J Psychiatry*, *178*(7), 599–610.

Appadurai, A. (1990). Disjuncture and difference in the global cultural economy. *Theory Cult Soc*, *7*(2), 295–310.

Arias, D., et al. (2016). Prayer camps and biomedical care in Ghana: is collaboration in mental health care possible?. *PLoS ONE, 11*(9), e0162305.

Barrett, R. J. (1998). The 'schizophrenic' and the liminal persona in modern society. *Cult Med Psychiatry, 22,* 465–494.

Bauer, S. M., et al. (2010). Culture and the prevalence of hallucinations in schizophrenia. *Compr Psychiatry, 52*(3), 319–325.

Beresford, P. (2016). The role of survivor knowledge in creating alternatives to psychiatry. In **Russo, J. & Sweeney, A.** (eds) *Searching for a rose garden: challenging psychiatry, fostering mad studies.* Monmouth, UK: PCCS Books, 25–34.

Bhabha, H. K. (1994). *The location of culture.* New York: Routledge.

Bidois, E. (2012). A cultural and personal perspective of psychosis. In **Geekie, J.**, et al. (eds) *Experiencing psychosis: personal and professional perspectives.* New York: Routledge, 35–43.

Biehl, J., Good, B., & Kleinman, A. (2007). *Subjectivity: ethnographic investigations.* Berkeley, CA: University of California Press.

Bromley, E. (2012). The texture of the real: experimentation and experience in schizophrenia. *Cult Med Psychiatry, 36,* 154–174.

Burns, J. K. & Tomita, A. (2015). Traditional and religious healers in the pathway to care for people with mental disorders in Africa: a systematic review and meta-analysis. *Soc Psychiatry Psychiatr Epidemiol, 50*(6), 867–877.

Chadwick, P. K. (2010). 'On not drinking soup with a fork': from spiritual experience to madness to growth—a personal journey. In **Clarke, I.** (ed.) *Psychosis and spirituality,* 2nd edition. Singapore: John Wiley & Sons, 65–73.

Cooper, J. & Sartorius, N. (1977). Cultural and temporal variations in schizophrenia: a speculation on the importance of industrialization. *Br J Psychiatry, 130,* 50–55.

Corin, E. & Lauzon, G. (1992). Positive withdrawal and the quest for meaning: the reconstruction of experience among schizophrenics. *Psychiatry (New York), 55*(3), 266–278.

Corin, E., Thara, R., & Padmavati, R. (2004). Living through a staggering world: the play of signifiers in early psychosis in South India. In **Jenkins, J. H. & Barrett, R. J.** (eds) *Schizophrenia, culture, and subjectivity: the edge of experience.* Cambridge: Cambridge University Press, 110–145.

DelVecchio Good, M.-J., et al. (2008). *Postcolonial disorders.* Berkeley, CA: University of California Press.

Desjarlais, R., et al. (1995). Dislocation. In **Desjarlais, R.**, et al. (eds) *World mental health: problems and priorities in low-income countries.* Oxford: Oxford University Press, 136–154.

Edgerton, R. B. & Cohen, A. (1994). Culture and schizophrenia: the DOSMD challenge. *Br J Psychiatry, 164,* 222–231.

Estroff, S. E. (1981). *Making it crazy: an ethnography of psychiatric clients in an American community.* Los Angeles, CA: University of California Press.

Farmer, P. (1999). Pathologies of power: rethinking health and human rights. *Am J Public Health, 89,* 1486–1496.

Gecici, O., et al. (2010). Phenomenology of delusions and hallucinations in patients with schizophrenia. *Bull Clin Psychopharmacol, 20,* 204–212.

Geekie, J., et al. (eds) (2012). *Experiencing psychosis: personal and professional perspectives.* New York: Routledge.

Goffman, E. (1963). *Stigma: notes on the management of spoiled identity.* Englewood Cliffs, NJ: Prentice Hall.

Good, B. J. (1997). Studying mental illness in context: local, global, or universal?. *Ethos, 25*(2), 230–248.

Griffith, J. L., Myers, N., & Compton, M. T. (2016). How can community religious groups aid recovery for individuals with psychotic illnesses?. *Community Ment Health J, 52*(7), 775–780.

Gureje, O., et al. (2005). Community study of knowledge of and attitude to mental illness in Nigeria. *Br J Psychiatry, 186*, 436–441.

Gureje, O., et al. (2006). Do beliefs about causation influence attitudes to mental illness?. *World Psychiatry, 5*(2), 104–107.

Gureje, O., et al. (2015). The role of global traditional and complementary systems of medicine in the treatment of mental health disorders. *Lancet Psychiatry, 2*(2), 168–177.

Gureje, O., et al. (2020). Effect of collaborative care between traditional and faith healers and primary health-care workers on psychosis outcomes in Nigeria and Ghana (COSIMPO): a cluster randomised controlled trial. *Lancet, 396*(10251), 612–622.

Halliburton, M. (2004). Finding a fit: psychiatric pluralism in South India and its implications for WHO studies of mental disorder. *Transcult Psychiatry, 41*, 80–98.

Harrison, G., et al. (2001). Recovery from psychotic illness: a 15- and 25-year follow-up study. *Br J Psychiatry, 178*, 506–517.

Harvey, P. D., et al. (2009). Performance-based measurement of functional disability in schizophrenia: a cross-national study in the United States and Sweden. *Am J Psychiatry, 166*(7), 821.

Hopper, K., et al. (1997). Homelessness, severe mental illness, and the institutional circuit. *Psychiatr Serv, 48*(5), 659–665.

Hopper, K. (2007). Rethinking social recovery in schizophrenia: what a capabilities approach might offer. *Soc Sci Med, 65*(5), 868–879.

Hopper, K., Wanderling, J., & Narayanan, P. (2007). To have and to hold: a cross-cultural inquiry into marital prospects after psychosis. *Glob Public Health, 2*(3), 257–280.

Howes, O. D. & Kapur, S. (2009). The dopamine hypothesis of schizophrenia: version III— the final common pathway. *Schizophr Bull, 35*(3), 549–562.

Jain, S. (2016). Cross-cultural psychiatry and the user/survivor movement in the context of global mental health. *Philos Psychiatry Psychol, 23*(3–4), 305–308.

Jenkins, J. H. (1988). Ethnopychiatric interpretations of schizophrenic illness: the problem of nervios within Mexican-American families. *Cult Med Psychiatry, 12*, 301–329.

Jenkins, J. H. & Barrett, R. J. (2004). Introduction. In Jenkins, J. H. and Barrett, R. J. (eds) *Schizophrenia, culture, and subjectivity: the edge of experience.* Cambridge: Cambridge University Press, 1–28.

Jenkins, J. H. & Carpenter-Song, E. A. (2008). Stigma despite recovery: strategies for living in the aftermath of psychosis. *Med Anthropol Q, 22*(4), 381–409.

Jenkins, J. H. & Karno, M. (1992). The meaning of expressed emotion: theoretical issues raised by cross-cultural research. *Am J Psychiatry, 149*, 9–21.

Jenkins, J. H. (2015). *Extraordinary conditions: culture and experience in mental illness.* University of California Press.

Jones, N., et al. (2016). 'Did I push myself over the edge?': complications of agency in psychosis onset and development. *Psychosis, 8*(4), 324–335.

Jones, N. & Kelly, T. (2015). Inconvenient complications: on the heterogeneities of madness and their relationship to disability. In **Spandler, H., Anderson, J., & Sapey, B.** (eds) *Madness distress and the politics of disablement.* Chicago, IL: Policy Press, 43–55.

Jones, N., Kelly, T., & Shattell, M. (2016). God in the brain: experiencing psychosis in the postsecular United States. *Transcult Psychiatry, 53*(4), 488–505.

Jones, N. & Luhrmann, T. M. (2016). Beyond the sensory: findings from an in-depth analysis of the phenomenology of 'auditory hallucinations' in schizophrenia. *Psychosis, 8*, 191–202.

Kelleher, I. & Cannon, M. (2011). Psychotic-like experiences in the general population: characterizing a high-risk group for psychosis. *Psychol Med, 41*(1), 1–6.

Kelly, B. D. (2005). Structural violence and schizophrenia. *Soc Sci Med, 61*(3), 721–730.

Kirkpatrick, B. & Galderisi, S. (2008). Deficit schizophrenia: an update. *World Psychiatry, 7*(3), 143–147.

Kirmayer, L. J. & Ban, L. (2013). Cultural psychiatry: research strategies and future directions. *Adv Psychosom Med, 33*, 97–114.

Kleinman, A. (1999). Experience and its moral modes: culture, human conditions, and disorder. In **Peterson, G. B.** (ed.) *The Tanner lectures on human values.* Salt Lake City, UT: University of Utah Press, 357–420.

Koelkebeck, K. & Wilhelm, C. (2014). Cross-cultural aspects of social cognitive abilities in schizophrenia. In **Lysaker, P. H., Dimaggio, G., & Brüne, M.** (eds) *Social cognition and metacognition in schizophrenia: psychopathology and treatment approaches.* Cambridge, MA: Academic Press, 29–47.

Koschorke, M., et al. (2017). Experiences of stigma and discrimination faced by family caregivers of people with schizophrenia in India. *Soc Sci Med, 178*(178), 66–77.

Larøi, F., et al. (2014). Culture and hallucinations: overview and future directions. *Schizophr Bull, 40*(Suppl_4), S213–S220.

Leff, J., et al. (1987). Expressed emotion and schizophrenia in north India. III. Influence of relatives' expressed emotion on the course of schizophrenia in Chandigarh. *Br J Psychiatry, 151*(2), 166–173.

Lende, D. H. & Downey, G. (eds) (2012). *The encultured brain: an introduction to neuroanthropology.* Boston, MA: MIT Press.

Lewis-Fernandez, R., et al. (2009). Significance of endorsement of psychotic symptoms by US Latinos. *J Nerv Ment Dis, 197*(5), 337.

Lewis, S., Hopper, K., & Healion, E. (2012). Partners in recovery: social support and accountability in a consumer-run mental health center. *Psychiatr Serv, 63*(1), 1–5.

Lopez, S. R., et al. (2009). Cultural variability in the manifestation of expressed emotion. *Fam Process, 48*(2), 179–194.

Luhrmann, T. (2001). *Of two minds: the growing disorder in American psychiatry.* New York: Vintage Books.

Luhrmann, T. M. (2007). Social defeat and the culture of chronicity: or, why schizophrenia does so well over there and so badly here. *Cult Med Psychiatry, 31*(2), 135–172.

Luhrmann, T. M. (2008). 'The street will drive you crazy': why homeless psychotic women in the institutional circuit in the United States say no to offers of help. *Am J Psychiatry*, *165*(1), 1–15.

Luhrmann, T. M., et al. (2015). Differences in voice-hearing experiences of people with psychosis in the USA, India and Ghana: interview-based study. *Br J Psychiatry*, *206*(1), 41–44.

Luhrmann, T. M., et al. (2015). Hearing voices in different cultures: a social kindling hypothesis. *Top Cogn Sci*, *7*(4), 646–663.

Luhrmann, T. & Marrow, J. (eds) (2016). *Our most troubling madness*. Los Angeles, CA: University of California Press.

Mattingly, C. (2014). *Moral laboratories: family peril and the struggle for a good life*. Los Angeles, CA: University of California Press.

Mead, S. & Hilton, D. (2003). Crisis and connection. *Psychiatr Rehabil J*, *27*(1), 87–94.

Morgan, C. & Hutchinson, G. (2010). The social determinants of psychosis in migrant and ethnic minority populations: a public health tragedy. *Psychol Med*, *1*, 705–709.

Myers, N. A. L. (2012). Toward an applied neuroanthropology of psychosis. *Ann Anthropol Pract*, *36*, 113–130.

Myers, N. A. L. (2015). Shared humanity among nonspecialist peer care providers for persons living with psychosis: implications for global mental health. In **Javier, I. & Escobar, M. D.** (eds) *Global mental health: anthropological perspectives*. Walnut Creek, CA: Left Coast Press, 325–340.

Myers, N. A. L. (2016). Recovery stories: an anthropological exploration of moral agency in stories of mental health recovery. *Transcult Psychiatry*, *53*(4), 427–444.

Myers, N. A. L. & Ziv, T. (2016). 'No one ever even asked me that before.' Autobiographical power, social defeat and recovery among African Americans with lived experiences of psychosis. *Med Anthropol Q*, *30*(3), 395–413.

Myers, N. L. (2011). Update: schizophrenia across cultures. *Curr Psychiatry Rep*, *13*(4), 305–311.

Myers, N. L. (2015). *Recovery's edge: an ethnography of mental health care and moral agency*. Nashville, TN: Vanderbilt University Press.

Myers, N. L. (2019). Beyond the 'crazy house': mental/moral breakdowns and moral agency in first-episode psychosis. *Ethos*, *47*(1), 13–34.

Myers, N. L. (2010). Culture, stress and recovery from schizophrenia: lessons from the field for global mental health. *Cult Med Psychiatry*, *34*(3), 500.

Ndetei, D. M., et al. (2011). Knowledge, attitude and practice (KAP) of mental illness among staff in general medical facilities in Kenya: practice and policy implications. *Afr J Psychiatry (Johannesbg)*, *14*(3), 225–235.

Nudel, C. (2009). *Firewalkers: madness, beauty and mystery*. Charlottesville, VA: VOCAL.

Van Os, J., et al. (2009). A systematic review and meta-analysis of the psychosis continuum: evidence for a psychosis proneness-persistence-impairment model of psychotic disorder. *Psychol Med*, *39*(2), 179–195.

Read, U. M. (2019). Rights as relationships: collaborating with faith healers in community mental health in Ghana. *Cult Med Psychiatry*, *43*(4), 613–635.

Rose, D. (2009). Collaboration. In **Wallcraft, J., Schrank, B., & Amering, M.** (eds) *Handbook of service user involvement in mental health research*. Chichester, UK: John Wiley and Sons, 169.

Rose, D. (2017). Service user/survivor-led research in mental health: epistemological possibilities. *Disabil Soc*, *32*(6), 773–789.

Russo, J. & Sweeney, A. (eds) (2016). *Searching for a rose garden: challenging psychiatry, fostering mad studies*. Monmouth, UK: PCCS Books.

Saravanan, B., et al. (2008). Perceptions about psychosis and psychiatric services: a qualitative study from Vellore, India. *Soc Psychiatry Psychiatr Epidemiol*, *43*(3), 231–238.

Sartorius, N. (2010). Short-lived campaigns are not enough. *Nature*, *468*(7321), 163–165.

Selten, J. P. & Cantor-Graae, E. (2005). Social defeat: risk factor for schizophrenia?. *Br J Psychiatry*, *187*(2), 101.

Sousa, A. J. (2016). Diagnostic neutrality in psychiatric treatment in North India. In Luhrmann, T. M. & Marrow, J. (eds) *Our most troubling madness: case studies in schizophrenia across cultures*. Berkeley, CA: University of California Press, 42–55.

Spandler, H., Anderson, J., & Sapey, B. (eds) (2015). *Madness, distress and the politics of disablement*. Bristol, UK: Policy Press, University of Bristol.

Strauss, G. P., et al. (2010). Periods of recovery in deficit syndrome schizophrenia: a 20-year multi-follow-up longitudinal study. *Schizophr Bull*, *36*(4), 788–799.

Thara, R., Kamath, S., & Kumar, S. (2003). Women with schizophrenia and broken marriages—doubly disadvantaged? Part I: patient perspective. *Int J Soc Psychiatry*, *49*(3), 233–240.

Thornicroft, G., et al. (2009). Global pattern of experienced and anticipated discrimination against people with schizophrenia: a cross-sectional survey. *Lancet*, *373*(9661), 408–415.

Ware, N. C., et al. (2007). Connectedness and citizenship. *Psychiatr Serv*, *58*(4), 469–475.

Ware, N. C., et al. (2008). A theory of social integration as quality of life. *Psychiatr Serv*, *59*(1), 27–33.

Warner, R. (2004). *Recovery from schizophrenia: psychiatry and political economy*, 3rd edition. London: Brunner-Routledge.

van der Watt, A. S. J., et al. (2018). The perceived effectiveness of traditional and faith healing in the treatment of mental illness: a systematic review of qualitative studies. *Soc Psychiatry Psychiatr Epidemiol*, *53*(6), 555–566.

Wexler, L., et al. (2013). Promoting positive youth development and highlighting reasons for living in northwest Alaska through digital storytelling. *Health Promot Pract*, *14*(4), 617–623.

Wright, A. G. (2012). Social defeat in recovery-oriented supported housing: moral experience, stigma, and ideological resistance. *Cult Med Psychiatry*, *36*(4), 660–678.

Yang, L. H., et al. (2009). 'Excessive thinking' as explanatory model for schizophrenia: impacts on stigma and 'moral' status in mainland China. *Schizophr Bull*, *36*(4), 836–845.

Zandi, T., et al. (2008). The need for culture sensitive diagnostic procedures. *Soc Psychiatry Psychiatr Epidemiol*, *43*(3), 244–250.

Zandi, T., et al. (2010). First contact incidence of psychotic disorders among native Dutch and Moroccan immigrants in the Netherlands: influence of diagnostic bias. *Schizophr Res*, *119*(1–3), 27–33.

van der Zeijst, M., et al. (2021). Ancestral calling, traditional health practitioner training and mental illness: an ethnographic study from rural KwaZulu-Natal, South Africa. *Transcult Psychiatry*, *58*(4), 471–485.

8

Services and systems of care for psychotic disorders: A global perspective

Ashok Malla and Srividya N. Iyer

Introduction

Psychotic disorders are arguably the most serious of all mental disorders. Although the annual incidence is relatively low (10–40 per 100,000) (McGrath et al., 2004), these disorders have a high lifetime prevalence of around 3.5% (Perala et al., 2007). Due to their onset predominantly in adolescence and young adulthood, their relapsing nature with a substantial proportion of individuals developing long-term disabling conditions, and relatively high need for long-term care and high levels of premature mortality, the social, family, and personal consequences of psychotic disorders are enormous. Despite the complexity of these disorders and their multifaceted impacts, pharmacological and multiple psychosocial treatments are effective for many. While access to mental health specialists and even to medication is limited in low- and middle-income countries (LMICs) (Lora et al., 2012; Morris et al., 2011), even in high-income countries (HICs), most patients receive only medication often without adequate psychosocial interventions and supports. This is tragic given that there is good evidence for the effectiveness of some relatively inexpensive family interventions in reducing relapse and hospitalization rates and in promoting social and functional recovery in patients with long-standing as well as first-episode schizophrenia (Pharoah et al., 2010; Pitschel-Walz et al., 2001); similar evidence exists in relation to case management (Dieterich et al., 2017), cognitive behavioural therapy (Bird et al., 2010; Fowler et al., 2009; Turner et al., 2014); social skills training (Almerie et al., 2015; Granholm et al., 2014; Turner et al., 2014); and employment support programmes (Bond, 2004; Bond & Drake, 2014; Killackey et al., 2008; Major et al., 2010; Waghorn et al., 2014). Much of this high-quality evidence for these specific interventions comes from trials conducted in HICs. In HICs, poor outcomes are associated, to some extent, with inadequate models and systems of care (Knapp et al., 2006; Priebe et al., 2005; WHO, 2008) that fail to provide timely access to the treatments and supports necessary to achieve and sustain personal and social recovery.

Only a properly designed system of care can integrate evidence-based treatments and ensure access and fidelity to such treatments and supports for all those in need. A brief historical review of the development of mental health services for psychotic disorders would assist us in understanding the current state of services for these disorders and in planning better services for the future.

In this chapter, we review (a) different models of treatment services, separately, for the later and the earlier phases of psychotic disorders and (b) how treatments are delivered within different systems of care in HICs and LMICs. We examine how the theoretical frameworks and practical implementations of these models are influenced by social, economic, cultural, and historical circumstances. Last, we discuss emerging concepts and innovations including the potential for bidirectional transfers of knowledge between HICs and LMICs.

Historical perspectives

Around the mid-twentieth century the process referred to as deinstitutionalization began in several countries in the Global North with the closure of large mental hospitals, triggered in part by economic and social factors (Pow et al., 2015) and facilitated by the introduction of newly discovered pharmacological treatments (Brill & Patton, 1962; Cancro, 2000; Deniker, 1978; Duval & Goldman, 2000). The former includes massive social changes in the 1950s and 1960s, exposés of the conditions in many long-stay asylums, increased affluence in the West, and, possibly, the experience of large-scale human suffering during the Second World War resulting in improved social consciousness about humane care of the mentally ill. This led to changes in mental healthcare legislation in most of the industrialized world. These legislations made deinstitutionalization a sanctioned reality, although non-institutional care had been initiated a decade or more earlier in India and Nigeria (Agarwal et al., 2004; Lambo, 1956).

A much earlier movement of social and moral awareness in the eighteenth century, led by Chiarugi (George, 1959), Pinel (Charland, 2008), Tuke (Laffey, 2003), Rush and others (Aldarondo, 2007), had raised hopes and standards of care for people with serious mental illness within some institutions. Unfortunately, this progressive trend soon dissipated partly because of the overcrowding of asylums to accommodate the larger numbers of new patients due to population growth and immigration (Hill & Laugharne, 2003; Shorter, 1998; Thompson, 1994). With the exception of a few private hospitals like Chestnut Lodge in the USA (McGlashan & Carpenter, 2007) and Ticehurst in England (Turner, 1992), care was primarily custodial, along with the introduction of some activities like gardening, farming, and laundry. The latter were designed to keep patients occupied and not necessarily to teach them skills for independent living.

Deinstitutionalization created a need to define and design a new system of care. A major initial task was to house people who had for years lived in institutional settings, with little independence in decision-making or ownership of their own care. In hospital environments, fixed daily regimens defined people's lives and were governed by rules set by the institutions and their agents (staff). Leaving the institution, therefore, became a major event in the lives of most institutionalized patients, who had little or no skills for independent living.

New patients seeking treatment and entering the system began to experience care mostly in the form of 'episodes' with brief hospital admissions, when either acutely ill or during crises such as those related to housing, aggression, or suicidal behaviour. Each such episode began to be treated as a distinct entity, often by clinicians and other staff who had little in the way of a long-term relationship with patients. Early community care consisted of such episodes of treatment offered increasingly in a hospital unit, situated in a general hospital, often followed by care focused mainly on medication maintenance that was offered in outpatient settings. The movement of care to general hospitals was driven by the desire to enhance the acceptance of mental illnesses as medical problems that ought to be treated in the same settings as general medical and surgical problems. However, in many jurisdictions (e.g. in parts of Canada) until recently, psychiatric and general hospitals continued to operate separately and concurrently, often with both overlapping as well as distinct roles and catering to different patient populations. In such circumstances psychiatric hospitals have often provided longer-term care or managed 'difficult-to-treat' patients such as those at risk of harming themselves or others. There is evidence that patients of lower socioeconomic status, with diagnoses of schizophrenia or who are admitted involuntarily tend to be admitted to mental hospitals more often when general and psychiatric hospitals coexist (Malla & Norman, 1983). General hospitals, on the other hand, tended to cater to larger proportions of patients with diagnoses of depression, anxiety, and personality disorders.

Beginnings of community care systems

In the 1970s, there was considerable effort in the UK to maintain contact with patients following their discharge from hospitals through home visits to group homes, created as part of the new system, or to individuals' private dwellings.

Such contacts often occurred for the provision of long-acting injectable medications by community nurses and/or visits by social workers addressing patients' financial, housing, and social welfare concerns. In most other jurisdictions, however, patients were expected to keep their own appointments at clinics attached to hospitals (Wasylenki et al., 1985). Given their diminished daily life management skills following multiple episodes of illness and hospitalizations, their impoverished lifestyles, and their lack of strong relationships with care providers (clinicians and family), many patients never went to their follow-up appointments (Wasylenki et al., 1985). Such interruption in care often led to readmission to hospital, resulting in what is now proverbially called a 'revolving door' phenomenon.

Models of care for patients with longstanding illness in high-income countries

Over several decades, from the beginning of deinstitutionalization in the UK, Europe, and North America, the need for patients with psychotic disorders to be integrated into their communities required a new approach to providing them care. Several models of community care have been used with varying results and mostly concentrating on the hospital treatment of acute episodes, medical follow-ups, and 'rehabilitation' following multiple episodes and cumulative disabilities. While different models have been effective in experimental conditions (Best & Bowie, 2017; Dieterich et al., 2017; Pharoah et al., 2010; Wykes, 2008), only a few have been successfully integrated within different systems of care (Eassom et al., 2014; Ince et al., 2016). The consistently low allocation of budgets to mental health across countries, but particularly in LMICs (WHO, 2018), has played a significant role in this regard. Variations in systems of care and in social and health policies are also likely to have facilitated or hindered large-scale implementation of these models in different ways. For example, psychotherapeutic, community integration, and employment interventions are often not included in packages of care covered by public healthcare systems (Fleischhacker et al., 2014).

In general, most patients have not benefited from models whose effectiveness is supported by evidence. Further, the overall impact on populations and communities has been limited, resulting in the relatively high prevalence of untreated or poorly treated psychosis, even in HICs (Large et al., 2008; Mossaheb et al., 2013).

A basic community care model required stable housing suited to patients' needs and skills; access to outpatient treatment; and episodic hospitalization, when necessary. Patients also needed to learn skills to survive in the community without full-time institutional support. This gave birth to the science and enterprise of psychiatric rehabilitation. Most programmes were designed for the rehabilitation of individuals who had spent long periods in hospitals and were in need of learning basic living and social skills to engage in society outside institutional settings. Interventions like life and social skills training were developed and delivered to patients, either in inpatient settings to prepare them for life in the community (Corrigan & Liberman, 1989; Spaulding et al., 2003; Sullivan et al., 1991) or in community settings after discharge from hospitals to facilitate their life in the community and prevent future hospital stays (Corrigan & Liberman, 1989). These models of care varied in their approaches and methods of delivery, but essentially focused on correcting deficits in skills (Kern et al., 2009). Substantial evidence was generated to support their effectiveness and such models were scaled up in different jurisdictions, albeit, to a limited degree. An extensive body of literature can be consulted for a thorough and detailed account of different models of psychiatric rehabilitation (Granholm et al., 2014; Krabbendam & Aleman, 2003; Liberman, 1994; Pankowski et al., 2016; Tungpunkom et al., 2012).

Many models of care and rehabilitation revolved around case management. The roles of case managers varied from pure brokerage for obtaining additional services, as required, to the actual delivery of direct clinical and social care (Ivezic et al., 2010) or to a combination of various tasks. The most influential models of case management were those that addressed the needs of the most seriously ill patients. These involved a high intensity of follow-up and a broad spectrum of services provided with a low case manager-to-patient ratio (Goodwin & Lawton-Smith, 2010; Stein & Test, 1980). Assertive community treatment (ACT) emerged as the model of case management with the strongest evidence (Dieterich et al., 2017; Ziguras & Stuart, 2000). ACT involves the provision of intensive case management (ratio of 1:10) within a multidisciplinary treatment team. The goal is to maintain patients with very high needs within the community through a home-based 24-hour service that addresses needs related to living in the community (housing, daily living skills); provides close supervision of and access to adequate medication (including clozapine); and psychiatric care. This is perhaps one of the few innovations in the care of those with longstanding mental illnesses that has been scaled up through incorporation into systems of care across multiple jurisdictions, especially in the USA (White et al., 2015) and Canada. Its uptake may be partly ascribable to the cost-effectiveness of the ACT model of care (Latimer, 2005), despite some evidence to the contrary (Clark et al., 1998; Slade et al., 2013). More recently there has been a decline in interest in ACT, possibly due to the changing needs of patients for whom ACT would have been deemed appropriate or, perhaps, the lack of continued substantiation of the impact and cost-effectiveness of ACT (Karow et al., 2012; Slade et al., 2013).

The impact of ACT in the UK and Europe has been relatively limited, at least in part, due to the better level of community care for patients with serious mental illness available, easier access to state benefits for disability, and universal access to healthcare. Within the UK, a comparison of intensive case management and the standard model of community care showed the intensive care model to have some advantage in terms of increasing social activity and reducing hospitalization but no differential effect on quality of life for patients, which remained relatively low for both models of care (Taylor et al., 1998).

As summarized in the systematic review by Folsom and Jeste (2008) with 33 studies all from HICs, schizophrenia is much more prevalent among homeless persons than in the larger population. With this has come an important recognition of the need for safe, affordable housing (McHugo et al., 2004). Among the better-known and evaluated approaches is Housing First (Tsemberis & Eisenberg, 2000), which prioritizes rapid, low-barrier re-housing for individuals who are homeless and who experience serious mental illnesses (e.g. schizophrenia) and/or other vulnerabilities. In schizophrenia specifically, there is high-quality evidence for its superior effectiveness on substance use outcomes compared with treatment-first approaches (Padgett et al., 2011); on medication adherence outcomes compared with usual care (Rezansoff et al., 2017); and on housing outcomes compared with usual care (Aubry et al., 2016).

Recovery vs. rehabilitation

Recently, there has been a proliferation of definitions, frameworks, and research on recovery. Two forms of recovery are reported (Drake & Whitley, 2014; Slade et al., 2008; Slade & Longden, 2015). Clinical recovery, often termed 'recovery *from* mental illness' (Davidson & Roe, 2007), involves sustained remission of positive and negative symptoms and, sometimes, return to work or school or social functioning, with the focus on the rates and determinants of clinical recovery (Jaaskelainen et al., 2013). Personal recovery, on the other hand, has its roots in consumer perspectives with a focus on subjective perceptions of living a satisfying or fulfilling life, sometimes, despite symptoms or other problems related to the illness. While there are both quantitative and qualitative studies exploring personal definitions and conceptions of recovery (Windell et al., 2012), much of the work on this topic has been autobiographical and qualitative in nature (Leamy et al., 2011; Whitley et al., 2015; Windell et al., 2015), emphasizing recovery as a personal journey, often using the term 'recovery *in* mental illness' (Davidson & Roe, 2007). Dimensions of personal recovery have included autonomy, hope, and agency and, importantly, participation in valued and functional roles such as gainful employment, social support, and community reintegration (Leamy et al., 2011; Windell et al., 2015). Across studies, personal definitions of recovery have tended to emphasize both freedom from illness as well as work and social roles (Windell et al., 2012; Windell et al., 2015). The results of these studies are in keeping with results from large quantitative studies that sustained symptom remission strongly predicts the achievement and maintenance of such roles (Jordan et al., 2014). It can thus be argued that to a large extent, clinical recovery facilitates personal recovery.

Currently, there is a growing consensus that mental health services for psychosis and other serious mental illnesses should be guided by a 'recovery orientation' (Whitley, 2014), the concept being adopted by many services with great alacrity. Simply being self-avowedly recovery-oriented, however, is unlikely to be enough to produce concrete results. In fact, recovery may be best promoted by maximizing the availability and uptake of evidence-based interventions and services that foster hope, are goals-focused, and facilitate engagement with valued activities and relationships (e.g. through supported employment). Much of the conceptualization of and research on personal recovery has occurred in high-income English-speaking countries (Slade et al., 2012). There is indeed a need to advance understanding of whether recovery is a valid concept and how it is defined in other geo-cultural contexts.

Another recent development in the recovery field has been a shift from deficit-focused service delivery models to a 'strengths-based' approach (Rapp & Goscha, 2011). The practice of this model involves the use of a strengths assessment and a personal recovery plan generated jointly by the service user and the service provider; utilization of naturally occurring and existing community (non-mental health) resources including supported housing, employment, education, and recreation; and shifting the venue of intervention by service providers to the community and away from the clinic office. While initial studies reported promising results, a recent systematic and meta-analysis has failed to show any advantages over other prevailing service delivery models (Ibrahim et al., 2014).

Interventions with impact on outcome and their inclusion in systems of care

Despite the efficacy of antipsychotic medications in treating positive psychotic symptoms for many (although not all) (Leucht et al., 2013), their effectiveness in achieving broader outcomes, including the prevention of relapses and rehospitalizations, social and housing stability, or improving community tenure has been limited (Hogarty & Ulrich, 1998). In some cases, the use of medications may have even limited the achievement of these important goals. Over the past few decades, innovations in individual interventions with moderate to strong effects on outcomes for patients with psychotic disorders have been developed.

Evidence has been particularly strong for the benefits of family interventions with more than 50 randomized clinical trials showing a strong impact on the reduction of relapse and rehospitalization rates when used in addition to antipsychotic medication (Pharoah et al., 2010). Different types of family interventions have, in general, incorporated a strong involvement of the family in the care of the individual, education of the family on various aspects of the illness, and teaching skills to families for dealing with various situations related to an individual's illness. Some have used a highly structured educational approach equipping families with knowledge about the illness combined with strong support to individual families in using this knowledge (Anderson et al., 1980). Others have emphasized communication skills (Asarnow et al., 1988; Goldstein, 1985) and behavioural interventions (Falloon et al., 1987). A particularly effective approach has involved groups of families and patients learning problem-solving strategies from each other (McFarlane et al., 1995). Despite such evidence, few patients receive the benefits of relatively simple forms of family interventions (Dixon et al., 2001; Lucksted et al., 2012). The reasons for this failure to incorporate family interventions as part of service delivery may include the lack of organizational support for training staff to offer family interventions; the historical institutional and professional suspicion of 'dysfunctional' families being the cause of schizophrenia; and discomfort among staff in institutional settings in dealing with families.

Social skills training has also been shown to improve outcomes in schizophrenia when delivered according to a well-defined and structured protocol (Almerie et al., 2015; Granholm et al., 2014; Guhne et al., 2012; Kurtz et al., 2015). It may be especially beneficial in preventing relapses when combined with family intervention (Hogarty et al., 1986). Yet, few patients are offered this effective skill to equip them to better manage their social and personal lives and prevent relapses.

More recently, a high level of evidence has accumulated for employment support programmes that place and support individuals with serious mental illness in competitive, open-market employment. Supported employment programmes have shown benefits in the form of higher rates of employment, more days worked and higher wages (Marshall et al., 2014). In some jurisdictions, supported employment has been incorporated into mental health policy with dedicated resources. However, for a majority of patients with psychotic disorders, this effective intervention remains out of reach and even unknown. For example, only 3% of patients have access to it (Bond & Drake, 2014) in the USA. Further, other forms of psychological interventions such as cognitive behavioural therapy (CBT for people with psychosis or CBTp) with moderate effect sizes compared to regular care (Garety, 2003; Hazell et al., 2016; Hofmann et al., 2012; Hutton & Taylor, 2014; Lecomte & Leclerc, 2013; Michail et al., 2017; Mueser & Noordsy, 2005; Turkington et al., 2017), and cognitive remediation (Best & Bowie, 2017; Revell et al., 2015; Wykes, 2008; Wykes, 2010), have established proven efficacy in psychotic disorders but are still not available to most patients. Psychological treatments are generally best integrated with or seen as part of a combination of treatments, along with other psychosocial interventions. More recently, innovations to increase access to psychological interventions are being piloted and show promise. These include low-intensity or brief CBT with comparable effect sizes to the more widely tested CBTp (Hazell et al., 2016); e-approaches to delivering therapy with evidence for feasibility and preliminary efficacy (Gaebel et al., 2016; Gottlieb et al., 2013); and self-help or self-guided psychological therapy approaches with preliminary evidence for acceptability and efficacy (Naeem et al., 2016; Scott et al., 2015). It is beyond the scope of this chapter to review psychological interventions in detail, and the reader is referred to the extensive literature available, especially on CBT (Dark et al., 2015; Haddock et al., 2014; Haglund et al., 2014; Ince et al., 2016; Ostergaard et al., 2014; Perry et al., 2015).

Models of care for individuals with long-standing illness in low- and middle-income countries

The biggest challenge in LMIC is the high prevalence of untreated serious mental illnesses like schizophrenia and other psychotic disorders. It is estimated that close to 20 million individuals suffer from schizophrenia in the world (James et al., 2018; Patel et al., 2007), with a majority of these naturally living in LMICs. Further, there has been a 19% increase in the prevalence of schizophrenia across the globe between 2005 and 2015 (GBD, 2016; Vos et al., 2016). Various factors could be contributing to this, including growth in population and ageing, variations in methodology across studies, and an increase in risk factors (Charlson et al., 2018; Simeone et al., 2015). Appallingly, the median global treatment gap is 69% (calculated as the proportion of people with a diagnosable disorder of schizophrenia who received mental healthcare in the past year) and as expected, the gap is higher in low-income countries (89%) compared with lower-middle-income (69%) and upper-middle-income countries (63%) (Lora et al., 2012).

Such a high level of untreated prevalence is the result, first and foremost, of poor or total lack of access to even minimal treatment (Institute of Medicine, 2001; de Jesus et al., 2009; Lora et al., 2012). In addition, a relatively large number of new cases emerge each year (incident cases) because in low- and middle-income countries, close to 50% of the population is under 25 years old and the onset of most mental disorders, including psychotic disorders, occurs mostly in the late teens and early twenties. Moreover, a considerable proportion of the population in LMIC (49%) lives in rural areas where access to effective resources is often poor to non-existent and where, in some countries (e.g. India), there are systems of unlicensed rural medical practitioners with little or no training and oversight who prescribe psychotropic medication (Ecks, 2013; Ecks, 2016; Ecks & Basu, 2014; Gautham et al., 2011; Nahar et al., 2017).

Applying different models of care to deliver treatment

The influence of cultural factors on the conceptualization, attribution, and treatment of mental disorders can pose additional challenges. For instance, magico-religious explanations of mental illness may prolong treatment delays and act as barriers to accessing and receiving appropriate care (Burns et al., 2011).

A workable system of care in LMIC may need to take into account the evidence for the effectiveness of certain treatments (e.g. medication; psychological interventions such as CBT). Although evidence for these treatments comes mostly from the West, there is evidence for models of psychosocial rehabilitation in schizophrenia in rural areas in India (Chatterjee et al., 2003; Chatterjee et al., 2009) as well as some overall support for effectiveness for psychosocial interventions (De Silva et al., 2013). While the evidence for the latter is based on studies of low quality, higher quality studies will need to provide further support and the interventions may need to be adapted to fit the contextual framework of culture, geography, and economy in LMIC. At the same time, there may be inherent strengths within traditional systems of care that are congruent with the prevailing local models of attribution of mental disorders. The latter can be leveraged to create a workable and cost-efficient system of care (Gureje et al., 2015b).

In LMIC, there are several large psychiatric institutions that were created in the mould of their counterparts in Europe and the UK during colonial occupation. However, they have been woefully inadequate in providing care to the vast majority of people with psychotic disorders. The little care they provided tended to be of low quality in crowded settings and, often, involved inhumane conditions (Murthy, 2017). It has become increasingly clear that LMIC will need to develop systems of care that are responsive to the real needs of people living in rural and crowded urban settings with very limited resources. The recent efforts of the World Health Organization under mhGap initiatives are attempting to address these serious deficiencies (WHO, 2015).

In most LMIC, the state provides very limited support and funding for the care of the mentally ill. There are also issues related to human rights abuses, particularly of the untreated seriously mentally ill (Poreddi et al., 2013). There is an acknowledged dearth of trained professionals (Bruckner et al., 2011) and the perceived effectiveness of antipsychotic medications alone is limited (Read, 2012). In this context, the traditional healers filling in such gaps in service must be acknowledged. While there is no strong evidence of their effectiveness in relation to treatment of schizophrenia, assessing their effectiveness poses its own challenges (Nortje et al., 2016). Thus, both out of necessity and in the interest of cultural congruity, mental health services in LMIC are being developed mostly around community rather than institutional care.

The important role of family and kinships in LMIC, the potential for mobilizing communities, and the use of relatively basic information technologies have recently spurred great innovation in providing care for patients with psychotic disorders. We will briefly review several programmes that, if scaled up, could go a long way to improving access to at least minimal but effective care for people with psychotic disorders. The examples described next include deployments of packages of care known to be effective in the West, the use of information technology to support service delivery, and the testing of custom-built models of care.

Community-based care programmes

Several demonstrations of the use of community-based programmes for the care of the seriously mentally ill have been reported. BasicNeeds, a non-governmental organization (NGO), introduced Mental Health and Development, a public-private partnered, community-based intervention which combines outpatient medical care with social support and economic opportunities through self-help groups in at least 11 LMICs. A small study in Kenya (de Menil et al., 2015) showed the successful implementation of this programme for 117 consecutively enrolled patients with schizophrenia and bipolar disorder with a follow-up of 10–20 months. The programme was cost-effective with the costs per healthy day gained being less than the agricultural minimum wage. Similarly, in Somalia (Odenwald et al., 2012), a small study tested the possibilities of home-based treatment for acute psychosis and a community-based relapse prevention intervention after the acute episode or for more long-term cases. The treatment package comprised psychoeducation, low-dose medication, home visits, and counselling. Most patients regularly used khat. The treatment package that was implemented produced significant improvement in long-term patients whose symptoms had remitted, but symptoms in patients treated initially for acute episodes tended to worsen over time. Nonetheless, most patients showed some improvement in functioning and communication and khat use was reduced in outpatients. The programme was regarded as feasible and practical for chronic remitted patients, although further evaluation of the model is needed as it is scaled up across diverse settings.

Integrating mental healthcare into primary and other forms of care

Several studies have shown the feasibility of integrating the provision of mental healthcare for psychotic disorders into primary care. In Nigeria, the mhGAP Intervention Guide (mhGAP-IG) was used to integrate mental health services into primary care and provide a cascade of training programmes for frontline mental health workers to serve a population of close to one million (Gureje et al., 2015a). A significant increase in the knowledge and capacity of frontline workers to find cases of and treat serious mental disorders such as major depression, psychosis, and substance abuse was reported. The impact on patient outcomes was not reported, although there was an increase in the number of cases identified. This was mainly a test of the feasibility of applying this model in a large population base and not an evaluation of outcomes.

The Programme for Improving Mental health (PRIME) was a multicounty project for the provision of affordable mental healthcare at the district level, using the mhGAP model. The purpose of the programme was to implement and scale up a package of care whose effectiveness was supported by established evidence (Lund et al., 2012). It demonstrated improvements in patient outcomes for depression, alcohol use disorders, and psychosis across diverse settings, although uptake of services was limited (de Menil et al., 2015; Gureje et al., 2015; Lund, 2018; Lund et al., 2016; Odenwald et al., 2012). The variety of strategies and processes involved in their implementation across five countries (Ethiopia, South Africa, Uganda, India, and Nepal) can be used to scale up similar programmes in other countries where resources are scarce (Lund, 2018; Lund et al., 2016).

Other studies have examined traditional methods of care for psychosis. In a Sudan study (Sorketti et al., 2013), patients with psychosis treated by traditional healers in their centres showed improvement in the level of symptoms at discharge. It is unclear if they were receiving any medications that could be considered antipsychotic as the patients' regular medications were stopped. The use of traditional healing centres needs further study, as the ingredients of traditional medicines are not fully known. Further, traditional healing practices unfortunately often involve practices such as chaining (Ofori-Atta et al., 2018), and little conclusive evidence exists for their effectiveness in treating severe mental disorders (Nortje et al., 2016).

Other community care-based programmes

In 2003, Chatterjee et al. reported significantly higher retention and disability reduction in persons with long-standing schizophrenia receiving community-based rehabilitation compared with outpatient care (OPC) in a resource-poor setting in India (Chatterjee et al., 2003). This was particularly true for persons who were fully compliant. The same research team later successfully scaled up this community rehabilitation programme with continued positive impacts in terms of service retention and disability reductions (Chatterjee et al., 2009). These promising findings fuelled a multicentre, parallel-group, randomized controlled trial (Chatterjee et al., 2014) of 'Community care for people with schizophrenia in India' (COPSI), wherein a collaborative community-based intervention was compared with standard facility-based care to test whether care could be successfully provided by community health workers under the supervision of specialists. Although results showed that community-based care produced a greater reduction in symptoms than facility-based care, there was no difference between these two models of delivery in terms of the proportion of patients who showed a magnitude of >20% reduction in symptoms. The experimental treatment service was, therefore, regarded as modestly more effective than the traditional facility-based model. Several other community-based rehabilitation and care models have been successfully applied in different rural settings in India (Keshavan et al., 2010; Rangaswamy et al., 2012b).

Models based on using non-professional mental health workers

Given the lack of professional resources within the mental health field in LMICs, especially specialists, the use of other professionals from other non-specialist health sectors (NSHWs) or other professionals with health roles (OPHRs) have been described as possibilities for filling service gaps. In addition, there have also been attempts at using lay health workers (LHWs) trained to provide mental healthcare at the community level to large sections of populations who would otherwise not have any access to mental healthcare. A review conducted recently (van Ginneken et al., 2013) identified 38 studies of task-sharing in mental health from 7 low-income and 15 middle-income countries. Of these, 22 used LHWs. Most of the studies did not address psychotic disorders, dealing primarily with depression and post-traumatic stress disorder. The use of non-specialist health sector workers has had impacts on treating depression, anxiety, and post-traumatic stress disorders, even in remote conflict-ridden areas in a LMIC environment (Malla et al 2019a, 2019b). There have been few reports of the impact of using LHWs or other professionals (teachers, primary care nurses, etc.) in the treatment of psychotic disorders (Balaji et al., 2012b).

Use of technology

Because specialist psychiatric resources are mostly situated in urban settings, 'tele-psychiatry' has been the most commonly used form of technology-enabled service delivery for patients with psychotic or other mental disorders in LMI countries. A review of the utilization and effectiveness of tele-psychiatry has shown that patients and providers are often satisfied with the service, with providers being more concerned than patients about the impact of such technology on the rapport between the patient and the treating clinician (Hubley et al., 2016). It is unclear how many of the studies reviewed were conducted in LMIC.

Tele-psychiatry is also comparable to face-to-face therapeutic interaction in terms of the reliability of clinical assessments and treatment outcomes. Studies using relatively sophisticated designs show that tele-psychiatry performs as well as, or better than, face-to-face interaction and may be more cost-effective (Hubley et al., 2016; Malhotra et al., 2015). The feasibility of using tele-psychiatry to make diagnoses and prescribe treatments in psychotic disorders has been demonstrated in at least a few studies in India (Malhotra et al., 2015; Thara et al., 2008; Thara, 2012). While concerns regarding confidentiality and legal repercussions may hinder its use in the HIC, these concerns appear to be expressed less often in LMIC.

Mental health services and programmes for the early phase of psychotic disorders

A recent promising development in service delivery has been the development, research, and scaling-up of early intervention services (EIS) following the onset of a psychotic disorder and, in some cases, in the state immediately prior to the onset of a full syndrome of psychosis. EIS essentially comprise of two components: one a comprehensive package of evidence-informed interventions adapted to a younger age and early stage of illness; and the other attempts at reducing delay in treatment. The intervention package comprises low-dose antipsychotic medication; family intervention; access to CBT, when indicated; and modified assertive case management (Malla et al., 2003; McGorry et al., 1996; Singh & Fisher, 2005). The latter is the primary mode of delivery of care with a recommended case manager–patient ratio of 1:20–22. Services such as skills training and supported employment and education interventions are additions recommended to be included in the package. Programmes are designed to be community-focused, recovery-oriented, and generally provide services for two to three years.

For the second component of EIS, attempts at reducing delay in treatment usually consist of making the service easily accessible through a combination of opening access without referrals from other layers of the system and providing rapid access to help-seeking individuals and their families. In addition, most programmes engage in some form of community education directed mostly at other parts of the mental health or general healthcare system and, in some cases, educational institutions. While there is evidence to support the impact of intervention to reduce duration of untreated psychosis (DUP) (Melle et al., 2004), such interventions have not been widely applied to EIS (Malla & McGorry, 2019).

While several national guidelines (Galletly et al., 2016; National Collaborating Centre for Mental Health, 2014) have been developed to identify the core features of an EIS, there are considerable variations across EIS, within and between different countries. Most experts in EIS delivery and research agree that case management, family intervention, CBT, low-dose medication, and a general orientation towards functional recovery are key ingredients of an EIS. It is also generally accepted that these services are best delivered by a team with varied expertise from different disciplines including a psychiatrist dedicated exclusively for the service. EIS are also expected to have a relatively open and easy entry system and to be well connected to resources and potential referral sources in the community. Similarities and differences between EIS are explored in a few survey-type studies. For example, a recent Canadian study (Nolin et al., 2016) showed that most services provide treatment and follow-up for two or three years, although some extended it to five years or even longer and few EI services have procedures in place for transferring patients to other types and levels of services. It is expected that in jurisdictions which are part of a national, regional, or provincial mental health policy, EIS are likely to have better-defined standards of care and would, therefore, exhibit greater similarity across services. Some attempts have been made to develop measures of fidelity to evaluate EIS (Addington et al., 2016).

The current development of EIS was based primarily on two related concepts. The first was the strong association between the duration of untreated psychosis (DUP) with poor clinical, social, and occupational outcomes (Marshall et al., 2005; Norman & Malla, 2001; Penttila et al., 2014; Perkins, 2006; Wyatt, 1991), an association that has been replicated in numerous studies and that is relatively independent of other factors, such as premorbid adjustment. The second is the hypothesis that there is a critical period of two to a maximum of five years following onset of psychosis, during which treatment has a greater positive impact (Birchwood et al., 1998). This is supported by evidence that long-term trajectories of outcome are established during this 'critical period' (Harrison et al., 2001; Harrison et al., 2009; Robinson et al., 1999).

By the end of the twentieth century, EIS development had become a reality in many publicly funded mental healthcare systems confined mostly to several HICs (e.g. Australia, the UK, Canada, Denmark, Norway, Hong Kong, and New Zealand).

Are these early intervention services effective?

Over the last two decades, the effectiveness of EIS of two years duration for treatment of first-episode psychosis (FEP) has been established through a number of controlled and uncontrolled studies, summarized in recent meta-analytic reviews (Correll et al., 2018; Harvey et al., 2007). Benefits are reported on rates of remission, relapse, substance abuse, functioning, housing, and residual positive and negative symptoms compared with regular care (Harvey et al., 2007; Marshall & Rathbone, 2011; Srihari et al., 2015). Evaluation of effectiveness of EIS has, however, been limited largely to the multimodal treatment component.

Although most of the earlier studies were conducted in countries with a publicly funded healthcare system, more recently this evidence base has been further supported by results from a pragmatic cluster randomized trial conducted in the USA (Kane et al., 2016), with a very different system of care. Recovery After an Initial Schizophrenia Episode Treatment Programme (RAISE-TP) used a model of care (NAVIGATE) comprising a combination of pharmacotherapy with a package of psychosocial interventions, very similar to EI models that had been operational in many other jurisdictions for the previous two decades. This programme did not include intensive case management or any active attempts at reducing DUP and was embedded within regular mental health services by increasing capacity and skills. Another USA study, involving randomization of patients and, unlike RAISE, not treatment clinics and including case management, also provided evidence to support the enhanced level of care for FEP in EIS (Srihari et al., 2015).

Other countries

Several other countries have attempted to set up EIS, mostly following international guidelines for EIS, including case management and other psychosocial interventions such as family intervention. These include Hong Kong (Chen et al., 2008; Chen et al., 2015; Tang et al., 2010; Wong et al., 2012) and Singapore (Verma et al., 2012). Both programmes have provided data suggesting improved patient outcomes, especially the programme in Hong Kong (Chan et al., 2015; Chang et al., 2017). Interestingly, the latter has succeeded in achieving results comparable to EIS elsewhere with a significantly higher case manager-to-patient ratio (1:80–100).

Apart from a few efforts on the part of service providers in LMIC to introduce EI, this remains confined to HIC because EI initially requires a high-intensity investment of resources. Further, the types of EI models that would be suitable in LMIC remain unexplored.

Given the extreme penury of mental health specialists, service development in LMIC generally has had the challenge of dealing with the very high prevalence of untreated psychotic disorders. However, several service delivery innovations with a community orientation, including the use of alternatives to professionals and of technology in recent years, may offer a unique opportunity for early intervention in LMIC at a relatively low cost.

Further, several studies have examined and confirmed the influence of delay in treatment in the LMIC context while others have examined variations in pathways to care. In general, a substantial proportion of patients with psychotic disorders go untreated for long periods of time resulting in relatively long DUP (e.g. mean 90 weeks), which, in turn, impacts clinical and functional outcome (Thirthalli et al., 2011). DUP and pathways to care are also likely influenced by prevailing models of attribution of symptoms and behaviours associated with psychosis. In the research programme, INTREPID (International Research Programme on Psychoses in Diverse Settings), the relative role and importance of traditional and folk providers as well as organized health services are being explored in identifying cases of psychosis (Morgan et al., 2015).

A few small-scale and pilot studies, often conducted in collaboration with established EIS programmes in the West, have reported encouraging results for both the feasibility of implementing EIS as well as subsequent FEP outcomes. The approach has often been a blend of EIS models in the West (e.g. concept of case management) and culturally compatible practices such as greater involvement of families and the latter's active role in delivering care (Balaji et al., 2012a; Keshavan et al., 2010; Rangaswamy et al., 2012a; Rangaswamy et al., 2012b). Family as a significant resource, given the high level of commitment and involvement, may be particularly important in the LMIC context for the development of EI services. Some reports have suggested that the use of family members as 'case managers' may not only be feasible but, at the very least, equally effective in treating psychotic disorders as is the use of professional case managers (Malakouti et al., 2009).

Based on an earlier pilot study (Iyer et al., 2010), a large collaborative mixed methods study comparing outcomes and underlying mechanisms to explain differences in outcomes in FEP patients between LMIC (SCARF, Chennai, India) and HIC (PEPP-Montréal, Canada) contexts has recently been completed. One of the principal objectives of this study was to conduct an in-depth examination of what families do and how they influence outcome in the two contexts. Preliminary results suggest significant differences, and some similarities, in the nature and extent of family involvement and provide insights into how culture and other environmental factors shape such involvement. These preliminary results also suggest that the development of EI services in the LMIC contexts must involve families as a resource, not only in shaping treatment but also in altering pathways to care. Some of the results from this study are now available in a few published articles (Malla et al., 2020; Iyer et al., 2021).

How long should early intervention services be continued?

Although the benefits of EIS at the end of two years of treatment and follow-up are well-established, some doubts have been raised about such benefits being sustained beyond the cessation of EIS. For example, at five-year follow-up to the OPUS-I study few differences remained in most outcome domains, including symptoms, between those who had received EIS initially for the first two years and those who had initially been randomized to regular care, once both groups had received three years of additional regular care (Bertelsen et al., 2008). In response to this, in an uncontrolled study in Canada better outcomes were observed at five years compared with the OPUS findings, when patients continued with the same psychiatrist and case management was made available only in crisis situations without other components of the EIS (Norman et al., 2011). Since then several randomized controlled trials (RCTs) have been conducted to compare the extension of EIS to three years in the Hong Kong EIS (Chang et al., 2015) or five years in OPUS-II in Denmark (Albert et al., 2017) and in Canada (Lutgens et al., 2015; Malla et al., 2017) with regular care following two years of EIS. The Hong Kong study showed improved clinical outcomes for the extended EIS patients compared with those in regular care on several clinical (e.g. negative symptoms) and social domains (Chang et al., 2015). The Canadian study also showed better outcomes in clinical domains (length of remission of positive and negative symptoms) in EIS patients compared with those in regular care (Malla et al., 2017). On the other hand, the OPUS study failed to show any difference on their primary outcome of negative symptoms (Albert et al., 2017).

Reducing DUP in EIS

A scientific basis for early intervention in psychotic disorders is the well-established relationship between DUP and outcome, with longer DUP being associated with poor outcomes. EIS that have actively sought to reduce DUP have used methods that are highly complementary. Reducing DUP requires interventions directed at the determinants of both the help-seeking and systemic phases of DUP (Bechard-Evans et al., 2007; Norman et al., 2004). Efforts to reduce help-seeking delay are usually directed at the entire community population with special emphasis on educational institutions and community non-health settings such as churches and other religious groups. Efforts to reduce systemic delay emphasize working closely with all potential sources of referral from health, social, educational, and other community sectors. The target for such system-focused interventions is to simplify pathways to care and provide rapid access to EIS for young people and their families without having to go through layers of primary and secondary care (for details, see Birchwood et al., 2013; Malla et al., 2005; Malla et al., 2010; Melle et al., 2004; Scholten et al., 2003).

Most EIS have generally focused on the content and comprehensiveness of treatment once patients make it to the service and not necessarily on addressing treatment delays through any intervention at the system level, with some exceptions (Malla et al., 2005; Malla et al., 2008; Malla et al., 2010; Malla et al., 2014; McGorry et al., 1996; Melle et al., 2004). For example, despite the widespread scaling up of EIS in England and Wales, a substantial proportion of patients have a DUP of greater than six months (Birchwood et al., 2013), because EIS have depended on the prevailing community mental health system for referrals. The division between child-adolescent and adult mental health services adds further complexity to delay in treatment (Singh et al., 2008). Consequently, many patients enter EIS with relatively long delays as observed in the RAISE study (median DUP of 74 weeks) (Kane et al., 2016) and the OPUS study (52 weeks) (Austin et al., 2015). Programmes that have made systematic efforts to reduce DUP have reported much shorter median DUPs (median 14 weeks at PEPP-Montréal; Iyer et al., 2015; and 4 weeks in the TIPS project in Norway; Melle et al., 2004).

Costs of early intervention

The value of EIS has been debated on the basis, among others, of the high upfront staffing costs required to provide high-intensity services (Castle & Singh, 2015; Pelosi & Birchwood, 2003; Malla & Pelosi, 2010). Mihalopoulos et al. (2012) argued that existing evidence, while not conclusive, does support EIS cost-effectiveness. This is based on the results of several studies conducted in different treatment environments and using varying methodologies (Goldberg et al., 2006; Hastrup et al., 2013; McCrone et al., 1998; McCrone et al., 2010; Mihalopoulos et al., 2009; Park et al., 2016). Most of these studies show considerable savings from improved employment and educational outcomes, homicides and suicides averted, and savings from reduced rates of hospitalizations. A British study reported a per-patient saving of £14,000 over a three-year period, using decision modelling to map care pathways for EIS and regular care (McCrone et al., 2009). Evidence of cost-effectiveness has been extended to longer duration of EIS, although such benefits seem to accrue for patients with a short DUP (Groff et al., 2022).

Scaling up early intervention services and challenges

Given the body of accumulated evidence on the effectiveness of EIS, several jurisdictions have scaled up EIS nationally (e.g. UK, Denmark, Singapore) or regionally (Ontario, British Columbia, Nova Scotia, Québec, and Yukon in Canada; a number of states in Australia). Most countries, even in the high-income context, have not incorporated EIS for psychotic disorders into their healthcare systems. There are significant challenges associated with the large-scale provision of EIS in many countries that are characterized by significant variations in geography and population density (rural and remote areas with low population numbers). Further, several groups of people, such as Indigenous populations in Canada, New Zealand, Australia, and the USA, have not benefited from EI services. In fact, their access to services may be no better, or even worse, than those living in LMICs. Models of EIS that would address such challenges have not been adequately tested. It also remains to be determined how these services are best structured or funded in different environments and how fidelity to EIS delivery can be maintained while adapting them to local contexts.

Emerging issues, challenges, and opportunities

Use of technology

The most commonly used technology is tele-psychiatry, both in the context of HIC and LMIC. Technology-delivered and technology-enhanced treatments are likely to be cost-effective. In addition, these may be more flexible and available to individuals in their own homes and, for remote areas, in their own communities. These are still being developed and evaluated (e.g. Horyzon RCT of a moderated online psychosocial therapy platform (Alvarez-Jimenez et al., 2013); studies using CBT being delivered via the internet (De Bruin et al., 2016)). The Health Technology Program (HTP) has recently been developed to provide in-person relapse prevention planning that directs the use of tailored, technology-based treatment based on CBT for psychosis, family psycho-education for schizophrenia, and prescriber decision support through an online-based programme that solicits information from patients (Brunette et al., 2016). Smartphones and computers are being used to deliver technology-based treatments. Another study found a high level of acceptance, feasibility, and satisfaction with HTP (Baumel et al., 2016). If replicated and then scaled up, this could go a long way to supplement the current poorly delivered non-pharmacological and other in-person interventions while also serving remote communities in HICs and large sections of populations in LMICs.

Learning from innovations in low resource contexts: the case of 'reverse engineering'

Several studies have provided new knowledge that can now be applied to many contexts in relatively higher resource environments, especially to vulnerable populations, those living in remote areas and, in particular, Indigenous peoples. The application of community care models in LMIC contexts has required utilization of non-professional community resources, and significant cultural adaptation taking into consideration models of attribution for mental disorders and incorporating traditional healing practices into models of care. Such approaches may be equally relevant for Indigenous populations in HIC settler colonial countries such as Australia and Canada with substantial Indigenous populations. Most Indigenous peoples have well-established traditional healing practices and land-based therapies that can be combined with adapted versions of interventions developed elsewhere. The remote nature of Indigenous communities also make them ideal for well-supported technology-enhanced services as long as they are adapted to their respective cultures.

Models of early intervention services in different contexts

While the dominant model thus far has been an independent specialized service, such a model is unlikely to serve all contexts, even within HI countries. Few alternate models have been described and fewer still tested. A systematic review revealed a paucity of such evaluations (Behan et al., 2017), although the RAISE study alluded to above could be considered one such model. Incorporating EIS within primary care or delivering it through primary or other forms of care with specialist support from other independent EIS may also need to be tested. An additional issue in the context of EIS is the potential treatment of individuals identified as being at clinical high risk (CHR) for psychosis for indicated pre-vention (Stain et al., 2019). While this is a logical step for early intervention, the vast majority of patients at CHR do not develop psychosis, and hence any interventions that are effective will need to have a significant advantage over no treatment and be risk neutral. Several pharmacological and psychological treat-ments have been shown to be equally effective in reducing the risk of conver-sion to psychosis (McGorry et al., 2013) and, at present, there is no agreement on any guidelines for treatment of CHR states. It is also important to establish if the CHR state is a common stage, as appears to be the case, that most individ-uals who develop a psychotic disorder go through (Shah et al., 2017).

Physical healthcare for people with psychotic disorders

It is beyond the scope of this chapter to address this extremely important issue, as it is now well-recognized that patients with psychotic disorders are among the most disadvantaged populations in terms of their physical health status (Casey et al., 2011; von Hausswolff-Juhlin et al., 2009). They have experi-enced no benefit to their physical health status while there have been very large improvements in the general health of the population in all contexts (Muir-Cochrane, 2006). All service delivery models for psychotic disorders must in-corporate attention to both prevention and treatment of medical problems such as infections, carcinomas, cardiovascular and respiratory diseases, diabetes, and other forms of metabolic disorders (Britvic et al., 2013; Galletly et al., 2012; Graham et al., 2014; Partti et al., 2015).

Stigma and the role of society and state

Social and service-based stigma are well recognized to be major barriers to seeking treatment as well as to recovery from psychotic disorders (Wood et al., 2017). There is also significant evidence for self-stigma (Vrbova et al., 2016; Watson et al., 2007) and anticipated discrimination (Lasalvia et al., 2013; Thornicroft et al., 2009). INDIGO (International Study of Discrimination and Stigma Outcomes), the largest cross-national study on stigma (732 participants with schizophrenia from 27 countries and 1,082 participants with depression from 35 countries) (Lasalvia et al., 2013; Thornicroft et al., 2009) has reported high rates of experienced discrimination across countries (>75%), with higher rates experienced by those with schizophrenia compared with depression.

While its importance is unquestionable, it is not within the scope of this re-port to pay adequate attention to this topic except to state that methods to re-duce stigma are likely very complex and their effectiveness difficult to judge (Wood et al., 2016). Although there has been a positive shift in people's attitudes towards mental illness in general, and depression in particular, such change has not been observed in relation to psychotic disorders. While large-scale campaigns are appealing to the public and well-meaning promoters, the evidence for their effectiveness is equivocal and generally they have little effect on stigma associated with psychotic disorders (Angermeyer et al., 2013; Evans-Lacko et al., 2014; Makowski et al., 2016; Thornicroft et al., 2016). Providing effective and timely treatment within a culture of care that is not stigmatizing and that promotes recovery may be the most effective approach to improving the status of persons with psychotic disorders and reducing stigma and discrimination.

Conclusion

The social, economic, and personal impacts of psychotic disorders can be reduced significantly through the provision of a myriad of evidence-based interventions and facilitation of recovery in ways that take into consideration the social, cultural, and economic context and use models of care suitable for the particular context. It will be essential to match that with a large injection of a humane approach; adequate legislation to protect individual human rights, including the right to receive adequate and timely treatment; integration of patient- and family-centred approaches; and adequate financial and intellectual resources.

Acknowledgement

The authors acknowledge the assistance of Bilal Issaoui-Mansouri in the preparation of this chapter, including multiple and extensive literature searches.

References

Addington, D. E., et al. (2016). Development and testing of the first-episode psychosis services fidelity scale. *Psychiatr Serv*, *67*(9), 1023–1025.

Agarwal, S. P., Goel, D. S., Services, I. D. G. o. H. (2004). *Mental health: an Indian perspective, 1946–2003*. New Delhi: Directorate General of Health Services, Ministry of Health & Family Welfare.

Albert, N., et al. (2017). Five years of specialised early intervention versus two years of specialised early intervention followed by three years of standard treatment for patients with a first episode psychosis: randomised, superiority, parallel group trial in Denmark (OPUS-II). *BMJ*, *356*, i6681.

Aldarondo, E. (2007). *Advancing social justice through clinical practice*. New Jersey, US: Lawrence Erlbaum.

Almerie, M. Q., et al. (2015). Social skills programmes for schizophrenia. *Cochrane Database Syst Rev*, (6), CD009006.

Alvarez-Jimenez, M., et al. (2013). On the HORYZON: moderated online social therapy for long-term recovery in first episode psychosis. *Schizophr Res*, *143*(1), 143–149.

Anderson, C. M., Hogarty, G. E., & Reiss, D. J. (1980). Family treatment of adult schizophrenic patients: a psycho-educational approach. *Schizophr Bull, 6*(3), 490–505.

Angermeyer, M. C., Matschinger, H., & Schomerus, G. (2013). Attitudes towards psychiatric treatment and people with mental illness: changes over two decades. *Br J Psychiatry, 203*(2), 146–151.

Asarnow, J. R., Goldstein, M. J., & Ben-Meir, S. (1988). Parental communication deviance in childhood onset schizophrenia spectrum and depressive disorders. *J Child Psychol Psychiatry, 29*(6), 825–838.

Aubry, T., et al. (2016). A multiple-city RCT of housing first with assertive community treatment for homeless Canadians with serious mental illness. *Psychiatr Serv, 67*(3), 275–281.

Austin, S. F., et al. (2015). Long-term trajectories of positive and negative symptoms in first episode psychosis: a 10-year follow-up study in the OPUS cohort. *Schizophr Res, 168*(1–2), 84–91.

Balaji, M., Chatterjee, S., Brennan, B., Rangaswamy, T., Thornicroft, G., & Patel, V. (2012a). Outcomes that matter: a qualitative study with persons with schizophrenia and their primary caregivers in India. *Asian J Psychiatr, 5*(3), 258–265.

Balaji, M., et al. (2012b). The development of a lay health worker delivered collaborative community based intervention for people with schizophrenia in India. *BMC Health Serv Res, 12*, 42.

Baumel, A., et al. (2016). Health technology intervention after hospitalization for schizophrenia: service utilization and user satisfaction. *Psychiatr Serv, 67*(9), 1035–1038.

Bechard-Evans, L., Schmitz, N., Abadi, S., Joober, R., King, S., & Malla, A. (2007). Determinants of help-seeking and system related components of delay in the treatment of first-episode psychosis. *Schizophr Res, 96*(1–3), 206–214.

Behan, C., Masterson, S., & Clarke, M. (2017). Systematic review of the evidence for service models delivering early intervention in psychosis outside the stand-alone centre. *Early Interv Psychiatry, 11*(1), 3–13.

Bertelsen, M., et al. (2008). Five-year follow-up of a randomized multicenter trial of intensive early intervention vs. standard treatment for patients with a first episode of psychotic illness: the OPUS trial. *Arch Gen Psychiatry, 65*(7), 762–771.

Best, M. W. & Bowie, C. R. (2017). A review of cognitive remediation approaches for schizophrenia: from top-down to bottom-up, brain training to psychotherapy. *Expert Rev Neurother, 17*(7), 713–723.

Birchwood, M., et al. (2013). Reducing duration of untreated psychosis: care pathways to early intervention in psychosis services. *Br J Psychiatry, 203*(1), 58–64.

Birchwood, M., Todd, P., & Jackson, C. (1998). Early intervention in psychosis. The critical period hypothesis. *Br J Psychiatry Suppl, 172*(33), 53–59.

Bird, V., Premkumar, P., Kendall, T., Whittington, C., Mitchell, J., & Kuipers, E. (2010). Early intervention services, cognitive-behavioural therapy and family intervention in early psychosis: systematic review. *Br J Psychiatry, 197*(5), 350–356.

Bond, G. R. & Drake, R. E. (2014). Making the case for IPS supported employment. *Adm Policy Ment Health, 41*(1), 69–73.

Bond, G. R. (2004). Supported employment: evidence for an evidence-based practice. *Psychiatr Rehabil J, 27*(4), 345–359.

Brill, H. & Patton, R. E. (1962). Clinical-statistical analysis of population changes in New York state mental hospitals since introduction of psychotropic drugs. *Am J Psychiatry*, *119*, 20–35.

Britvic, D., et al. (2013). Metabolic issues in psychotic disorders with the focus on first-episode patients: a review. *Psychiatr Danub*, *25*(4), 410–415.

Bruckner, T. A., et al. (2011). The mental health workforce gap in low- and middle-income countries: a needs-based approach. *Bull World Health Organ*, *89*(3), 184–194.

Brunette, M. F., et al. (2016). Coordinated technology-delivered treatment to prevent rehospitalization in schizophrenia: a novel model of care. *Psychiatric Serv*, *67*(4), 444–447.

Burns, J. K., Jhazbhay, K., Kidd, M., & Emsley, R. A. (2011). Causal attributions, pathway to care and clinical features of first-episode psychosis: a South African perspective. *Int J Soc Psychiatry*, *57*(5), 538–545.

Cancro, R. (2000). The introduction of neuroleptics: a psychiatric revolution. *Psychiatr Serv*, *51*(3), 333–335.

Casey, D. A., Rodriguez, M., Northcott, C., Vickar, G., & Shihabuddin, L. (2011). Schizophrenia: medical illness, mortality, and aging. *Int J Psychiatry Med*, *41*(3), 245–251.

Castle, D. J. & Singh, S. P. (2015). Early intervention in psychosis: still the 'best buy'? *Br J Psychiatry*, *207*(4), 288–292.

Chan, S. K. W., et al. (2015). 10-year outcome study of an early intervention program for psychosis compared with standard care service. *Psychol Med*, *45*(6), 1181–1193.

Chang, W. C., et al. (2015). Optimal duration of an early intervention programme for first-episode psychosis: randomised controlled trial. *Br J Psychiatry*, *206*(6), 492–500.

Chang, W. C., et al. (2017). Sustainability of treatment effect of a 3-year early intervention programme for first-episode psychosis. *Br J Psychiatry*, *211*(1), 37–44.

Charland, L. C. (2008). A moral line in the sand: Alexander Crichton and Philippe Pinel on the psychopathology of the passions. In **Zachar L. C. C. a. P.** (ed.) *Fact and value in emotion*. Amsterdam, NL: John Benjamins Publishing Company, 15–35.

Charlson, F. J., et al. (2018). Global epidemiology and burden of schizophrenia: findings from the global burden of disease study 2016. *Schizophr Bull*, *44*(6), 1195–1203.

Chatterjee, S., et al. (2014). Effectiveness of a community-based intervention for people with schizophrenia and their caregivers in India (COPSI): a randomised controlled trial. *Lancet*, *383*(9926), 1385–1394.

Chatterjee, S., Patel, V., Chatterjee, A., & Weiss, H. A. (2003). Evaluation of a community-based rehabilitation model for chronic schizophrenia in rural India. *Br J Psychiatry*, *182*(1), 57–62.

Chatterjee, S., Pillai, A., Jain, S., Cohen, A., & Patel, V. (2009). Outcomes of people with psychotic disorders in a community-based rehabilitation programme in rural India. *Br J Psychiatry*, *195*(5), 433–439.

Chen, E. Y., et al. (2015). Three-year community case management for early psychosis: a randomised controlled study. *Hong Kong Med J*, *21* Suppl 2, 23–26.

Chen, E. Y., Wong, G. H., Lam, M. M., Chiu, C. P., & Hui, C. L. (2008). Real-world implementation of early intervention in psychosis: resources, funding models and evidence-based practice. *World Psychiatry*, *7*(3), 163–164.

Clark, R. E., et al. (1998). Cost-effectiveness of assertive community treatment versus standard case management for persons with co-occurring severe mental illness and substance use disorders. *Health Serv Res, 33*(5 Pt 1), 1285–1308.

Cohen, B. (2006). Urbanization in developing countries: current trends, future projections, and key challenges for sustainability. *Technol Soc, 28*(1), 63–80.

Correll, C. U., et al. (2018). Comparison of early intervention services vs. treatment as usual for early-phase psychosis: a systematic review, meta-analysis, and meta-regression. *JAMA Psychiatry, 75*(6), 555–565.

Corrigan, P. W. & Liberman, R. P. (1989). Social rehabilitation of schizophrenia. *West J Med, 151*(3), 316–317.

Craig, T. K., et al. (2015). The effects of an Audio Visual Assisted Therapy Aid for Refractory auditory hallucinations (AVATAR therapy): study protocol for a randomised controlled trial. *Trials, 16*, 349.

Dark, F., Whiteford, H., Ashkanasy, N. M., Harvey, C., Crompton, D., & Newman, E. (2015). Implementing cognitive therapies into routine psychosis care: organisational foundations. *BMC Health Serv Res, 15*, 310.

Davidson, L. & Roe, D. (2007). Recovery from versus recovery in serious mental illness: one strategy for lessening confusion plaguing recovery. *J Ment Health, 16*(4), 459–470.

De Bruin, E. J., van Steensel, F. J., & Meijer, A. M. (2016). Cost-effectiveness of group and internet cognitive behavioral therapy for insomnia in adolescents: results from a randomized controlled trial. *Sleep, 39*(8), 1571–1581.

de Jesus, M. J., Razzouk, D., Thara, R., Eaton, J., & Thornicroft, G. (2009). Packages of care for schizophrenia in low- and middle-income countries. *PLoS Med, 6*(10), e1000165.

de Menil, V., et al. (2015). Cost-effectiveness of the mental health and development model for schizophrenia-spectrum and bipolar disorders in rural Kenya. *Psychol Med, 45*(13), 2747–2756.

De Silva, M. J., Cooper, S., Li, H. L., Lund, C., & Patel, V. (2013). Effect of psychosocial interventions on social functioning in depression and schizophrenia: meta-analysis. *Br J Psychiatry, 202*(4), 253–260.

Deniker, P. (1978). Impact of neuroleptic chemotherapies on schizophrenic psychoses. *Am J Psychiatry, 135*(8), 923–927.

Dieterich, M., Irving, C. B., Bergman, H., Khokhar, M. A., Park, B., & Marshall, M. (2017). Intensive case management for severe mental illness. *Cochrane Database Syst Rev, 1*, CD007906.

Dixon, L., et al. (2001). Evidence-based practices for services to families of people with psychiatric disabilities. *Psychiatr Serv, 52*(7), 903–910.

Drake, R. E. & Whitley, R. (2014). Recovery and severe mental illness: description and analysis. *Can J Psychiatry, 59*(5), 236–242.

Duval, A. M. & Goldman, D. (2000). The new drugs (chlorpromazine and reserpine): administrative aspects. 1956. *Psychiatr Serv, 51*(3), 327–331.

Eassom, E., Giacco, D., Dirik, A., & Priebe, S. (2014). Implementing family involvement in the treatment of patients with psychosis: a systematic review of facilitating and hindering factors. *BMJ Open, 4*(10), e006108.

Ecks, S. & Basu, S. (2014). 'We always live in fear': antidepressant prescriptions by unlicensed doctors in India. *Cult Med Psychiatry, 38*(2), 197–216.

Ecks, S. (2016). Commentary: ethnographic critiques of global mental health. *Transcult Psychiatry*, *53*(6), 804–808.

Ecks, S. (2013). *Eating drugs: psychopharmaceutical pluralism in India*. New York, US: NYU Press.

Evans-Lacko, S., Corker, E., Williams, P., Henderson, C., & Thornicroft, G. (2014). Effect of the time to change anti-stigma campaign on trends in mental-illness-related public stigma among the English population in 2003–13: an analysis of survey data. *Lancet Psychiatry*, *1*(2), 121–128.

Falloon, I. R. H., Boyd, J. L., & McGill, C. W. (1987). *Family care of schizophrenia: a problem-solving approach to the treatment of mental illness*. New York, US: Guilford Press.

Fleischhacker, W. W., et al. (2014). Schizophrenia—time to commit to policy change. *Schizophr Bull*, *40*(Suppl_3), S165–S194.

Folsom, D. & Jeste, D. V. (2008). Schizophrenia in homeless persons: a systematic review of the literature. *Acta Psychiatr Scand*, *105*(6), 404–413.

Fowler, D., et al. (2009). Cognitive behaviour therapy for improving social recovery in psychosis: a report from the ISREP MRC Trial Platform Study (Improving Social Recovery in Early Psychosis). *Psychol Med*, *39*(10), 1627–1636.

Gaebel, W., et al. (2016). European Psychiatric Association (EPA) guidance on the quality of eMental health interventions in the treatment of psychotic disorders. *Eur Arch Psychiatry Clin Neurosci*, *266*(2), 125–137.

Galletly, C., et al. (2016). Royal Australian and New Zealand College of Psychiatrists clinical practice guidelines for the management of schizophrenia and related disorders. *Aust N Z J Psychiatry*, *50*(5), 410–472.

Galletly, C. A., et al. (2012). Cardiometabolic risk factors in people with psychotic disorders: the second Australian national survey of psychosis. *Aust N Z J Psychiatry*, *46*(8), 753–761.

Garety, P. A. (2003). The future of psychological therapies for psychosis. *World Psychiatry*, *2*(3), 147–152.

Gautham, M., Binnendijk, E., Koren, R., & Dror, D. M. (2011). 'First we go to the small doctor': first contact for curative health care sought by rural communities in Andhra Pradesh & Orissa, India. *Indian J Med Res*, *134*(5), 627.

GBD (2016). Global, regional, and national incidence, prevalence, and years lived with disability for 310 diseases and injuries, 1990–2015: a systematic analysis for the Global Burden of Disease Study 2015. *Lancet*, *388*(10053), 1545–1602.

George, M. (1959). Vincenzo Chiarugi (1759–1820) and his psychiatric reform in Florence in the late 18th century (on the occasion of the bi-centenary of his birth). *J Hist Med Allied Sci*, *14*(10), 424–433.

Goldberg, K., et al. (2006). Impact of a specialized early intervention service for psychotic disorders on patient characteristics, service use, and hospital costs in a defined catchment area. *Can J Psychiatry*, *51*(14), 895–903.

Goldstein, M. J. (1985). Family factors that antedate the onset of schizophrenia and related disorders: the results of a fifteen year prospective longitudinal study. *Acta Psychiatr Scand Suppl*, *319*, 7–18.

Goodwin, N. & Lawton-Smith, S. (2010). Integrating care for people with mental illness: the care programme approach in England and its implications for long-term conditions management. *Int J Integr Care*, *10*, e040.

Gottlieb, J. D., Romeo, K. H., Penn, D. L., Mueser, K. T., & Chiko, B. P. (2013). Web-based cognitive-behavioral therapy for auditory hallucinations in persons with psychosis: a pilot study. *Schizophr Res, 145*(1–3), 82–87.

Graham, K. L., Carson, C. M., Ezeoke, A., Buckley, P. F., & Miller, B. J. (2014). Urinary tract infections in acute psychosis. *J Clin Psychiatry, 75*(4), 379–385.

Granholm, E., Holden, J., Link, P. C., & McQuaid, J. R. (2014). Randomized clinical trial of cognitive behavioral social skills training for schizophrenia: improvement in functioning and experiential negative symptoms. *J Consult Clin Psychol, 82*(6), 1173–1185.

Groff, M., et al. (2021). Economic evaluation of extended early intervention service vs regular care following 2 years of early intervention: secondary analysis of a randomized controlled trial. *Schizophr Bull, 47*(2), 465–473.

Guhne, U., Weinmann, S., Arnold, K., Becker, T., & Riedel-Heller, S. (2012). [Social skills training in severe mental illness--is it effective?]. *Psychiatr Prax, 39*(8), 371–380.

Gureje, O., Abdulmalik, J., Kola, L., Musa, E., Yasamy, M. T., & Adebayo, K. (2015a). Integrating mental health into primary care in Nigeria: report of a demonstration project using the mental health gap action programme intervention guide. *BMC Health Serv Res, 15*, 242.

Gureje, O., Nortje, G., Makanjuola, V., Oladeji, B. D., Seedat, S., & Jenkins, R. (2015b). The role of global traditional and complementary systems of medicine in the treatment of mental health disorders. *Lancet Psychiatry, 2*(2), 168–177.

Haddock, G., Eisner, E., Boone, C., Davies, G., Coogan, C., & Barrowclough, C. (2014). An investigation of the implementation of NICE-recommended CBT interventions for people with schizophrenia. *J Ment Health, 23*(4), 162–165.

Haglund, M., Cabaniss, D., Kimhy, D., & Corcoran, C. M. (2014). A case report of cognitive behavioural therapy for social anxiety in an ultra-high risk patient. *Early Interv Psychiatry, 8*(2), 176–180.

Harrison, G., Croudace, T., Mason, P., Glazebrook, C., & Medley, I. (2009). Predicting the long-term outcome of schizophrenia. *Psychol Med, 26*(4), 697–705.

Harrison, G., et al. (2001). Recovery from psychotic illness: a 15- and 25-year international follow-up study. *Br J Psychiatry, 178*(6), 506–517.

Harvey, P. O., Lepage, M., & Malla, A. (2007). Benefits of enriched intervention compared with standard care for patients with recent-onset psychosis: a metaanalytic approach. *Can J Psychiatry, 52*(7), 464–472.

Hastrup, L. H., et al. (2013). Cost-effectiveness of early intervention in first-episode psychosis: economic evaluation of a randomised controlled trial (the OPUS study). *Br J Psychiatry, 202*(1), 35–41.

Hazell, C. M., Hayward, M., Cavanagh, K., & Strauss, C. (2016). A systematic review and meta-analysis of low intensity CBT for psychosis. *Clin Psychol Rev, 45*, 183–192.

Hill, S. A. & Laugharne, R. (2003). Mania, dementia and melancholia in the 1870s: admissions to a Cornwall asylum. *J R Soc Med, 96*(7), 361–363.

Hofmann, S. G., Asnaani, A., Vonk, I. J., Sawyer, A. T., & Fang, A. (2012). The efficacy of cognitive behavioral therapy: a review of meta-analyses. *Cognit Ther Res, 36*(5), 427–440.

Hogarty, G. E., et al. (1986). Family psychoeducation, social skills training, and maintenance chemotherapy in the aftercare treatment of schizophrenia. I. One-year effects of a controlled study on relapse and expressed emotion. *Arch Gen Psychiatry, 43*(7), 633–642.

Hogarty, G. E. & Ulrich, R. F. (1998). The limitations of antipsychotic medication on schizophrenia relapse and adjustment and the contributions of psychosocial treatment. *J Psychiatr Res*, **32**(3–4), 243–250.

Hubley, S., Lynch, S. B., Schneck, C., Thomas, M., & Shore, J. (2016). Review of key telepsychiatry outcomes. *World J Psychiatry*, *6*(2), 269–282.

Hulsbosch, A. M., Nugter, M. A., Tamis, P., & Kroon, H. (2017). Videoconferencing in a mental health service in the Netherlands: a randomized controlled trial on patient satisfaction and clinical outcomes for outpatients with severe mental illness. *J Telemed Telecare*, *23*(5), 513–520.

Hutton, P. & Taylor, P. J. (2014). Cognitive behavioural therapy for psychosis prevention: a systematic review and meta-analysis. *Psychol Med*, *44*(3), 449–468.

Ibrahim, N., Michail, M., & Callaghan, P. (2014). The strengths based approach as a service delivery model for severe mental illness: a meta-analysis of clinical trials. *BMC Psychiatry*, *14*, 243.

Ince, P., Haddock, G., & Tai, S. (2016). A systematic review of the implementation of recommended psychological interventions for schizophrenia: rates, barriers, and improvement strategies. *Psychol Psychother*, *89*(3), 324–350.

Institute of **Medicine**, et al. (2001). *Neurological, psychiatric, and developmental disorders: meeting the challenge in the developing world*. Washington DC: National Academies Press.

Ivezic, S. S., Muzinic, L., & Filipac, V. (2010). Case management—a pillar of community psychiatry. *Psychiatr Danub*, *22*(1), 28–33.

Iyer, S., Jordan, G., MacDonald, K., Joober, R., & Malla, A. (2015). Early intervention for psychosis: a Canadian perspective. *J Nerv Ment Dis*, *203*(5), 356–364.

Iyer, S., et al. (2020). Context and contact: a comparison of patient and family engagement with early intervention services for psychosis in India and Canada. *Psychol Med*, 1–10. doi:10.1017/S0033291720003359

Iyer, S. N., Mangala, R., Thara, R., & Malla, A. K. (2010). Preliminary findings from a study of first-episode psychosis in Montreal, Canada and Chennai, India: comparison of outcomes. *Schizophr Res*, *121*(1–3), 227–233.

Jaaskelainen, E., et al. (2013). A systematic review and meta-analysis of recovery in schizophrenia. *Schizophr Bull*, **39**(6), 1296–1306.

James, S. L., et al. (2018). Global, regional, and national incidence, prevalence, and years lived with disability for 354 diseases and injuries for 195 countries and territories, 1990–2017: a systematic analysis for the Global Burden of Disease Study 2017. *Lancet*, *392*(10159), 1789–1858.

Jones, M., Kruger, M., & Walsh, S. M. (2016). Preparing non-government organization workers to conduct health checks for people with serious mental illness in regional Australia. *J Psychiatr Ment Health Nurs*, *23*(5), 247–254.

Jordan, G., Lutgens, D., Joober, R., Lepage, M., Iyer, S. N., & Malla, A. (2014). The relative contribution of cognition and symptomatic remission to functional outcome following treatment of a first episode of psychosis. *J Clin Psychiatry*, *75*(6), e566–e572.

Kane, J. M., et al. (2016). Comprehensive versus usual community care for first-episode psychosis: 2-year outcomes from the NIMH RAISE early treatment program. *Am J Psychiatry*, *173*(4), 362–372.

Karow, A., et al. (2012). Cost-effectiveness of 12-month therapeutic assertive community treatment as part of integrated care versus standard care in patients with schizophrenia treated with quetiapine immediate release (ACCESS trial). *J Clin Psychiatry*, *73*(3), e402–e408.

Kern, R. S., Glynn, S. M., Horan, W. P., & Marder, S. R. (2009). Psychosocial treatments to promote functional recovery in schizophrenia. *Schizophr Bull*, *35*(2), 347–361.

Keshavan, M. S., Shrivastava, A., & Gangadhar, B. N. (2010). Early intervention in psychotic disorders: challenges and relevance in the Indian context. *Indian J Psychiatry*, *52*(Suppl 1), S153–S158.

Killackey, E., Jackson, H. J., & McGorry, P. D. (2008). Vocational intervention in first-episode psychosis: individual placement and support v. treatment as usual. *Br J Psychiatry*, *193*(2), 114–120.

Knapp, M., McDaid, D., & Mossialos, E. (2006). *Mental health policy and practice across Europe*. London: McGraw-Hill Education.

Krabbendam, L. & Aleman, A. (2003). Meta-analyses of randomized controlled trials of social skills training and cognitive remediation. *Psychol Med*, *33*(4), 756, author reply 758.

Kurtz, M. M., Mueser, K. T., Thime, W. R., Corbera, S., & Wexler, B. E. (2015). Social skills training and computer-assisted cognitive remediation in schizophrenia. *Schizophr Res*, *162*(1–3), 35–41.

Laffey, P. (2003). Psychiatric therapy in Georgian Britain. *Psychol Med*, *33*(7), 1285–1297.

Lambo, T. A. (1956). Neuropsychiatric observations in the western region of Nigeria. *Br Med J*, *2*(5006), 1388.

Large, M., Farooq, S., Nielssen, O., & Slade, T. (2008). Relationship between gross domestic product and duration of untreated psychosis in low- and middle-income countries. *Br J Psychiatry*, *193*(4), 272–278.

Lasalvia, A., et al. (2013). Global pattern of experienced and anticipated discrimination reported by people with major depressive disorder: a cross-sectional survey. *Lancet*, *381*(9860), 55–62.

Latimer, E. (2005). Economic considerations associated with assertive community treatment and supported employment for people with severe mental illness. *J Psychiatry Neurosci*, *30*(5), 355–359.

Leamy, M., Bird, V., Le Boutillier, C., Williams, J., & Slade, M. (2011). Conceptual framework for personal recovery in mental health: systematic review and narrative synthesis. *Br J Psychiatry*, *199*(6), 445–452.

Lecomte, T. & Leclerc, C. (2013). Implementing cognitive behaviour therapy for psychosis. In Hagen, R., et al. (eds) *CBT for psychosis: a symptom-based approach*. London: Routledge, 144.

Leucht, S., et al. (2013). Comparative efficacy and tolerability of 15 antipsychotic drugs in schizophrenia: a multiple-treatments meta-analysis. *Lancet*, *382*(9896), 951–962.

Liberman, R. P. (1994). Psychosocial treatments for schizophrenia. *Psychiatry*, *57*(2), 104–114.

Lora, A., Kohn, R., Levav, I., McBain, R., Morris, J., & Saxena, S. (2012). Service availability and utilization and treatment gap for schizophrenic disorders: a survey in 50 low- and middle-income countries. *Bull World Health Organ*, *90*(1), 47–54, 54A–54B.

Lucksted, A., McFarlane, W., Downing, D., & Dixon, L. (2012). Recent developments in family psychoeducation as an evidence-based practice. *J Marital Fam Ther*, *38*(1), 101–121.

Lund, C., et al. (2012). PRIME: a programme to reduce the treatment gap for mental disorders in five low- and middle-income countries. *PLoS Med, 9*(12), e1001359.

Lund, C., Tomlinson, M., & Patel, V. (2016). Integration of mental health into primary care in low- and middle-income countries: the PRIME mental healthcare plans. *Br J Psychiatry, 208*(Suppl 56), s1–3.

Lund, C. (2018). Improving quality of mental health care in low-resource settings: lessons from PRIME. *World Psychiatry, 17*(1), 47.

Lutgens, D., et al. (2015). A five-year randomized parallel and blinded clinical trial of an extended specialized early intervention vs. regular care in the early phase of psychotic disorders: study protocol. *BMC Psychiatry, 15*, 22.

Major, B. S., Hinton, M. F., Flint, A., Chalmers-Brown, A., McLoughlin, K., & Johnson, S. (2010). Evidence of the effectiveness of a specialist vocational intervention following first episode psychosis: a naturalistic prospective cohort study. *Soc Psychiatry Psychiatr Epidemiol, 45*(1), 1–8.

Makowski, A. C., et al. (2016). Changes in beliefs and attitudes toward people with depression and schizophrenia—results of a public campaign in Germany. *Psychiatry Res, 237*, 271–278.

Malakouti, S. K., et al. (2009). Case-management for patients with schizophrenia in Iran: a comparative study of the clinical outcomes of Mental Health Workers and Consumers' Family Members as case managers. *Community Ment Health J, 45*(6), 447–452.

Malhotra, S., Chakrabarti, S., Shah, R., Mehta, A., Gupta, A., & Sharma, M. (2015). A novel screening and diagnostic tool for child and adolescent psychiatric disorders for telepsychiatry. *Indian J Psychol Med, 37*(3), 288–298.

Malla, A., et al. (2020). Comparison of clinical outcomes following 2 years of treatment of first-episode psychosis in urban early intervention services in Canada and India. *Br J Psychiatry, 217*(3), 514–520.

Malla, A., et al. (2019a). Testing the effectiveness of implementing a model of mental healthcare involving trained lay health workers in treating major mental disorders among youth in a conflictridden low- middle income environment: Part II Results. *Can J Psychiatry, 64*(9), 630–637.

Malla, A., et al. (2019b). A model of mental health care involving trained lay health workers for treatment of major mental disorders among youth in a conflict-ridden low-middle in- come environment: Part I Adaptation and implementation. *Can J Psychiatry, 64*(9), 621–629.

Malla, A. & McGorry, P. (2019). Early intervention in psychosis in young people: a population and public health perspective. *Am J Public Health, 109*, S181–S184.

Malla, A., et al. (2017). Comparing three-year extension of early intervention service to regular care following two years of early intervention service in first-episode psychosis: a randomized single blind clinical trial. *World Psychiatry, 16*(3), 278–286.

Malla, A., et al. (2014). A controlled evaluation of a targeted early case detection intervention for reducing delay in treatment of first episode psychosis. *Soc Psychiatry Psychiatr Epidemiol, 49*(11), 1711–1718.

Malla, A., Lal, S., Vracotas, N. C., Goldberg, K., & Joober, R. (2010). Early intervention in psychosis: specialized intervention and early case identification. *L'Encephale, 36* Suppl 3, S38–S45.

Malla, A., Norman, R., Bechard-Evans, L., Schmitz, N., Manchanda, R., & Cassidy, C. (2008). Factors influencing relapse during a 2-year follow-up of first-episode psychosis in a specialized early intervention service. *Psychol Med, 38*(11), 1585–1593.

Malla, A., Norman, R., McLean, T., Scholten, D., & Townsend, L. (2003). A Canadian programme for early intervention in non-affective psychotic disorders. *Aust N Z J Psychiatry, 37*(4), 407–413.

Malla, A., Norman, R., Scholten, D., Manchanda, R., & McLean, T. (2005). A community intervention for early identification of first episode psychosis: impact on duration of untreated psychosis (DUP) and patient characteristics. *Soc Psychiatry Psychiatr Epidemiol, 40*(5), 337–344.

Malla, A. & Norman, R. M. (1983). Mental hospital and general hospital psychiatric units: a comparison of services within the same geographic area. *Psychol Med, 13*(2), 431–439.

Malla, A. & Pelosi, A. J. (2010). Is treating patients with first-episode psychosis cost-effective? *Can J Psychiatry, 55*(1), 3–7, discussion 8.

Marshall, M., Lewis, S., Lockwood, A., Drake, R., Jones, P., & Croudace, T. (2005). Association between duration of untreated psychosis and outcome in cohorts of first-episode patients: a systematic review. *Arch Gen Psychiatry, 62*(9), 975–983.

Marshall, M. & Rathbone, J. (2011). Early intervention for psychosis. *Cochrane Database Syst Rev,* (6), CD004718.

Marshall, T., et al. (2014). Supported employment: assessing the evidence. *Psychiatr Serv, 65*(1), 16–23.

McCrone, P., Craig, T. K., Power, P., & Garety, P. A. (2010). Cost-effectiveness of an early intervention service for people with psychosis. *Br J Psychiatry, 196*(5), 377–382.

McCrone, P., Knapp, M., & Dhanasiri, S. (2009). Economic impact of services for first-episode psychosis: a decision model approach. *Early Interv Psychiatry, 3*(4), 266–273.

McCrone, P., Thornicroft, G., Parkman, S., Nathaniel-James, D., & Ojurongbe, W. (1998). Predictors of mental health service costs for representative cases of psychosis in south London. *Psychol Med, 28*(1), 159–164.

McFarlane, W. R., et al. (1995). Multiple-family groups and psychoeducation in the treatment of schizophrenia. *Arch Gen Psychiatry, 52*(8), 679–687.

McGlashan, T. H. & Carpenter, W. T. (2007). Identifying unmet therapeutic domains in schizophrenia patients: the early contributions of Wayne Fenton from Chestnut Lodge. *Schizophr Bull, 33*(5), 1086–1092.

McGorry, P. D., Edwards, J., Mihalopoulos, C., Harrigan, S. M., & Jackson, H. J. (1996). EPPIC: an evolving system of early detection and optimal management. *Schizophr Bull, 22*(2), 305–326.

McGorry, P. D., et al. (2009). Intervention in individuals at ultra-high risk for psychosis: a review and future directions. *J Clin Psychiatry, 70*(9), 1206–1212.

McGorry, P. D., et al. (2013). Randomized controlled trial of interventions for young people at ultra-high risk of psychosis: twelve-month outcome. *J Clin Psychiatry, 74*(4), 349–356.

McGorry, P. D., et al. (2002). Randomized controlled trial of interventions designed to reduce the risk of progression to first-episode psychosis in a clinical sample with subthreshold symptoms. *Arch Gen Psychiatry, 59*(10), 921–928.

McGrath, J., Saha, S., Welham, J., El Saadi, O., MacCauley, C., & Chant, D. (2004). A systematic review of the incidence of schizophrenia: the distribution of rates and the influence of sex, urbanicity, migrant status and methodology. *BMC Med*, *2*, 13.

McHugo, G. J., et al. (2004). A randomized controlled trial of integrated versus parallel housing services for homeless adults with severe mental illness. *Schizophr Bull*, *30*(4), 969–982.

Melle, I., et al. (2004). Reducing the duration of untreated first-episode psychosis: effects on clinical presentation. *Arch Gen Psychiatry*, *61*(2), 143–150.

Michail, M., Birchwood, M., & Tait, L. (2017). Systematic review of cognitive-behavioural therapy for social anxiety disorder in psychosis. *Brain Sci*, *7*(5), 45.

Mihalopoulos, C., Harris, M., Henry, L., Harrigan, S., & McGorry, P. (2009). Is early intervention in psychosis cost-effective over the long term? *Schizophr Bull*, *35*(5), 909–918.

Mihalopoulos, C., McCrone, P., Knapp, M., Johannessen, J. O., Malla, A., & McGorry, P. (2012). The costs of early intervention in psychosis: restoring the balance. *Aust N Z J Psychiatry*, *46*(9), 808–811.

Morgan, C., et al. (2015). Searching for psychosis: INTREPID (1): systems for detecting untreated and first-episode cases of psychosis in diverse settings. *Soc Psychiatry Psychiatr Epidemiol*, *50*(6), 879–893.

Morris, J., et al. (2011). Treated prevalence of and mental health services received by children and adolescents in 42 low-and-middle-income countries. *J Child Psychol Psychiatry*, *52*(12), 1239–1246.

Mossaheb, N., et al. (2013). Duration of untreated psychosis in a high-income versus a low- and middle-income region. *Aust N Z J Psychiatry*, *47*(12), 1176–1182.

Mueser, K. T. & Noordsy, D. L. (2005). Cognitive behavior therapy for psychosis: a call to action. *Clin Psychol (New York)*, *12*(1), 68–71.

Muir-Cochrane, E. (2006). Medical co-morbidity risk factors and barriers to care for people with schizophrenia. *J Psychiatr Ment Health Nurs*, *13*(4), 447–452.

Murthy, R. S. (2017). National mental health survey of India 2015–2016. *Indian J Psychiatry*, *59*(1), 21–26.

Naeem, F., et al. (2016). Cognitive Behavior Therapy for psychosis based Guided Self-help (CBTp-GSH) delivered by frontline mental health professionals: results of a feasibility study. *Schizophr Res*, *173*(1–2), 69–74.

Nahar, P., Kannuri, N. K., Mikkilineni, S., Murthy, G., & Phillimore, P. (2017). At the margins of biomedicine: the ambiguous position of 'registered medical practitioners' in rural Indian healthcare. *Sociol Health Illn*, *39*(4), 614–628.

National Collaborating Centre for Mental Health/National Institute for Health and Clinical Excellence (2014). *Psychosis and schizophrenia in adults: treatment and management: updated edition 2014*. London, UK: National Institute for Health and Care Excellence.

Nolin, M., Malla, A., Tibbo, P., Norman, R., & Abdel-Baki, A. (2016). Early intervention for psychosis in Canada: what is the state of affairs? *Can J Psychiatry*, *61*(3), 186–194.

Norman, R., Malla, A., Verdi, M., Hassall, L., & Fazekas, C. (2004). Understanding delay in treatment for first-episode psychosis. *Psychol Med*, *34*(2), 255–266.

Norman, R. M. & Malla, A. K. (2001). Duration of untreated psychosis: a critical examination of the concept and its importance. *Psychol Med*, *31*(3), 381–400.

Norman, R. M., Manchanda, R., Malla, A. K., Windell, D., Harricharan, R., & Northcott, S. (2011). Symptom and functional outcomes for a 5 year early intervention program for psychoses. *Schizophr Res*, *129*(2–3), 111–115.

Nortje, G., Oladeji, B., Gureje, O., & Seedat, S. (2016). Effectiveness of traditional healers in treating mental disorders: a systematic review. *Lancet Psychiatry*, *3*(2), 154–170.

Odenwald, M., et al. (2012). A pilot study on community-based outpatient treatment for patients with chronic psychotic disorders in Somalia: change in symptoms, functioning and co-morbid khat use. *Int J Ment Health Syst*, *6*(1), 8.

Ofori-Atta, A., Attafuah, J., Jack, H., Baning, F., & Rosenheck, R. (2018). Joining psychiatric care and faith healing in a prayer camp in Ghana: randomised trial. *Br J Psychiatry*, *212*(1), 34–41.

Ostergaard Christensen T, et al. (2014). Cognitive remediation combined with an early intervention service in first episode psychosis. *Acta Psychiatr Scand*, *130*(4), 300–310.

Padgett, D. K., Stanhope, V., Henwood, B. F., & Stefancic, A. (2011). Substance use outcomes among homeless clients with serious mental illness: comparing housing first with treatment first programs. *Community Ment Health J*, *47*(2), 227–232.

Pankowski, D., Kowalski, J., & Gaweda, L. (2016). The effectiveness of metacognitive training for patients with schizophrenia: a narrative systematic review of studies published between 2009 and 2015. *Psychiatr Pol*, *50*(4), 787–803.

Park, A. L., McCrone, P., & Knapp, M. (2016). Early intervention for first-episode psychosis: broadening the scope of economic estimates. *Early Interv Psychiatry*, *10*(2), 144–151.

Partti, K., et al. (2015). Lung function and respiratory diseases in people with psychosis: population-based study. *Br J Psychiatry*, *207*(1), 37–45.

Patel, V., et al. (2007). Treatment and prevention of mental disorders in low-income and middle-income countries. *Lancet*, *370*(9591), 991–1005.

Pelosi, A. J. & Birchwood, M. (2003). Is early intervention for psychosis a waste of valuable resources? *Br J Psychiatry*, *182*, 196–198.

Penttila, M., Jaaskelainen, E., Hirvonen, N., Isohanni, M., & Miettunen, J. (2014). Duration of untreated psychosis as predictor of long-term outcome in schizophrenia: systematic review and meta-analysis. *Br J Psychiatry*, *205*(2), 88–94.

Perala, J., et al. (2007). Lifetime prevalence of psychotic and bipolar I disorders in a general population. *Arch Gen Psychiatry*, *64*(1), 19–28.

Perkins, D. O. (2006). Review: longer duration of untreated psychosis is associated with worse outcome in people with first episode psychosis. *Evid Based Ment Health*, *9*(2), 36.

Perry, Y., et al. (2015). The development and implementation of a pilot CBT for early psychosis service: achievements and challenges. *Early Interv Psychiatry*, *9*(3), 252–259.

Pharoah, F., Mari, J., Rathbone, J., & Wong, W. (2010). Family intervention for schizophrenia. *Cochrane Database Syst Rev*, (12), CD000088.

Pitschel-Walz, G., Leucht, S., Bauml, J., Kissling, W., & Engel, R. R. (2001). The effect of family interventions on relapse and rehospitalization in schizophrenia—a meta-analysis. *Schizophr Bull*, *27*(1), 73–92.

Poreddi, V., Ramachandra, Reddemma, K., & Math, S. B. (2013). People with mental illness and human rights: a developing countries perspective. *Indian J Psychiatry*, *55*(2), 117–124.

Pow, J. L., Baumeister, A. A., Hawkins, M. F., Cohen, A. S., & Garand, J. C. (2015). Deinstitutionalization of American public hospitals for the mentally ill before and after the introduction of antipsychotic medications. *Harv Rev Psychiatry, 23*(3), 176–187.

Priebe, S., et al. (2005). Reinstitutionalisation in mental health care: comparison of data on service provision from six European countries. *BMJ, 330*(7483), 123–126.

Priebe, S., et al. (2016). Effectiveness of one-to-one volunteer support for patients with psychosis: protocol of a randomised controlled trial. *BMJ Open, 6*(8), e011582.

Priebe, S., et al. (2013). Effectiveness and cost-effectiveness of body psychotherapy in the treatment of negative symptoms of schizophrenia—a multi-centre randomised controlled trial. *BMC Psychiatry, 13*, 26.

Rangaswamy, T., Mangala, R., Mohan, G., Joseph, J., & John, S. (2012a). Early intervention for first-episode psychosis in India. *East Asian Arch Psychiatry, 22*(3), 94–99.

Rangaswamy, T., Mangala, R., Mohan, G., Joseph, J., & John, S. (2012b). Intervention for first episode psychosis in India—the SCARF experience. *Asian J Psychiatry, 5*(1), 58–62.

Rapp, C. A. & Goscha, R. J. (2011). *The strengths model: a recovery-oriented approach to mental health services.* New York, US: Oxford University Press.

Read, U. (2012). 'I want the one that will heal me completely so it won't come back again': the limits of antipsychotic medication in rural Ghana. *Transcult Psychiatry, 49*(3–4), 438–460.

Revell, E. R., Neill, J. C., Harte, M., Khan, Z., & Drake, R. J. (2015). A systematic review and meta-analysis of cognitive remediation in early schizophrenia. *Schizophr Res, 168*(1–2), 213–222.

Rezansoff, S. N., Moniruzzaman, A., Fazel, S., McCandless, L., Procyshyn, R., & Somers, J. M. (2017). Housing first improves adherence to antipsychotic medication among formerly homeless adults with schizophrenia: results of a randomized controlled trial. *Schizophr Bull, 43*(4), 852–861.

Robinson, D., et al. (1999). Predictors of relapse following response from a first episode of schizophrenia or schizoaffective disorder. *Arch Gen Psychiatry, 56*(3), 241–247.

Scholten, D. J., et al. (2001, April). Early intervention in psychosis: the impact of a novel approach to early case detection. In *Schizophrenia Research* (**Vol. 49**, No. 1-2, pp. 41–42).

Scholten, D., et al. (2003). Removing barriers to treatment of first episode psychotic disorders. *Can J Psychiatry, 48*(8), 561–565.

Scott, A. J., Webb, T. L., & Rowse, G. (2015). Self-help interventions for psychosis: a meta-analysis. *Clin Psychol Rev, 39*, 96–112.

Shah, J. L., Crawford, A., Mustafa, S. S., Iyer, S. N., Joober, R., & Malla, A. K. (2017). Is the clinical high-risk state a valid concept? Retrospective examination in a first-episode psychosis sample. *Psychiatr Serv, 68*(10), 1046–1052.

Shorter, E. (1998). *A history of psychiatry: from the era of the asylum to the age of prozac.* New Jersey: Wiley.

Simeone, J. C., Ward, A. J., Rotella, P., Collins, J., & Windisch, R. (2015). An evaluation of variation in published estimates of schizophrenia prevalence from 1990–2013: a systematic literature review. *BMC Psychiatry, 15*(1), 193.

Singh, S. P. & Fisher, H. L. (2005). Early intervention in psychosis: obstacles and opportunities. *Adv Psychiatr Treat, 11*(1), 71–78.

Singh, S. P., Paul, M., Ford, T., Kramer, T., & Weaver, T. (2008). Transitions of care from child and adolescent mental health services to adult mental health services (TRACK Study): a study of protocols in Greater London. *BMC Health Serv Res, 8,* 135.

Slade, E. P., McCarthy, J. F., Valenstein, M., Visnic, S., & Dixon, L. B. (2013). Cost savings from assertive community treatment services in an era of declining psychiatric inpatient use. *Health Serv Res, 48*(1), 195–217.

Slade, M., Amering, M., & Oades, L. (2008). Recovery: an international perspective. *Epidemiol Psichiatr Soc, 17*(2), 128–137.

Slade, M., et al. (2012). International differences in understanding recovery: systematic review. *Epidemiol Psichiatr Sci, 21*(4), 353–364.

Slade, M. & Longden, E. (2015). Empirical evidence about recovery and mental health. *BMC Psychiatry, 15,* 285.

Sorketti, E. A., Zainal, N. Z., & Habil, M. H. (2013). The treatment outcome of psychotic disorders by traditional healers in central Sudan. *Int J Social Psychiatry, 59*(4), 365–376.

Spaulding, W. D., Sullivan, M. E., & Poland, J. S. (2003). *Treatment and rehabilitation of severe mental illness.* New York: Guilford Press.

Srihari, V. H., et al. (2015). First-episode services for psychotic disorders in the U.S. public sector: a pragmatic randomized controlled trial. *Psychiatr Serv, 66*(7), 705–712.

Stain, H. J., Mawn, L., Common, S., Pilton, M., & Thompson, A. (2019). Research and practice for ultra-high risk for psychosis: a national survey of early intervention in psychosis services in England. *Early Interv Psychiatry, 13*(1), 47–52.

Stein, L. I. & Test, M. A. (1980). Alternative to mental hospital treatment. I. Conceptual model, treatment program, and clinical evaluation. *Arch Gen Psychiatry, 37*(4), 392–397.

Sullivan, M. E., Richardson, C. E., & Spaulding, W. D. (1991). University-state hospital collaboration in an inpatient psychiatric rehabilitation program. *Community Ment Health J, 27*(6), 441–453.

Tang, J. Y. M., et al. (2010). Early intervention for psychosis in Hong Kong—the EASY programme. *Early Interv Psychiatry, 4*(3), 214–219.

Taylor, R. E., Leese, M., Clarkson, P., Holloway, F., & Thornicroft, G. (1998). Quality of life outcomes for intensive versus standard community mental health services. PRiSM Psychosis Study. 9. *Br J Psychiatry, 173,* 416–422.

Thara, R., John, S., & Rao, K. (2008). Telepsychiatry in Chennai, India: the SCARF experience. *Behav Sci Law, 26*(3), 315–322.

Thara, R. (2012). Using mobile telepsychiatry to close the mental health gap. *Curr Psychiatry Rep, 14*(3), 167–168.

Thirthalli, J., Channaveerachari, N. K., Subbakrishna, D. K., Cottler, L. B., Varghese, M., & Gangadhar, B. N. (2011). Prospective study of duration of untreated psychosis and outcome of never-treated patients with schizophrenia in India. *Indian J Psychiatry, 53*(4), 319–323.

Thompson, J. W. (1994). Trends in the development of psychiatric services, 1844–1994. *Hosp Community Psychiatry, 45*(10), 987–992.

Thornicroft, G., Brohan, E., Rose, D., Sartorius, N., & Leese, M. (2009). Global pattern of experienced and anticipated discrimination against people with schizophrenia: a cross-sectional survey. *Lancet, 373*(9661), 408–415.

Thornicroft, G., et al. (2016). Evidence for effective interventions to reduce mental-health-related stigma and discrimination. *Lancet, 387*(10023), 1123–1132.

Tsemberis, S. & Eisenberg, R. F. (2000). Pathways to housing: supported housing for street-dwelling homeless individuals with psychiatric disabilities. *Psychiatr Serv, 51*(4), 487–493.

Tungpunkom, P., Maayan, N., & Soares-Weiser, K. (2012). Life skills programmes for chronic mental illnesses. *Cochrane Database Syst Rev*, 1, CD000381.

Turkington, D., Spencer, H., Lebert, L., & Dudley, R. (2017). Befriending: active placebo or effective psychotherapy? *Br J Psychiatry, 211*(1), 5–6.

Turner, D. T., van der Gaag, M., Karyotaki, E., & Cuijpers, P. (2014). Psychological interventions for psychosis: a meta-analysis of comparative outcome studies. *Am J Psychiatry, 171*(5), 523–538.

Turner, T. H. (1992). A diagnostic analysis of the casebooks of Ticehurst House asylum, 1845–1890. *Psychol Med Monogr Suppl, 21*, 1–70.

van Ginneken, N., et al. (2013). Non-specialist health worker interventions for the care of mental, neurological and substance-abuse disorders in low- and middle-income countries. *Cochrane Database Syst Rev*, (11), CD009149.

Verma, S., Poon, L. Y., Subramaniam, M., Abdin, E., & Chong, S. A. (2012). The Singapore Early Psychosis Intervention Programme (EPIP): a programme evaluation. *Asian J Psychiatr, 5*(1), 63–67.

von Hausswolff-Juhlin, Y., Bjartveit, M., Lindstrom, E., & Jones, P. (2009). Schizophrenia and physical health problems. *Acta Psychiatr Scand Suppl*, (438), 15–21.

Vos, T., et al. (2016). Global, regional, and national incidence, prevalence, and years lived with disability for 310 diseases and injuries, 1990–2015: a systematic analysis for the Global Burden of Disease Study 2015. *Lancet, 388*(10053), 1545–1602.

Vrbova, K., et al. (2016). Self-stigma and schizophrenia: a cross-sectional study. *Neuropsychiatr Dis Treat, 12*, 3011–3020.

Waghorn, G., Dias, S., Gladman, B., Harris, M., & Saha, S. (2014). A multi-site randomised controlled trial of evidence-based supported employment for adults with severe and persistent mental illness. *Aust Occup Ther J, 61*(6), 424–436.

Wasylenki, D., Goering, P., Lancee, W., Fischer, L., & Freeman, S. J. (1985). Psychiatric aftercare in a metropolitan setting. *Can J Psychiatry, 30*(5), 329–336.

Watson, A. C., Corrigan, P., Larson, J. E., & Sells, M. (2007). Self-stigma in people with mental illness. *Schizophr Bull, 33*(6), 1312–1318.

Where next with psychiatric illness? (Editorial) (1988). *Nature, 336*(6195), 95–96.

White, D. A., Luther, L., Bonfils, K. A., & Salyers, M. P. (2015). Essential components of early intervention programs for psychosis: available intervention services in the United States. *Schizophr Res, 168*(1–2), 79–83.

Whitley, R., Palmer, V., & Gunn, J. (2015). Recovery from severe mental illness. *CMAJ, 187*(13), 951–952.

Whitley, R. (2014). Introducing recovery. *Can J Psychiatry, 59*(5), 233–235.

Windell, D., Norman, R., & Malla, A. K. (2012). The personal meaning of recovery among individuals treated for a first episode of psychosis. *Psychiatr Serv, 63*(6), 548–553.

Windell, D. L., Norman, R., Lal, S., & Malla, A. (2015). Subjective experiences of illness recovery in individuals treated for first-episode psychosis. *Soc Psychiatry Psychiatr Epidemiol, 50*(7), 1069–1077.

Wong, G. H., et al. (2012). Developments in early intervention for psychosis in Hong Kong. *East Asian Arch Psychiatry*, *22*(3), 100–104.

Wood, L., Byrne, R., Burke, E., Enache, G., & Morrison, A. P. (2017). The impact of stigma on emotional distress and recovery from psychosis: the mediatory role of internalised shame and self-esteem. *Psychiatry Res*, *255*, 94–100.

Wood, L., Byrne, R., Varese, F., & Morrison, A. P. (2016). Psychosocial interventions for internalised stigma in people with a schizophrenia-spectrum diagnosis: a systematic narrative synthesis and meta-analysis. *Schizophr Res*, *176*(2–3), 291–303.

World Health Organization (WHO) (2018). *Mental health atlas 2017*. Geneva: World Health Organization.

World Health Organization (WHO) (2008). *Policies and practices for mental health in Europe: meeting the challenges*. Geneva: WHO Regional Office for Europe.

World Health Organization (WHO) (2015). *WHO guidelines approved by the guidelines review committee. Update of the mental health gap action programme (mhGAP) guidelines for mental, neurological and substance use disorders, 2015*. Geneva: World Health Organization.

Wyatt, R. J. (1991). Neuroleptics and the natural course of schizophrenia. *Schizophr Bull*, *17*(2), 325–351.

Wykes, T. (2010). Cognitive remediation therapy needs funding. *Nature*, *468*(7321), 165–166.

Wykes, T. (2008). Review: cognitive remediation improves cognitive functioning in schizophrenia. *Evid Based Ment Health*, *11*(4), 117.

Yung, A. R., et al. (2003). Psychosis prediction: 12-month follow up of a high-risk ('prodromal') group. *Schizophr Res*, *60*(1), 21–32.

Ziguras, S. J. & Stuart, G. W. (2000). A meta-analysis of the effectiveness of mental health case management over 20 years. *Psychiatr Serv*, *51*(11), 1410–1421.

9

Human rights and psychosis

Ursula M. Read and Erminia Colucci

Introduction

Human rights abuses of people with mental illness have been documented throughout the world in psychiatric institutions and in traditional and faith-based healing centres and private family homes (Drew et al., 2011; Kleinman, 2009; Rugkasa, 2016). These include the use of mechanical restraints, seclusion rooms and locked wards, enforced medication and unmodified electro-convulsive treatment (i.e. without anaesthetic), beatings, coercion, and neglect. People with psychosis are commonly the target of such abuses. Unusual or disruptive behaviours and popular perceptions of psychosis can provoke harsh responses and demands for containment and control. Despite early speculations that stigma might be lower in 'non-Western' societies (Littlewood et al., 2007), discrimination against people with psychosis has now been consistently demonstrated globally (Gerlinger et al., 2013; Thornicroft et al., 2009). In many languages psychosis comes closest to what is termed 'madness', indicating a condition which lies outside shared human experience and threatens person-hood (Cohen et al., 2016). Psychosis is commonly associated with irrational, dangerous or immoral traits or behaviour including the use of psychoactive substances such as cannabis or the manipulation of evil forces through witch-craft, sorcery, curses, or spirit possession (Cohen et al., 2016).

Education and social contact are key approaches utilized to address stigma against persons with mental illness (Thornicroft, et al., 2016). However, studies in high-income countries have shown that while psychosis may increasingly be considered as an illness with physiological, social, or psychological origins, this by itself does not necessarily reduce discrimination and exclusion (Read et al., 2006; Schomerus et al., 2012). Furthermore, human rights abuses are not simply the outcome of individual attitudes and behaviours but are embedded in dis-criminatory structures and laws (UNHRC, 2019). While cultural perspectives and beliefs may play a part, difficulties in accessing effective support and treat-ment alongside poverty and infrastructural factors have been demonstrated to underlie harsh responses to people with severe mental illness (Asher et al., 2017;

Patel & Bhui, 2018; Read et al., 2009). Involuntary detention and treatment are permitted under the laws of high and low-income countries (Sashidharan et al., 2019) and in many jurisdictions persons deemed to be of 'unsound mind' are denied civil or legal status and hence are unable to marry, vote, or own property (for example, Davar, 2012). Experiences of psychosis also intersect with historical inequalities and structural discrimination. Persons from disadvantaged groups, including migrants and ethnic minorities, are among those most likely to be diagnosed with psychosis and to be subject to discrimination, compulsory treatment and detention, and other human rights violations (Barnett et al., 2019; Bourque et al., 2011; Halvorsrud et al., 2018; Pearce et al., 2019).

Psychosis can be viewed as the paradigmatic condition to highlight the dilemmas and controversies surrounding the relationship between human rights and mental health. The concept of human rights is the outcome of historical, social, and cultural influences and there are longstanding debates regarding the balance between individual rights and communal responsibilities (Kirmayer, 2012). In the case of psychosis, there can be differing views of rights from the perspective of the person affected, the family and community, and mental health practitioners (Rosen et al., 2012). Such questions come to the fore in relation to the potential impact of psychosis on decision-making and the ethics of coercion in mental healthcare (Szmukler, 2015; Szmukler, 2019). People diagnosed with psychotic illnesses are most likely to be subject to involuntary detention and treatment in psychiatric hospitals or other institutions (Raboch et al., 2010). This can be based solely on the judgement that a person is deemed to suffer from a psychotic illness (Wickremsinhe, 2018) and reflects an assumption that persons with psychosis lack the ability to make decisions and are thus deprived of legal capacity (Szmukler, 2015). Worldwide, most mental health legislation, even that which makes explicit reference to human rights, permits involuntary confinement and treatment where there is deemed to be a 'risk of harm' to self or others (Saya et al., 2019; Wang & Colucci, 2017; Wickremsinhe, 2018). Such risks are associated with symptoms such as paranoia, delusions and hallucinations, and suicidal ideation. There are enduring debates between those who argue that withholding treatment in the absence of consent violates the right to health (Freeman et al., 2015; Maj, 2011), and those who assert that all involuntary treatment constitutes a human rights violation (Minkowitz, 2007). Involuntary admission and treatment are traumatic and humiliating and may jeopardize recovery and increase stigma and exclusion (Tingleff et al., 2017). Some activists with lived experience of psychosis describe themselves as 'survivors' of state-sponsored psychiatric coercion and critique the medicalization of their experience (Oaks, 2012). By contrast, many advocates in low-income countries with limited mental health services argue that a lack of access to psychiatric treatment breaches their right to health (Copeland et al., 2012; Jenkins et al., 2011).

Protecting the human rights of people with mental illness has been a central concern in campaigns to improve mental healthcare worldwide. These have centred around the development of rights-based legislation and policy, a shift to community-based services, and the participation of people with lived experience of mental illness, alongside families and civil society groups (Drew et al., 2011; Funk et al., 2006; Puschner et al., 2019; Wallcraft et al., 2011). In some settings, there are efforts to introduce monitoring and regulation of healing centres and promote collaboration with mental health services (Gureje et al., 2015) as explored by the co-authors in Ghana and Indonesia (Read, 2019; Colucci, 2021a, 2021b; Kpobi, in press).[1] Despite these initiatives, coercion and confinement remain central tools in psychiatric practice. Records are unavailable or unreliable in many settings. However, involuntary admission has increased in several European states including the UK, France, Spain, and the Netherlands (Sheridan Rains et al., 2019). Alongside this is sustained neglect in which people with psychosis are deprived of needed care and support, including medical care, secure housing, and opportunities for decent work and social inclusion (Kelly, 2005; Ebuenyi et al., 2018; UNHRC, 2019). People with psychosis experience poor physical health and premature mortality due to a combination of multilevel factors including iatrogenic effects of medication, social and economic conditions, and untreated physical conditions (De Hert et al., 2011; Liu et al., 2017; Maj, 2009; Suetani et al., 2015). Kelly (2005) has argued that the combination of such factors constitutes structural violence, operating to systematically exclude people with psychosis from full participation in civic and social life.

This chapter starts with an outline of the history of global initiatives to protect the human rights of people with psychotic illness. This is followed by an overview of three major approaches: legislative reform, community-based mental healthcare, and advocacy. We consider the opportunities and challenges presented by these approaches, specifically in relation to psychosis. The final section describes innovations to address human rights abuses in low-resource settings and three case studies illustrating different approaches including the reform of mental health legislation in Ghana, mental health service user advocacy in Indonesia, and recovery-focused interventions and peer support in Uganda.

Outline of the history of human rights in relation to psychosis

Coercion, neglect, and abuse in asylums across the world cast a long shadow over the history of psychiatry, and people with psychosis are among those who have suffered most severely (Desjarlais et al., 1995). However, in settings where there were few formal psychiatric institutions, people considered afflicted by madness remained in the custody of family networks or religious or traditional facilities (Cohen et al., 2013; Keller, 2005). As in the 'mad houses' of Europe, which predated the asylum era (Porter, 2006), forms of restraint such as chaining were likely widespread in such facilities. Those few asylums which were inaugurated in Europe's colonies functioned primarily as sites for the detention of vagrant 'lunatics' (Mahone, 2006; Swartz, 2010). After the end of the colonial period, community-based mental health services were promoted by the WHO and a new generation of psychiatrists working within emerging postcolonial states (Heaton, 2013). This was in line with the move towards deinstitutionalization in the US and Europe, which began in the 1950s (Fakhoury & Priebe, 2002; Thornicroft & Bebbington, 1989). Opposition to compulsory psychiatric detention and treatment in the US took inspiration from the Civil Rights movement, with people who had experienced involuntary confinement self-organizing to advocate for their rights (Testa & West, 2010).

However, confinement and neglect within psychiatric institutions has persisted. In the late 1980s a media exposé of appalling conditions in the psychiatric hospital on the Greek island of Leros (Giannakopoulos & Anagnostopoulos, 2016) led to a UN inquiry and publication of the UN Principles for the Protection of Persons with Mental Illness and for the Improvement of Mental Health Care (the MI Principles) (United Nations, 1991). These enshrined many of the principles that govern current recommendations for the protection of human rights in mental health care including a preference for community-based care (Mari & Thornicroft, 2010; Lancet Global Mental Health Group, 2007). However, the MI Principles permitted involuntary treatment (including seclusion and mechanical restraint) in cases where the patient was deemed to lack capacity and where there was a likelihood of serious harm to the patient or others and/ or the person's mental health was likely to deteriorate without treatment. For this reason, the MI Principles proved controversial among user groups. The MI Principles were also not legally binding and difficult to enforce.

Whereas these earlier initiatives had primarily been concerned with human rights in Europe and North America, a report on 'world mental health' published in 1995 by a prominent group of anthropologists and psychiatrists at Harvard University (Desjarlais et al., 1995) focused attention on stigma, neglect, and abuse in developing countries from Latin America to Asia. Both this report and the subsequent WHO World Health Report *Mental Health: New Understanding, New Hope* (WHO, 2001) promoted the provision of mental health services within primary care rather than specialized institutions as a means to protect human rights. The same year in which the World Health

Report was published, a fire at a shrine in Erwardi, India led to the deaths of several people being treated for mental illness who were chained to stakes and unable to escape (Murthy, 2001). Like Leros, this brought international attention, this time focused on human rights abuses within traditional healing centres rather than hospitals. Since then reports have highlighted human rights abuses of persons with psychotic illness across the globe as well as exposing the continuing failures of psychiatric institutions. Following the publication of the World Health Report, the WHO Mental Health Division began to promote legislative reform and in 2005 produced a *Resource Book on Mental Health, Human Rights and Legislation* (WHO, 2005). This built on the MI Principles to provide guidelines for member states on the development of rights-based mental health legislation.

The UN Convention on the Rights of Persons with Disabilities (CRPD), which came into force in 2008, brought mental health under the umbrella of 'disability rights' (United Nations, 2006). Where the MI Principles were predominantly concerned with protecting people from harm, so-called negative or first-generation rights (Cresswell, 2009), the CRPD is concerned with also promoting and protecting 'positive' or second-generation rights such as social and economic participation and the right to education, work, and family life, as well as political and civil rights, such as the right to vote and participate in public life (Wildeman, 2013). The Convention also compels signatories to take action to prevent persons with disabilities from 'cruel, inhuman or degrading treatment or punishment' (Article 15) and 'exploitation, violence and abuse' (Article 16). The adoption of the UN CRPD and its ratification by nearly 200 countries worldwide has been seen to promise greater human rights protection for people with mental disorders. Like other UN conventions, implementation is monitored by a designated committee, the Committee on the Rights of Persons with Disabilities. Signatory states are obliged to provide regular reports to the Committee and where the Convention is seen to be contravened, persons affected can seek legal redress from national judicial bodies and the UN (Wildeman, 2013). Unlike the MI Principles, the CRPD drew on close consultation with mental health service users who argued that all forms of coercive treatment represented a human rights violation. A General Comment on Article 12 asserted that 'substitute decision-making regimes' including guardianship and 'forced treatment' must be abolished since they represent a denial of legal capacity. This has provoked protests from psychiatrists who argue that withholding treatment in the absence of consent could undermine the person's right to treatment and care (Freeman et al., 2015; Wildeman, 2013).

Despite these controversies, the discourse on human rights in relation to mental illness is now integral to international mental health policies and initiatives, including the UN, WHO, and the World Psychiatric Association (Maj, 2011). An article in *Nature* in 2011 on 'grand challenges' for mental health research, included identifying ways to reduce stigma and social exclusion and improve access to care (Collins et al., 2011). Human rights, along with universal health coverage and evidence-based practice, were one of three cross-cutting principles in the WHO Mental Health Action Plan which was first published in 2013 (WHO, 2013). The plan, which initially spanned 2013–2020, was later extended to 2030 and the principles expanded to six, with human rights remaining the second principle after universal health coverage (WHO, 2021). Additional principles included empowerment of persons with mental disorders and psychosocial disabilities, alongside life-course and multi-sectoral approaches. The plan states that strategies, actions, and interventions should promote and protect the rights of people with mental disorders in line with the UN CRPD and other international and regional human rights instruments. The WHO QualityRights initiative also aims to promote human rights within mental health services worldwide (Funk & Drew Bold, 2020). Nonetheless, significant challenges remain in fulfilling these ideals. Many psychiatric institutions, particularly in low- and middle-income countries (LMIC), are poorly equipped and staff lack training and resources to respond humanely and safely to people in crisis (Nadkarni et al., 2015). Low staff numbers and morale, lack of essential resources, and decrepit infrastructure are all likely to exacerbate human rights abuses (Jack et al., 2015). Aside from continuing debates around coercion (Szmukler, 2015), a narrow focus on scaling up access to treatment can detract from the structural inequalities and injustice which threaten the rights of people with psychosis to full inclusion and participation in all aspects of society (Burns et al., 2014; UNHRC, 2019).

Legislative reform

The reform of mental health legislation has been promoted as essential to protect human rights and regulate the activities of psychiatric services and other actors such as the police, families, and traditional and faith healers (WHO, 2005). In many states legislation is lacking or concerned primarily with governing involuntary admission and treatment, rather than promoting social, cultural, and economic rights (Wickremsinhe, 2018). In settings where legislation is absent, outdated, or poorly implemented, admission to psychiatric institutions is often the decision of medical personnel, the police, or family members, with obvious potential for abuse. In many LMICs, mental health legislation has been inherited from the 'lunacy' laws of colonial regimes (Mahone, 2006). The 2021 WHO Comprehensive Mental Health Action Plan aims for 80% of countries to have developed or updated their mental health legislation in line with international and regional human rights instruments by 2030 (WHO 2021). Since the turn of the millennium, several states including India, Ghana, South Africa, China, and, most recently, Nigeria, have engaged in legislative reform (Adepoju, 2023; Doku, 2012; Duffy & Kelly, 2019; Hussey & Mannan, 2016; Lund et al., 2012). However, there is wide variation in the extent to which mental health legislation is fully concordant with the UN CRPD and psychiatrists have continued to resist the complete removal of powers to enforce treatment (Duffy & Kelly, 2019; Xie, 2012). Even where reform has taken place, most laws retain 'exceptions' where involuntary treatment can be legally permissible, putting the legislation in conflict with the CRPD. As argued by Puras and Gooding (2019), the risk is that exceptions slide into becoming the norm. The framing of psychotic breakdown as a 'psychiatric emergency' can be used to justify the deprivation of rights in the interests of safety and the need for an urgent response.

Legal provisions that aim to protect human rights have often proved problematic to implement in practice, particularly where infrastructural and resource capacity is insufficient (Dudley et al., 2012; Hussey & Mannan, 2016). There may be limited access to legal representation or designated persons to enable supported decision-making as mandated under legislation which aims for compliance with the UN CRPD (Duffy & Kelly, 2019). As in other arenas, the passing of legislation or signing of conventions is insufficient in itself to protect human rights—there is a need for training and infrastructure, substantial investment in mental health and social services, and coordinated action by mental health professionals and advocacy organizations, alongside social and cultural change (Bartlett, 2010; Irmansyah et al., 2009). There is also a danger that legislation may be used primarily, and most effectively, as a means to enforce treatment rather than protect human rights (Spandler & Calton, 2009:248). Appeals against involuntary detention are rarely successful (Gosney & Lomax, 2017; Lund et al., 2012) and in practice legislation may reinforce inequalities and human rights abuses. Historically disadvantaged or minority groups, for example Black patients in the UK, are much more likely to be forcibly detained (Barnett et al., 2019) and less likely to win appeals (Nilforooshan et al., 2009). The extension of legally permitted forms of compulsion to community-based settings, such as community treatment orders (CTOs), is also highly controversial. CTOs involve significant deprivation of civil liberties through surveillance, coercion, and enforced medication, yet there is little evidence of their effectiveness in improving functioning, reducing symptoms, or preventing hospital admission (Kisely & Hall, 2014). While the WHO insists that hospital admission must serve a 'therapeutic purpose', i.e. not undertaken solely for custodial purposes (WHO, 2005), practices of confinement, such as 'seclusion rooms', can be recast as therapy as in the notion of 'isolement therapeutique' in France (Velpry & Eyraud, 2014) and 'time out' in the UK and US (Brodwin & Velpry, 2014). Similarly, an emphasis on disease-specific effects of antipsychotics, although based on questionable evidence, disguises their primary use as sedation (Moncrieff, 2013). The inherent paternalism of mental health services and power imbalances in clinical relationships risk forms of coercion being exercised even outside the legislative framework. This can range from a person not realizing they have a right to refuse treatment (WHO, 2005), to the use of threats, inducements, and persuasion. There is also what Szmukler (2015) calls psychiatry's 'coercive shadow' in which people may submit to treatment for fear of compulsion. Russo and Wallcraft (2011:218) point out that 'The context in which psychiatric treatment happens, and its potential to turn into forced treatment, means that the legal definition of coercion is much narrower than the coercion actually exerted'.

More fundamentally, it has been argued that the ways in which mental health legislation is framed, in which involuntary treatment can be predicated solely on the diagnosis of a mental disorder and 'preventive detention' can be justified on the grounds of risk, is inherently discriminatory since such provisions do not apply to other illnesses or disabilities. Szmukler and others (2014) advocate for a 'Fusion Law' based on decision-making capacity and 'best interests' regardless of cause. They argue that psychosis, which often follows a fluctuating course, does not fit easily with notions of 'disability', nor with legislation designed for persons with long-term or degenerative conditions which affect capacity, such as intellectual disabilities or dementia. As a consequence, some advocate the use of 'advance directives' in which people state their preferences for treatment and support in the event of a relapse (Duffy & Kelly, 2019; Saya et al., 2019). Others argue that 'legislative tinkering' evades the need for systemic change in the culture and practice of psychiatry (Sashidharan et al., 2019). This includes greater dialogic engagement with service users and families, investment in community-based crisis supports, and social interventions, enabling supported decision-making and addressing social determinants (Funk & Drew, 2019; Sashidharan et al., 2019; Sugiura et al., 2020).

Deinstitutionalization and community care

As previously outlined, deinstitutionalization began as a response to abuses within asylums and routine and prolonged confinement (Thornicroft & Bebbington, 1989). The discovery of chlorpromazine as a treatment for psychosis in the 1950s also promised more effective pharmacological treatment (Cohen et al., 2013). Community-based services and integrating mental health into primary healthcare became integral to WHO policy from the 1970s (Sartorius & Harding, 1983). Since the emergence of global mental health there has been renewed focus on 'task-shifting' to scale up access to treatment (Mendenhall et al., 2014; Patel et al., 2011). The WHO's mhGAP programme was developed to train non-specialist health workers in LMIC to identify mental disorders, including psychosis, and to treat and refer where needed (WHO, 2016). However, the vision of mental health in primary care has been poorly realized due to overstretched health services, limited funding, and lack of specialist workers to receive referrals and provide supervision (Jacob, 2017; Petersen et al., 2011). Community mental healthcare remains limited and uneven (Thornicroft et al., 2016). Lessons from the PRIME study underscore the need for supervision and support for non-specialist workers as well as adequate funding (Davies & Lund, 2017). This is particularly important, to provide quality community-based care for people with psychotic illness who often have complex support needs.

While more people with psychosis are living within communities than confined in institutions, there are concerns regarding the neglect and abandonment of people with psychosis, who may become homeless and isolated, vulnerable to stigma, social exclusion, exploitation, and abuse (Dudley et al., 2012). Where families provide the majority of care, without adequate support they may face additional stresses. Hussey and Manan (2016) argue that the Chinese mental health act effectively pushed care back into the hands of families who were not provided with any additional support. This led to the paradoxical effect of hospital admissions increasing because families were unable to cope. In some countries such as India, the closure of state-sponsored psychiatric hospitals has been accompanied by a rise in private facilities which are poorly regulated and can offer substandard and sometimes inhumane care (Davar, 2012). In 2016 in South Africa, in an attempt to cut costs and meet policy targets for deinstitutionalization, 1,711 people with severe mental illness and complex care needs were hurriedly transferred from long-stay specialist facilities to ill-equipped NGO-run homes. A total of 143 people died and many others were neglected and abused in what became known as the Life Edisimeni tragedy. Conditions in the homes included overcrowding, poor hygiene, insufficient food, a lack of qualified staff, and a lack of access to medicines (Durojaye & Agaba, 2018). A policy focus on community-based services has deflected investment and innovation from psychiatric hospitals where many people with psychosis will receive treatment in times of crisis, and where the risks of human rights violations are highest (Cohen & Minas, 2017). One consequence is that people with psychotic illness are increasingly dealt with by the criminal justice system and deprived of needed support and care (Fazel & Seewald, 2012; Gostin, 2008).

Concerns have also been expressed that community care policies and practice are often constructed around what Brodwin has called the 'assemblage of compliance' (2010), in particular with medication regimes (Spandler & Calton, 2009:248). This is evident in the introduction of CTOs and 'assertive treatment' (Kisely et al., 2017). While the use of involuntary treatment is predicated on arguments regarding the 'right to health' there are serious and potentially irreversible iatrogenic harms from psychopharmaceuticals, particularly those used for psychosis, including tardive dyskinesia, diabetes, weight gain, cardiac problems, and metabolic syndrome. Such disabling and stigmatizing effects may prevent social inclusion and participation (Spandler & Calton, 2009:251), have a major impact on quality of life, and considerably shorten the life span. The risk of such harms is likely to be higher where there is lack of supervision or regular review, assessment is cursory, and prescriptions may be inaccurate (Silove & Ward, 2014). A tendency to rely on high doses of antipsychotics to manage challenging behaviours, polypharmacy, and lack of access to non-pharmacological interventions, can all impact the quality of community-based care and the promotion of human rights (Patel & Bhui, 2018).

Furthermore, rights to health are indivisible from social, economic, civil, and political rights (UNHRC, 2019). For people with psychosis to live well in the community, decent housing and employment are paramount, alongside opportunities for broader social inclusion. However, these are often neglected as secondary to psychiatric intervention. As Dudley and colleagues (Dudley et al., 2012) point out, 'deinstitutionalization' and 'community care' are empty alternatives to coercion if there is not governmental, institutional, and community support for the full participation of those living in society (p. 50). Campaigners have argued not only for the right to be free from coercive treatment, but also for the right to access forms of support which lie outside the medical model of psychosis (Spandler & Calton, 2009). Innovative approaches such as 'Housing First' in Canada (Padgett et al., 2011) suggest ways in which funding and services could be re-purposed away from a narrow focus on treatment. Since its emergence in the 1990s (Anthony, 1993) there is an increasing policy emphasis on recovery-oriented approaches within mental health services, though to date this is primarily in high-income countries. This has been conceptualized as a collaborative approach between service users and mental health workers, which aims to foster connectedness, hope, meaning, empowerment, and identity through aspects such as peer support and involvement in meaningful social roles (Leamy et al., 2011). However, there are fears of the co-option of the recovery ethos which may reduce it to technical, service-focused interventions, rather than a radical approach to the organization of services and the relationship between services users and health professionals (Slade et al., 2014). There is also relatively little known about what recovery could mean in diverse settings (Slade et al., 2012). Emerging research from countries in the Global South and with minoritized ethnic groups in high-income settings suggests an emphasis on the value of work, relationships, and spirituality in perceptions of recovery and inclusion (Gopal et al., 2020; Leamy et al., 2011; McDonough & Colucci, 2019; Price-Robertson et al., 2016; Read et al., 2020; Yang et al., 2014).

Peer support, advocacy, and NGOs

The involvement of 'service users' or 'experts by experience' is now widely promoted in mental health policy and the delivery of services in recognition of what Cresswell (2009) calls 'experiential rights'. Activists within longstanding movements such as the World Network of Users and Survivors of Psychiatry (WNUSP) and Mindfreedom International claim recognition for the diversity of human experience, including 'madness', and have often taken a strongly antipsychiatry stance based on personal experience of enforced treatment (Oaks, 2012; Copeland et al., 2012). Since the 1990s the Hearing Voices Movement (Corstens et al., 2014), Soteria (Calton et al., 2008), and more recently Open Dialogue (Seikkula et al., 2001), among others, have argued for attention to the value and meaning of psychotic experience and for non-medical approaches including participatory interventions and alternatives to hospitalization. Self-advocacy and peer support have enormous potential to promote the human rights of people with psychosis. Activists have successfully challenged harmful and exclusionary practices, and persons with lived experience of psychosis are increasingly engaged in advocacy, peer support, research, and policy development. Over the last decade, self-advocacy and peer support has emerged within low-income settings. International campaigns aim to increase the involvement of service users and civil society groups in mental health policy and services and implementation of the CRPD (Funk et al., 2006; Kleintjes et al., 2013; Puschner et al., 2019).

However, there are risks that efforts to involve service users remain tokenistic and their influence on policy development can be constrained by established power imbalances (Ryan et al., 2019). There is also a danger that some forms of service user representation may exclude those in positions of relative disadvantage such as people with communication difficulties, people from minority groups, and those who do not conform to conventional narratives of disability, recovery, or 'survivorship' (Woods et al., 2019). As in the wider area of 'patient rights', there is an assumption that identities and solidarity can cohere around a disability or pathology to serve as a platform for support and advocacy. However, this is far from self-evident, particularly in relation to psychosis. Psychosis is not readily comparable to physical impairment and, under a disability rights model, arguments for social inclusion are predicated on the person accepting a diagnosis and the need for treatment. Some argue that their experiences do not constitute an illness at all but are on the continuum of human experience as meaningful responses to problems of living, trauma, racism, and spiritual or existential crisis (Spandler & Calton, 2009).

In low-income countries, where there are fewer formal services to support recovery and inclusion for people with severe mental illness (Iemmi et al., 2016), it has been argued that support needs can be met by families, communities, and civil society organizations, such as faith-based organizations and NGOs (Nguyen et al., 2019; Thornicroft et al., 2016; WHO, 2013). In recent years there has been an increase in the activities of NGOs in mental health in LMIC, often with an explicit rights focus. BasicNeeds, for example, frames access to sustainable livelihoods and social inclusion within a rights-based approach (Lund et al., 2013; Raja et al., 2012). However, stigma surrounding mental illness may reduce available support from families and communities. In addition, social, political, and economic changes can impact on the availability and sustainability of support, particularly in poorer communities where resources are already overstretched. Migration, relationship breakdown, and household poverty can all impact on the viability of family care (Duncan et al., 2011; MacGregor, 2018; Read, 2019; Thrush & Hyder, 2014). Furthermore, families and community agencies often operate in paternalistic ways that work to restrict the choices of people with psychosis (Zhu et al., 2018). Communities, NGOs, and civil society organizations may struggle to provide sustainable high-quality interventions without the support of health and social care systems (Thara et al., 2008). A lack of coordination between agencies, differing perspectives on human rights, proliferation of organizations, and divergence of perspectives may hinder communication and collaboration (Copeland et al., 2012). There are also challenges in monitoring and evaluating NGO interventions (Dudley et al., 2012).

Case studies

The following section provides examples of initiatives to promote and protect the human rights of people with psychosis in Ghana, Uganda, and Indonesia. These illustrate some of the issues discussed earlier. We highlight the aims of these projects and the successes and challenges in implementing them.

Mental health law reform in Ghana

Ghana has been the focus of considerable concern regarding the human rights of persons with mental illness after the publication of damning reports exposing conditions in healing churches (prayer camps) and shrines, including the widespread use of chaining, shackling, and forced fasting (CHRI, 2008; Ssengooba, 2012; United Nations, 2014).[2] Poor sanitation, overcrowding, and the punitive use of medication and seclusion in psychiatric hospitals were also noted. The most common diagnosis in these facilities is schizophrenia (Mental Health Authority, 2018). Colonial lunacy ordinances were replaced in 1978, but the new legislation was more concerned with regulating involuntary treatment than protecting and promoting broader rights (Lund et al., 2012). With support from the WHO, a new mental health act was passed in 2012 after several years of negotiation (Doku, 2012). The same year Ghana ratified the UN CRPD. The act makes ambitious commitments to protect the rights of persons with mental illness including establishing a visiting committee to oversee the activities of 'non-orthodox' healers and a shift to community-based mental healthcare. Despite this, the act permits involuntary treatment and substitute decision-making in cases where there is deemed to be a risk of harm or deterioration in health, albeit accompanied by rights of appeal through a mental health tribunal. The act has been widely praised and taken as an example of best practice for the African region (Alem & Manning, 2016). Since the passage of the act, there has been an expansion of community-based mental healthcare, with mental health workers in hospitals and clinics nationwide. As part of their role, they are mandated to conduct outreach to traditional and faith-based healers with the aim of reducing chaining and other abuses and to join forces in the care of people with mental illness (Draicchio, 2020; Read, 2019).

However mental health financing remains a low priority for the Ghanaian government and dedicated funding, mandated in the act, has yet to materialize. The psychiatric hospitals struggle to meet their running costs and lack basic supplies. The tribunal and visiting committee were not inaugurated until November 2022 with technical support from the Ghana Somubi Dwumadie programme funded by the UK government. There is resentment among some nurses who see the Mental Health Act as promoting patients' over nurses' rights, allowing patients to refuse treatment, and exposing nurses to greater risks (Read & Sakyi, 2017). Despite the proliferation in numbers, in the absence of ring-fenced funding most community mental health workers do not have access to transport, fuel, or telecommunications to visit more remote communities (Opare et al., 2020). Interventions, whether in hospital or the community, are primarily focused on dispensing medication (Agyapong et al., 2016) and enforced tranquilization remains commonplace (Jack et al., 2015). Indeed, this has become the point of entry for collaboration with healers where chemical sedation by mental health workers is framed as removing the need for chains (Read, 2019; Yaro et al., 2020). However, without transport and funding, nurses' efforts to establish such partnerships have been piecemeal and human rights abuses such as chaining continue (McVeigh, 2020; Read, 2019). In addition, pharmaceuticals are often unavailable in public health facilities and families must meet the cost on the open market as well as fees for hospital admission. This results in a high economic burden and associated stress for families (Opoku-Boateng et al., 2017). Many discontinue using mental health services and (re)turn to traditional and faith healers. In the absence of funding and infrastructure to fully implement the Mental Health Act, it has been deployed to forcibly detain homeless people suspected of mental illness in the psychiatric hospital (Read, 2020). This was justified under clauses of the act which permit emergency control and treatment of 'persons found in public places' judged to be 'highly aggressive or showing out of control behaviour'. These operations, which echo practices under the colonial lunacy ordinance, continue the function of psychiatry as a form of social control (Read, 2020).

The experiences of Ghana show that legislation alone can only go so far in protecting the human rights of people with psychosis without funding and infrastructure for implementation and a commitment to change at all levels. Indeed face-to-face mediation may be more acceptable than legal compulsion where there is a need to maintain vital care networks (Read, 2019). The introduction of WHO QualityRights in Ghana has gone some way to increase awareness of human rights and alternatives to coercion but significant investment in mental health and social services is needed to make a sustained impact (Funk & Drew Bold, 2020).

In recent years there has been growing involvement of persons with lived experience of psychotic illness as mental health advocates. They have opened up conversations on mental health on social and broadcast media, challenging stigma and discrimination and asserting their rights to be included as equal citizens. To date this advocacy has had limited reach beyond the English-speaking middle-classes in the urban centres. The challenge therefore is to reach the most excluded and engage policymakers and communities to ensure rights enshrined in the UN CRPD and the Mental Health Act are protected. This is not only in the arena of negative rights such as freedom from coercive treatment but also to promote social inclusion through, for example, ensuring workplaces make reasonable accommodations (Read et al., 2020).

Free from *pasung* in Indonesia

The Human Rights Watch report 'Living in Hell' (Human Rights Watch, 2016) highlighted that persons with mental illness, particularly schizophrenia and other psychotic disorders, face stigma and discrimination in Indonesia and are at risk of becoming victims of *pasung*. In Bahasa Indonesia, *pasung* literally means 'tie' or 'bind' and refers to forms of restraint or containment such as chaining and caging traditionally used in Indonesia for 'criminals, crazy and dangerously aggressive people' (Broch, 2001:303). Although the Indonesian government has banned *pasung* since 1977, it is estimated that in 2013 more than 57,000 people with psychosocial disability, mostly in rural Indonesia, were living under some form of *pasung* at the hands of their own families, traditional and religious healers, and psychiatric or social care institutions (Ministry of Health of the Republic of Indonesia, 2014; Diatri, 2014; Human Rights Watch, 2016). Most of the '*pasung* victims' received a diagnosis of schizophrenia (Minas & Diatri, 2008) and the duration of *pasung* ranges from three months to 30 years (Puteh et al., 2011; Suryani et al., 2011). As also shown in the ethnographic documentary 'Breaking the Chains' (Colucci, 2015; Colucci, 2016), *pasung* is usually the result of an inadequate mental health system; unaffordable, ineffective, and difficult to access treatments; uncoordinated if not conflicting therapeutic approaches to 'mental healthcare' (i.e. traditional/spiritual vs. biomedical interventions); and a general lack of reinforcement of human rights and health legislations (Anto & Colucci, 2015; Irmansyah et al., 2009; Minas & Diatri, 2008; Puteh et al., 2011).

Pasung and abusive treatment of people with mental illness breaches national as well as international legislation, including the CRPD which was ratified by the Indonesian government in 2011. The Indonesian government has recognized *pasung* as an 'inhuman and discriminatory' treatment and has committed to its elimination through a programme called *Indonesia Bebas Pasung* (Indonesia Free from *Pasung*). This initiative by the Indonesian Ministry of Health followed the localized programme *Aceh Bebas Pasung*, which was initiated by the governor of Aceh in 2010. The programme focuses on raising awareness about mental health and *pasung*, integrating mental healthcare into primary healthcare by providing psychotropic medication within *puskesmas* (i.e. primary healthcare centres), training health workers to identify and diagnose basic mental disorders, and creating community mental health teams that act as a coordination mechanism between the Department of Health and other departments at the provincial and district levels to monitor and facilitate the release of people from *pasung* (Ministry of Health of the Republic of Indonesia, 2014). These components were implemented in a stepped manner, starting with regulation and problem mapping in 2010, followed by capacity building to strengthen human resources, psychotropic drug distribution and building commitment from the multiple sectors involved (MHInnovation, 2016). Six major enabling elements were identified that needed to be developed to ensure the successful implementation and sustainability of this programme including:

legislation and policy; adequate financing; intersectoral collaboration; advocacy and community (including service users and family) empowerment; and human resource development (MHInnovation, 2016).

Despite the launch of these programmes across the country and the protections available in legislation, including the Mental Health Act passed in 2014 and the recent Law No. 8/2016 on Persons with Disabilities, violations of the basic rights of people with mental illness remain widespread. The Indonesian government has missed its target to eradicate *pasung* by 2020 (the original deadline was 2014, then moved to 2017) due also to the lack of funding (currently only 1% of the total health budget) and human resources (Diatri, 2014). For instance, the ministerial decree regulating primary and community health centres mandates that all centres provide mental health services. However, only about 30% of over 9,000 *puskesmas* across the country have programmes for mental health and this often consists of only one nurse with basic mental health training and shortage or absence of psychotropic drugs (Human Rights Watch, 2016). Furthermore, the recent mental health and disability legislation still fails to guarantee full legal capacity for persons with psychosocial disabilities and to meet the standards set by CRPD (Human Rights Watch, 2016).

The prevalence of mental illness in Indonesia is high (estimated at 11% for the entire country) with an estimated one million people with psychosis (Diatri, 2014). There are only 48 mental health institutions concentrated mainly in four provinces (Diatri, 2016), and community/primary mental healthcare is understaffed and under-resourced. Therefore, the use of *pasung* seems unlikely to subside without intensive education campaigns, community-based initiatives, and substantial investments in mental health services. Nevertheless, the recent legal advancements and *Bebas Pasung* programmes are of great significance because they are examples of the actions necessary to eliminate such human rights abuses and governments assuming responsibility for taking those actions. To date, 21 out of 34 provinces have launched their *Bebas Pasung* activities, in addition to the 12 'rapid response' teams attached to 20 *pantis* (social care institutions run by the Social Affairs Ministry) across the country that conduct community outreach activities, reaching more than 8,000 people in *pasung* (Diatri, 2016; Human Rights Watch, 2016).

As observed by Puteh and colleagues, the *Bebas Pasung* programmes represent 'an important mental health and human rights initiative that can serve to inform similar efforts in other parts of Indonesia and other LMICs where restraint and confinement of the mentally ill is receiving insufficient attention' (2011:1). However, 'top down' approaches that focus on the development of legislation and policies to protect human rights and provide better mental healthcare have a limited impact on their own (Irmansyah et al., 2009), especially when legislation is not tied to significant government investment in appropriate decentralized services (Nurjannah et al., 2015) and community education programmes. The new Indonesian national mental health plan currently under development will hopefully address some of these challenges.

Peer support in Uganda

As mentioned previously, recovery is an approach that has gained some credibility in promoting the human rights and social inclusion of people with psychosis in high-income countries but is poorly tested in LMIC.[3]

Ugandan mental health services have taken steps to introduce the recovery approach in collaboration with the Butabika East London Link (BELL) in the UK, a longstanding link between the East London NHS Foundation Trust and Butabika Hospital, the largest psychiatric hospital in Uganda. The link was established in 2004 with the aim of developing the capacity of Ugandan mental health services to offer high-quality treatment. A key initiative of this link has been the Brain Gain programme, funded by the British Department for International Development (DFID), which focused on the introduction of Peer Support Work (PSW) alongside existing mental health services. The first Brain Gain project in 2011 trialled the concept of PSW predominantly in community-based settings. Brain Gain 2 in 2014 was scaled up to include more clients and operate in ward environments and more thorough efforts were made to evaluate the impact. This included an analysis of readmission rates, as well as the impact on disability, satisfaction, and social outcomes. With a greater presence and role within Butabika Hospital, there was recognition that for PSW to be effective, an environment that welcomed the expertise of people with lived experience of mental illness, including psychosis, would need to be fostered.

To this end, the Brain Gain 2 programme included the development of the Butabika Recovery College (BREC). Recovery colleges were initially developed in the US and introduced into UK mental health services in the last decade. They employ an educational rather than therapeutic orientation, and focus on developing skills, rather than highlighting deficits. They involve people with experience of mental illness, including psychosis, as peer tutors who share their skills (Perkins et al., 2012). BREC was designed to offer a focal point by which service users could develop a curriculum of training and education related to recovery and the skills to deliver this. Brain Gain 2 provided a group of UK service users and staff trainers to coproduce sessions on key recovery topics and training, including adult learning, lesson planning, and evaluation skills.

Educators, clinicians, and service users linked to Lancaster University in the UK were enlisted to develop a process by which Ugandan service users could clarify their own perspective of recovery (Parker, 2015). The initial 'listening event' highlighted key concerns in recovery in Uganda. Recovery was deemed to be about 'freedom' to make choices and opportunities to participate in family and community life. The impact of alienation from economic opportunity also loomed large with poverty seen as a major hindrance to recovery. Not being able to meet responsibilities to others and helping to financially support family members was particularly problematic as was generally not being productive. Attention was also paid to ensuring families are knowledgeable about mental health and involved in the process of recovery and support. There were several aspects of religious teachings and spirituality that participants identified as being helpful in recovery, including belief in a divine plan, perseverance, and being equal in the eyes of God. It was also recognized that working collaboratively with religious leaders might be a positive way to empower communities to support participants with mental health problems effectively. Other key elements of recovery included raising awareness of mental health issues at all levels of society, from local communities to political leaders, challenging stigma and discrimination, influencing policy, and being included in decision-making.

Since its inception, the BREC has delivered weekly classes to over 1,000 patients, the majority of whom have experiences of psychotic illness, and 240 staff at Butabika Hospital. They demonstrate a fluency not only in describing the experience of recovery from a local perspective, but skills and capacity to teach and explore these subjects in more depth. Peer trainers provide a weekly timetable of sessions, including a Hearing Voices group, and also assist with transporting inpatients to attend the college. Alongside the peer trainers of the BREC, there have been several cohorts of peer support workers trained. The training was provided by UK health and service user professionals in conjunction with peer workers/peer trainers from the Brain Gain 1 pilot. Peer support workers regularly visit the Butabika Hospital to link with patients whom they then follow up with in the community, usually making at least three visits to a person's home following discharge.

The hostility of some mental health workers during the initial pilot has faded and for the most part, the Peer Support Workers are a welcome part of the hospital team. They have also developed a close working relationship with the Community Recovery Team which provides community-based mental healthcare in Kampala and staff and peer support workers often visit clients together. That said, PSW is often perceived by senior health workers as a singular intervention, rather than a source of expertise that could transform the hospital system and the Ministry of Health has yet to commit to providing equitable remuneration to peer support workers. Several service user leaders are included on the management team for Brain Gain 2. However, they are confined to the Brain Gain programme rather than the institution at large. Peer support workers and peer trainers at BREC have recently set up 'Peer Nation', an independent service user group.[4] Significant human rights concerns remain. Bullying and violence towards patients are endemic within the overcrowded wards of Butabika Hospital. Peer support workers and peer trainers have highlighted these injustices and are involved in actions to advocate for change. Peer support workers have also identified instances of churches using physical restraint and have provided education and advocacy for people to access mental health services if needed.

Overall, the implementation of a recovery-oriented approach in the Ugandan setting has yielded a steady increase in staff and institutional support for service user leadership in challenging stigma and poor practice. The impact is being felt farther afield as peer trainers have gone on to train staff and service users in other regions of the country. Early reports suggest that these newly trained peer support workers have been active in promoting a compassionate and positive approach to mental healthcare. Not only has the approach yielded promising direct outcomes but the ownership by service users of key activities of delivery and dissemination is congruent with Ugandan recovery narratives of the need for empowerment and thus may have secondary benefits for those involved. The impact of the programme is being formally evaluated alongside other peer support interventions in LMIC as part of the UPSIDES project (Puschner et al., 2019).

Conclusion

This chapter has provided an overview of human rights concerns for people with psychotic illness and various initiatives to address these by international agencies, national governments, and communities, including people with lived experience of mental illness. It is evident that significant challenges remain. Coercive responses remain institutionalized within psychiatric services and in some countries are increasing rather than declining (Sheridan Rains et al., 2019). In other contexts, people with psychosis continue to be routinely chained and neglected. Mental health financing remains a low priority for many governments and rising inequality exposes marginalized and disadvantaged groups to the greatest risk of both coercion and neglect. The initiatives outlined in this chapter, including greater involvement of people with lived experience of mental illness at all levels of mental health research, policy development, service delivery, and advocacy, suggest positive directions for addressing these concerns. Meeting the vision of rights described in the UN CRPD requires a more honest engagement with the 'ethical limits' (Brodwin & Velpry, 2014) of psychiatric treatments. Ultimately protecting and promoting the human rights of people with psychosis goes beyond reducing coercion and improving access to treatment, to holistic action to address the social and structural determinants of mental health and ensure the promotion and protection of social, economic, political, and civil rights (UNHRC, 2019).

Notes

1. 'Together for Mental Health' is funded through the ESRC/AHRC Global Challenges Research Fund (Grant Ref: ES/S00114X/1). The co-authors, who are partially funded through this grant, gratefully acknowledge their support. For more information see https://movie-ment.org/together4mh/.

2. This section is based on research conducted in Ghana by the first author and Lionel Sakyi in 2015–16 for the European Research Council project 'From International to Global: Knowledge, Diseases and the Postwar Government of Health' (grant number: 340510), in 2017–19 as part of the Mental Health and Justice project funded by the Wellcome Trust (grant number: 203376/Z/16/Z) and in 2019 by both authors and Lily Kpobi as part of 'Together for Mental Health' (see note 1).

3. This section was written with Cerdic Hall, Nurse Consultant, Camden and Islington NHS Foundation Trust, Butabika East London Link.

4. http://www.peernation.org Home 1.

References

Adepoju, P. (2023). New legislation to overhaul mental health care in Nigeria. *Lancet*, *401*(10373), 257.

Agyapong, V. I., et al. (2016). Task shifting-perception of stake holders about adequacy of training and supervision for community mental health workers in Ghana. *Health Policy Plan*, *31*(5), 645–655.

Alem, A. & Manning, C. (2016). Coercion in community mental health care: African perspectives. In **Molodynski, A., Rugkasa, J., & Burns, T.** (eds) *Coercion in community mental health care: international perspectives*. Oxford: Oxford University Press, Chapter 19, 301–314.

Anthony, W. A. (1993). Recovery from mental illness: the guiding vision of the mental health service system in the 1990s. *Int J Psychosoc Rehabilitation*, *16*(4), 11–23.

Anto, S. G. & Colucci, E. (2015). Free from pasung: a story of chaining and freedom in Indonesia told through painting, poetry and narration. *World Cult Psychiatry Res Rev*, *10*(34), 149–167.

Asher, L., et al. (2017). 'I cry every day and night, I have my son tied in chains': physical restraint of people with schizophrenia in community settings in Ethiopia. *Global Health*, *13*(1), 47.

Barnett, P. E., et al. (2019). Ethnic variations in compulsory detention under the Mental Health Act: a systematic review and meta-analysis of international data. *Lancet Psychiatry*, *6*(4), 305–317.

Bartlett, P. (2010). Thinking about the rest of the world: mental health and rights outside the 'first world'. In McSherry, B. & Weller, P. (eds) *Re-thinking rights-based mental health law*. Oxford: Oxford Academic, 397–418.

Bourque, F., van der Ven, E., & Malla, A. (2011). A meta-analysis of the risk for psychotic disorders among first- and second-generation immigrants. *Psychol Med*, *41*(5), 897–910.

Broch, H. B. (2001). The villagers' reactions towards craziness: an Indonesian example. *Transcult Psychiatry*, *38*(3), 275–305.

Brodwin, P. (2010). The assemblage of compliance in psychiatric case management. *Anthropol Med*, *17*(2), 129–143.

Brodwin, P. & Velpry, L. (2014). The practice of constraint in psychiatry: emergent forms of care and control. *Cult Med Psychiatry*, *38*(4), 524–526.

Burns, J. K., Tomita, A., & Kapadia, A. S. (2014). Income inequality and schizophrenia: increased schizophrenia incidence in countries with high levels of income inequality. *Int J Soc Psychiatry*, *60*(2), 185–196.

Calton, T., et al. (2008). A systematic review of the Soteria paradigm for the treatment of people diagnosed with schizophrenia. *Schizophr Bull*, *34*(1), 181–192.

CHRI (2008). *Human rights violations in prayer camps and access to mental health in Ghana*. Accra: Commonwealth Human Rights Initiative Africa.

Cohen, A, Patel, V., & Minas, H. (2013). A brief history of global mental health. In Prince, M. J., Cohen, A., Minas, H., & Patel, V. (eds) *Global mental health: principles and practice*. Oxford: Oxford University Press, Chapter 1, 3–26.

Cohen, A., & Minas, H. (2017). Global mental health and psychiatric institutions in the 21st century. *Epidemiol Psychiatr Sci*, *26*(1), 4–9.

Cohen, A., et al. (2016). Concepts of madness in diverse settings: a qualitative study from the INTREPID project. *BMC Psychiatry*, *16*(1), 388.

Colucci, E. (2021a). *Harmoni: Healing together*. London: Royal Anthropological Institute/Movie-ment.

Colucci, E. (2021b). *Nkabom: A little medicine, a little prayer*. London: Royal Anthropological Institute/Movie-ment.

Colucci, E. (2015). *Breaking the chains*. London: Royal Anthropological Institute/Movie-ment

Colucci, E. (2016). 'Breaking the chains': ethnographic film-making in mental health. *Lancet Psychiatry 3*(6), 509–510.

Copeland, J., et al. (2012). The role of world associations and the United Nations. In Dudley, M., Silove, D., & Gale, F. (eds) *Mental health and human rights*. Oxford: Oxford University Press, Chapter 32, 554–565.

Corstens, D., E., et al. (2014). Emerging perspectives from the hearing voices movement: implications for research and practice. *Schizophr Bull*, *40* Suppl 4, S285–S294.

Cresswell, M. (2009). Psychiatric survivors and experiential rights. *Soc Policy Soc*, *8*(02), 231–243.

Davar, B V. (2012). Legal frameworks for and against people with psychosocial disabilities. *Econ Polit Wkly*, *47*(52), 123–131.

Davies, T. & Lund, C. (2017). Integrating mental health care into primary care systems in low—and middle-income countries: lessons from PRIME and AFFIRM. *Glob Ment Health*, *4*, e7.

De Hert, M, C. U., et al. (2011). Physical illness in patients with severe mental disorders. I. Prevalence, impact of medications and disparities in health care. *World Psychiatry*, 10(1), 52–77.

Desjarlais, R., et al. (1995). *World mental health: problems and priorities in low-income countries*. New York; Oxford: Oxford University Press.

Diatri, H. (2014). Indonesia aims to free the mentally ill from their shackles. *The Conversation*. Retrieved from https://theconversation.com/indonesia-aims-to-free-the-mentally-ill-from-their-shackles-30078

Diatri, H. (2016). How can Indonesia free the mentally ill from shackles once and for all? *The Conversation*. Retrieved from https://theconversation.com/how-can-indonesia-free-the-mentally-ill-from-shackles-once-and-for-all-57185

Doku, V. C. K. (2012). Implementing the Mental Health Act in Ghana: any challenges ahead? *Ghana Med J*, 46(4), 241–250.

Draicchio, C. (2020). 'Extraordinary conditions' and experiments with collaboration in 'zones of social abandonment'. Mental health care between psychiatry and prayer camps in rural Ghana. *Politique Africaine*, 157, 165–182.

Drew, N., et al. (2011). Human rights violations of people with mental and psychosocial disabilities: an unresolved global crisis. *Lancet*, 378(9803), 1664–1675.

Dudley, M., Silove, D., & Gale, F. (2012). Mental health, human rights, and their relationship: an introduction. In **Dudley, M., Silove, D., & Gale, F.** (eds) *Mental health and human rights*. Oxford: Oxford University Press.1–49.

Duffy, R. M. & Kelly, B. D. (2019). India's Mental Healthcare Act, 2017: content, context, controversy. *Int J Law Psychiatry*, 62, 169–178.

Duncan, M., Swartz, L., & Kathard, H. (2011). The burden of psychiatric disability on chronically poor households: part 1 (costs). *S Afr J Occup Ther*, 41(3), 55–63.

Durojaye, E. & Agaba, D. K. (2018). Contribution of the health ombud to accountability: the life Esidimeni tragedy in South Africa. *Health Hum Rights*, 20(2), 161–168.

Ebuenyi, I. D., et al. (2018). Barriers to and facilitators of employment for people with psychiatric disabilities in Africa: a scoping review. *Glob Health Action*, 11(1), 1463658.

Fakhoury, W. & Priebe, S. (2002). The process of deinstitutionalization: an international overview. *Curr Opin Psychiatry*, 15(2), 187–192.

Fazel, S. & Seewald, K. (2012). Severe mental illness in 33,588 prisoners worldwide: systematic review and meta-regression analysis. *Br J Psychiatry*, 200(5), 364–373.

Freeman, M. C., et al. (2015). Reversing hard won victories in the name of human rights: a critique of the General Comment on Article 12 of the UN Convention on the Rights of Persons with Disabilities. *Lancet Psychiatry*, 2(9), 844–850.

Funk, M. & Drew Bold, N. (2020). WHO's quality rights initiative: transforming services and promoting rights in mental health. *Health Hum Rights*, 22(1), 69–75.

Funk, M. & Drew, N. (2019). Practical strategies to end coercive practices in mental health services. *World Psychiatry*, 18(1), 43–44.

Funk, M., et al. (2006). Advocacy for mental health: roles for consumer and family organizations and governments. *Health Promot Int*, 21(1), 70–75.

Gerlinger, G., et al. (2013). Personal stigma in schizophrenia spectrum disorders: a systematic review of prevalence rates, correlates, impact and interventions. *World Psychiatry*, 12(2), 155–164.

Giannakopoulos, G., & Anagnostopoulos, D. C. (2016). Psychiatric reform in Greece: an overview. *BJPsych Bull, 40*(6), 326–328.

Gopal, S., et al. (2020). What constitutes recovery in schizophrenia? Client and caregiver perspectives from South India. *Int J Soc Psychiatry, 66*(2), 118–123.

Gosney, P. & Lomax, P. (2017). Re: mental health: patients and service in crisis. *BMJ, 356*, j1141.

Gostin, L. O. (2008). 'Old' and 'new' institutions for persons with mental illness: treatment, punishment or preventive confinement? *Public Health, 122*(9), 906–913.

Gureje, O., et al. (2015). The role of global traditional and complementary systems of medicine in the treatment of mental health disorders. *Lancet Psychiatry, 2*(2), 168–177.

Halvorsrud, K., et al. (2018). Ethnic inequalities and pathways to care in psychosis in England: a systematic review and meta-analysis. *BMC Med, 16*(1), 223.

Heaton, M. M. (2013). *Black skin, white coats: Nigerian psychiatrists, decolonization, and the globalization of psychiatry.* Athens: Ohio University Press.

Human Rights Watch (2016). *Living in hell: abuses against people with psychosocial disabilities in Indonesia.* New York: Human Rights Watch.

Hussey, M. M. & Mannan, H. (2016). China's mental health law: analysis of core concepts of human rights and inclusion of vulnerable groups. *DCID, 26*(4), 117–137.

Iemmi, V., et al. (2016). Community-based rehabilitation for people with physical and mental disabilities in low- and middle-income countries: a systematic review and meta-analysis. *J Dev Eff, 8*(3), 368–387.

Irmansyah, I., Prasetyo, Y. A., & Minas, H. (2009). Human rights of persons with mental illness in Indonesia: more than legislation is needed. *Int J Ment Health Syst, 3*(1), 14.

Jack, H., et al. (2015). Aggression in mental health settings: a case study in Ghana. *Bull World Health Organ, 93*(8), 587–588.

Jacob, K. S. (2017). Mental health services in low-income and middle-income countries. *Lancet Psychiatry, 4*(2), 87–89.

Jenkins, R., et al. (2011). Social, economic, human rights and political challenges to global mental health. *Ment Health Fam Med, 8*(2), 87–96.

Keller, R. C. (2005). Pinel in the Maghreb: liberation, confinement, and psychiatric reform in French North Africa. *Bull Hist Med, 79*(3), 459–499.

Kelly, B. D. (2005). Structural violence and schizophrenia. *Soc Sci Med, 61*(3), 721–730.

Kirmayer, L. J. (2012). Culture and context in human rights. In Dudley, M., Silove, D., & Gale, F. (eds) *Mental health and human rights: vision, praxis and courage.* Oxford: Oxford University Press, Chapter 4, 95–112.

Kisely, S. & Hall, K. (2014). An updated meta-analysis of randomized controlled evidence for the effectiveness of community treatment orders. *Can J Psychiatry, 59*(10), 561–564.

Kisely, S. R., Campbell, L. A., & O'Reilly, R. (2017). Compulsory community and involuntary outpatient treatment for people with severe mental disorders. *Cochrane Database Syst Rev, 3*, CD004408.

Kleinman, A. (2009). Global mental health: a failure of humanity. *Lancet, 374*(9690), 603–604.

Kleintjes, S., Lund, C., & Swartz, L. (2013). Organising for self-advocacy in mental health: experiences from seven African countries. *Afr J Psychiatry (Johannesbg), 16*(3), 187–195.

Kpobi, L., et al. (in press). 'We are all working toward one goal. We want people to become well': a visual exploration of what promotes successful collaboration between community mental health workers and healers in Ghana. *Transcultural Psychiatry*.

Lancet Global Mental Health Group (2007). Scale up services for mental disorders: a call for action. *Lancet*, *370*(9594), 1241–1252.

Leamy, M., et al. (2011). Conceptual framework for personal recovery in mental health: systematic review and narrative synthesis. *Br J Psychiatry*, *199*(6), 445–452.

Littlewood, R., Jadhav, S., & Ryder, A. G. (2007). A cross-national study of the stigmatization of severe psychiatric illness: historical review, methodological considerations and development of the questionnaire. *Transcult Psychiatry*, *44*(2), 171–202.

Liu, N. H., et al. (2017). Excess mortality in persons with severe mental disorders: a multilevel intervention framework and priorities for clinical practice, policy and research agendas. *World Psychiatry*, *16*(1), 30–40.

Lund, C., et al. (2013). Outcomes of the mental health and development model in rural Kenya: a 2-year prospective cohort intervention study. *Int Health*, *5*(1), 43–50.

Lund, C., et al. (2012). Protecting the rights of the mentally ill in poorly resourced settings: experiences from four African countries. In Dudley, M., Silove, D., & Gale, F. (eds) *Mental health and human rights, vision, praxis and courage*. Oxford: Oxford University Press.527–537.

MacGregor, H. (2018). Mental health and the maintenance of kinship in South Africa. *Medical Anthropology*, *37*(7), 597–610.

Mahone, S. (2006). Psychiatry in the East African colonies: a background to confinement. *Int Rev Psychiatry*, *18*(4), 327–332.

Maj, M. (2009). Physical health care in persons with severe mental illness: a public health and ethical priority. *World Psychiatry*, *8*(1), 1–2.

Maj, M. (2011). The rights of people with mental disorders: WPA perspective. *Lancet*, *378*(9802), 1534–1535.

Mari, J. J. & Thornicroft, G. (2010). Principles that should guide mental health policies in low- and middle-income countries. *Rev Bras Psiquiatr*, *32*(3), 210–211.

McDonough, S. & Colucci, E. (2019). People of immigrant and refugee background sharing experiences of mental health recovery: reflections and recommendations on using digital storytelling. *Vis Commun*, *20*(1), 1470357218820651.

McVeigh, T. (2020). 'All we can offer is the chain': the scandal of Ghana's shackled sick. *The Guardian*, 3 Feb 2020. Retrieved from https://www.theguardian.com/global-developm ent/2020/feb/03/all-we-can-offer-is-the-chain-the-scandal-of-ghanas-shackled-sick

Mendenhall, E., et al. (2014). Acceptability and feasibility of using non-specialist health workers to deliver mental health care: stakeholder perceptions from the PRIME district sites in Ethiopia, India, Nepal, South Africa, and Uganda. *Soc Sci Med*, *118*, 33–42.

Mental Health Authority (2018). 2017 annual report.

Mental Health Innovation Network. Chain-free pasung program. Retrieved from http://www.mhinnovation.net/innovations/chain-free-pasung-program

Minas, H. & Diatri, H. (2008). Pasung: physical restraint and confinement of the mentally ill in the community. *Int J Ment Health Syst*, *2*(1), 8.

Ministry of Health of the Republic of Indonesia (2014). 'Stop Stigma and Discrimination to People with "Mental Disorder"'. 'Menuju Indonesia Bebas Pasung (Towards a shackle-free Indonesia)'.

Minkowitz, T. (2007). The United Nations convention on the rights of persons with disabilities and the right to be free from noncensensual psychiatric interventions. *Syracuse Journal of International Law and Commerce, 34*(2), 405–428.

Moncrieff, J. (2013). *The bitterest pills: the troubling story of antipsychotic drugs.* London: Palgrave Macmillan.

Murthy, S. R. (2001). Lessons from the Erwadi tragedy for mental health care in India. *Indian J Psychiatry, 43*(4), 362–366.

Nadkarni, A., et al. (2015). The management of adult psychiatric emergencies in low-income and middle-income countries: a systematic review. *Lancet Psychiatry, 2*(6), 540–547.

Nguyen, T., et al. (2019). Informal mental health interventions for people with severe mental illness in low and lower middle-income countries: a systematic review of effectiveness. *Int J Soc Psychiatry, 65*(3), 194–206.

Nilforooshan, R., Amin, R., & Warner, J. (2009). Ethnicity and outcome of appeal after detention under the Mental Health Act 1983. *Psychiatr Bull, 33*(8), 288–290.

Nurjannah, I., et al. (2015). Human rights of the mentally ill in Indonesia. *Int Nurs Rev, 62*(2), 153–161.

Oaks, D. W. (2012). Whose voices should be heard? The role of mental health consumers, psychiatric survivors, and families. In **Dudley, M., Silove, D., & Gale, F.** (eds) *Mental health and human rights: vision, praxis, and courage.* Oxford: Oxford University Press, Chapter 33, 566–577.

Opare, F. Y., et al. (2020). 'We try our best to offer them the little that we can' coping strategies of Ghanaian community psychiatric nurses: a qualitative descriptive study. *BMC Nurs, 19,* 56.

Opoku-Boateng, Y. N., et al. (2017). Economic cost and quality of life of family caregivers of schizophrenic patients attending psychiatric hospitals in Ghana. *BMC Health Serv Res, 17*(Suppl 2), 697.

Padgett, D. K., et al. (2011). Substance use outcomes among homeless clients with serious mental illness: comparing housing first with treatment first programs. *Commun Ment Health J, 47*(2), 227–232.

Patel, V., et al. (2011). A renewed agenda for global mental health. *Lancet, 378*(9801), 1441–1442.

Patel, V. & Bhui, K. (2018). Unchaining people with mental disorders: medication is not the solution. *Br J Psychiatry, 212*(01), 6–8.

Pearce, J., et al. (2019). Perceived discrimination and psychosis: a systematic review of the literature. *Soc Psychiatry Psychiatr Epidemiol, 54*(9), 1023–1044.

Perkins, R., et al. (2012). *Recovery colleges.* London: Centre for Mental Health; Mental Health Network NHS Confederation.

Petersen, I., Lund, C., & Stein, D. J. (2011). Optimizing mental health services in low-income and middle-income countries. *Curr Opin Psychiatry, 24*(4), 318–323.

Porter, R. (2006). *Madmen: a social history of madhouses, mad-doctors and lunatics.* Stroud: Tempus Publishing Limited. Original edition, 1987.

Price-Robertson, R., Obradovic, A., & Morgan, B. (2016). Relational recovery: beyond individualism in the recovery approach. *Adv Ment Health*, *15*(2), 108–120.

Puras, D., & Gooding, P. (2019). Mental health and human rights in the 21st century. *World Psychiatry*, *18*(1), 42–43.

Puschner, B., et al. (2019). Using peer support in developing empowering mental health services (UPSIDES): background, rationale and methodology. *Ann Glob Health*, *85*(1), 53.

Puteh, I., Marthoenis, M., & Minas, H. (2011). Aceh free pasung: releasing the mentally ill from physical restraint. *Int J Ment Health Syst*, 5, 10.

Raboch, J., et al. (2010). Use of coercive measures during involuntary hospitalization: findings from ten European countries. *Psychiatr Serv*, *61*(10), 1012–1017.

Raja, S., et al. (2012). Integrating mental health and development: a case study of the BasicNeeds Model in Nepal. *PLOS Med*, *9*(7), e1001261.

Read, J., et al. (2006). Prejudice and schizophrenia: a review of the 'mental illness is an illness like any other' approach. *Acta Psychiatr Scand*, *114*(5), 303–318.

Read, U. M. (2019). 'It is left to me and my God': precarity, responsibility and social change in family care for mental illness in Ghana. *Africa Today*, *65*(3), 3–28.

Read, U. M. (2020). 'Clearing the streets': enacting human rights in mental health care in Ghana. In Gaudilliere, J.-P., Beaudevin, C., Gradmann, C., Lovell, A. M., & Pordié, L. (eds) *Global health and the new world order: historical and anthropological approaches to a changing regime of governance*. Manchester: Manchester University Press, 103–129.

Read, U. M., Adiibokah, E., & Nyame, S. (2009). Local suffering and the global discourse of mental health and human rights: an ethnographic study of responses to mental illness in rural Ghana. *Global Health*, *5*(1), 13.

Read, U. M. & Sakyi, L. (2017). The right to care: mobilising rights in the care of people with mental illness in Ghana. Canadian Anthropology Society/International Union of Anthropological and Ethnographic Sciences Conference. Canada: University of Ottawa.

Read, U. M, Sakyi, L., & Abbey, W. (2020). Exploring the potential of a rights-based approach to work and social inclusion for people with lived experience of mental illness in Ghana. *Health Hum Rights*, *22*(1), 91–104.

Read, U. M. (2019). Rights as relationships: collaborating with faith healers in community mental health in Ghana. *Cult Med*, *43*(4), 613–635.

Rosen, A., Rosen, T., & McGorry, P. (2012). The human rights of people with severe and persistent mental illness. In Dudley, M., Silove, D., & Gale, F. (eds) *Mental health and human rights*. Oxford: Oxford University Press, 297.

Rugkasa, J. (2016). Family carers and coercion in the community. In Molodynski, A., Rugkasa, J., & Burns, J. (eds) *Coercion in community mental health care: international perspectives*. Oxford: Oxford University Press, 161–178.

Russo, J. & Wallcraft, J. (2011). Resisting variables—service user/survivor perspectives on researching coercion. In Kallert, T. W., Mezzich, J. E., & Monahan, J. (eds) *Coercive treatment in psychiatry: clinical, legal and ethical aspects*. Hoboken, NJ: John Wiley & Sons, 213–234.

Ryan, G. K., et al. (2019). Service user involvement in global mental health: what have we learned from recent research in low and middle-income countries? *Curr Opin Psychiatry*, *32*(4), 355–360.

Sartorius, N. & Harding, T. W. (1983). The WHO collaborative study on strategies for extending mental health care, I: the genesis of the study. *Am J Psychiatry, 140*(11), 1470–1473.

Sashidharan, S. P., Mezzina, R., & Puras, D. (2019). Reducing coercion in mental healthcare. *Epidemiol Psychiatr Sci, 28*(6), 605–612.

Saya, A., et al. (2019). Criteria, procedures, and future prospects of involuntary treatment in psychiatry around the world: a narrative review. *Front Psychiatry, 10*, 271.

Schomerus, G., et al. (2012). Evolution of public attitudes about mental illness: a systematic review and meta-analysis. *Acta Psychiatr Scand, 125*(6), 440–452.

Seikkula, J., Alakare, B., & Aaltonen, J. (2001). Open dialogue in psychosis I: an introduction and case illustration. *J Constr Psychol, 14*(4), 247–265.

Sheridan Rains, L., et al. (2019). Variations in patterns of involuntary hospitalisation and in legal frameworks: an international comparative study. *Lancet Psychiatry, 6*(5), 403–417.

Silove, D. & Ward, P. B. (2014). Challenges in rolling out interventions for schizophrenia. *Lancet, 383*(9926), 1362–1364.

Slade, M., et al. (2014). Uses and abuses of recovery: implementing recovery-oriented practices in mental health systems. *World Psychiatry, 13*(1), 12–20.

Slade, M., et al. (2012). International differences in understanding recovery: systematic review. *Epidemiol Psychiatr Sci, 21*(4), 353–364.

Spandler, H. & Calton, T. (2009). Psychosis and human rights: conflicts in mental health policy and practice. *Soc Policy Soc, 8*(02), 245–256.

Ssengooba, M. (2012). 'Like a death sentence': abuses against persons with mental disabilities in Ghana. Human rights watch. Retrieved from https://www.hrw.org/report/2012/10/02/death-sentence/abuses-against-persons-mental-disabilities-ghana

Suetani, S., Whiteford, H. A., & McGrath, J. J. (2015). An urgent call to address the deadly consequences of serious mental disorders. *JAMA Psychiatry, 72*(12), 1166–1167.

Sugiura, K., et al. (2020). An end to coercion: rights and decision-making in mental health care. *Bull World Health Organ, 98*(1), 52–58.

Suryani, L. K., Lesmana, C. B., & Tiliopoulos, N. (2011). Treating the untreated: applying a community-based, culturally sensitive psychiatric intervention to confined and physically restrained mentally ill individuals in Bali, Indonesia. *Eur Arch Psychiatry Clin Neurosci, 261* Suppl 2, S140–S144.

Swartz, S. (2010). The regulation of British colonial lunatic asylums and the origins of colonial psychiatry, 1860–1864. *Hist Psychol, 13*(2), 160–177.

Szmukler, G. (2015). Compulsion and 'coercion' in mental health care. *World Psychiatry, 14*(3), 259–261.

Szmukler, G. (2019). 'Capacity', 'best interests', 'will and preferences' and the UN convention on the rights of persons with disabilities. *World Psychiatry, 18*(1), 34–41.

Szmukler, G., Daw, R., & Callard, F. (2014). Mental health law and the UN convention on the rights of persons with disabilities. *Int J Law Psychiatry, 37*(3), 245–252.

Testa, M. & West, S. G. (2010). Civil commitment in the United States. *Psychiatry, 7*(10), 30–40.

Thara, R., et al. (2008). Community mental health in India: a rethink. *Int J Ment Health Syst, 2*(1), 11.

Thornicroft, G., et al. (2009). Global pattern of experienced and anticipated discrimination against people with schizophrenia: a cross-sectional survey. *Lancet, 373*(9661), 408–415.

Thornicroft, G., Deb, T., & Henderson, C. (2016). Community mental health care worldwide: current status and further developments. *World Psychiatry, 15*(3), 276–286.

Thornicroft, G. & Bebbington, P. (1989). Deinstitutionalisation—from hospital closure to service development. *Br J Psychiatry, 155*(6), 739–753.

Thornicroft, G., et al. (2016). Evidence for effective interventions to reduce mental-health-related stigma and discrimination. *Lancet, 387*(10023), 1123–1132.

Thrush, A. & Hyder, A. A. (2014). The neglected burden of caregiving in low- and middle-income countries. *Disabil Health J, 7*(3), 262–272.

Tingleff, E. B., et al. (2017). 'Treat me with respect'. A systematic review and thematic analysis of psychiatric patients' reported perceptions of the situations associated with the process of coercion. *J Psychiatr Ment Health Nurs, 24*(9–10), 681–698.

UNHRC (2019). Report of the Special Rapporteur on the Right of Everyone to the Enjoyment of the Highest Attainable Standard of Physical and Mental Health.

United Nations (1991). Principles for the Protection of Persons with Mental Illness and the Improvement of Mental Health Care. Office of the High Commissioner for Human Rights, Resolution 46/119.

United Nations (2006). Convention on the Rights of Persons with Disabilities and Optional Protocol.

United Nations (2014). Report of the Special Rapporteur on torture and other cruel, inhuman or degrading treatment or punishment, Juan E. Méndez. Addendum: Mission to Ghana. United Nations General Assembly Human Rights Council.

Velpry, L. & Eyraud, B. (2014). Confinement and psychiatric care: a comparison between high-security units for prisoners and for difficult patients in France. *Cult Med Psychiatry, 38*(4), 550–577.

Wallcraft, J., et al. (2011). Partnerships for better mental health worldwide: WPA recommendations on best practices in working with service users and family carers. *World Psychiatry, 10*(3), 229–236.

Wang, D. W. L. & Colucci, E. (2017). Should compulsory admission to hospital be part of suicide prevention strategies? *BJPsych Bull, 41*(3), 169–171.

Weich, S., et al. (2017). Variation in compulsory psychiatric inpatient admission in England: a cross-classified, multilevel analysis. *Lancet Psychiatry, 4*(8), 619–626.

WHO (2013). *Mental health action plan 2013–2020.* Geneva: World Health Organization.

WHO (2016). *mhGAP intervention guide for mental, neurological and substance use disorders in non-specialized health settings. Version 2.0.* Geneva: World Health Organization.

WHO. (2021). *Comprehensive mental health action plan 2013–2030.* Geneva, World Health Organization.

Wickremsinhe, M. N. (2018). Emergency involuntary treatment law for people with mental disorders: a comparative analysis of legislation in LMICs. *Int J Law Psychiatry, 56*, 1–9.

Wildeman, S. (2013). Protecting rights and building capacities: challenges to global mental health policy in light of the convention on the rights of persons with disabilities. *J Law Med Ethics, 41*(1), 48–73.

Woods, A., Hart, A., & Spandler, H. (2019). The recovery narrative: politics and possibilities of a genre. *Cult Med Psychiatry, 46*(2), 221–247.

Xie, B. (2012). Where is the path to recovery when psychiatric hospitalization becomes too difficult? *Shanghai Arch Psychiatry, 24*(1), 38–40.

Yang, L. H., et al. (2014). 'What matters most:' a cultural mechanism moderating structural vulnerability and moral experience of mental illness stigma. *Soc Sci Med, 103*(0), 84–93.

Yaro, P. B., et al. (2020). Stakeholders' perspectives about the impact of training and sensitization of traditional and spiritual healers on mental health and illness: A qualitative evaluation in Ghana. *Int J Soc Psychiatry, 66*(5), 476–484.

Zhu, J., et al. (2018). Guan (care/control): an ethnographic understanding of care for people with severe mental illness from Shanghai's urban communities. *Cult Med Psychiatry, 42*(1), 92–111.

Part II

Psychosis by Place

10

Ribeirão Preto, Brazil: Incidence and risks

Cristina Marta Del-Ben, Rosana Shuhama, and Paulo Rossi Menezes

Introduction

The majority of epidemiological studies regarding schizophrenia and other psychotic disorders have been carried out in high-income countries (HICs). Data from low- and middle-income countries (LMICs) are still very sparse, even with evidence showing that the burden caused by schizophrenia is around four times higher in LMICs than in HICs (Charlson et al., 2018).

Brazil is a middle-income country with continental dimensions. The fifth-largest country in the world, Brazil is composed of 5,570 municipalities distributed in 26 states, with massive economic and social inequalities, especially for those from minority groups. Moreover, differently from some European countries, in LMICs, such as Brazil, living in small cities may be associated with higher levels of social deprivation and economic adversities. As discussed elsewhere (see Chapters 1–3), there is evidence pointing to a role of social context as a risk factor for psychosis (Charlson et al., 2018).

In Brazil, few programmes of research have focused on the epidemiology of psychoses. In the early 2000s, the incidence of first-episode psychosis was estimated in a study conducted in the city of São Paulo (Menezes et al., 2007). The metropolitan region of São Paulo has a population of approximately 18 million inhabitants, and the geographic area under study covered a population of around 1,200,000 people, being economically very heterogeneous. At that time, all public and private mental health services that could offer psychiatric care to individuals residing in the geographic areas under study were contacted, and individuals with potential first-episode psychosis were identified. Standardized diagnostic assessment interviews were conducted, whenever possible, when the diagnosis of a first-episode psychosis was confirmed. In the case of a refusal to be interviewed, the diagnosis was made by consensus with all the information available from medical records and key informants.

Three hundred and sixty-seven people with first-episode psychosis were identified during the 2002–2005 period, with incidence rates of 15.8/100,000 (95% CI = 14.3–17.6) person-years at risk for all psychoses, and 10.0/100,000 (95% CI = 8.7–11.4) for non-affective psychoses. These rates were much lower than expected for a large metropolis such as the city of São Paulo, considering results showing a greater risk for psychosis in residents of more densely popu-lated areas (Jongsma et al., 2018). Taken together, these data suggested that some biological vulnerability and/or social and environmental risk factors may not operate in Brazil and possibly other LMICS in the same way as in wealthy countries.

Ten years later, the incidence of psychosis was estimated in and around Ribeirão Preto, the capital city of the 13th Regional Health Department of the State of São Paulo, which is located 320 km from São Paulo city. The study con-ducted in Ribeirão Preto was named STREAM, an acronym for 'Schizophrenia and Other Psychoses Translational Research: Environment and Molecular Biology' (Del-Ben et al., 2019), which, in turn, is part of the international con-sortium 'European Network of National Schizophrenia Networks Studying Gene-Environment Interactions' (EU-GEI) (Gayer-Anderson et al., 2020).

The aim of the STREAM study was to estimate the incidence of psychosis in the Ribeirão Preto catchment area and to investigate possible interactions between social and biological factors in the occurrence of psychotic disorders. The São Paulo Research Foundation funded the study.

Ribeirão Preto

The Ribeirão Preto catchment area has a territorial area of 10,367,436 km^2, comprised of 26 municipalities, with a total population of 1,327,989 inhabit-ants (Brazilian Census, https://cidades.ibge.gov.br/). This set of municipalities is characterized by heterogeneous demographic and economic parameters, promising to be a useful context for investigating several risk factors for psych-osis, which may be either specific to Brazil and LMICs more generally, or may operate in directions different from those observed in wealthy countries. In particular, Ribeirão Preto, the host city of the catchment area, where almost half of the region's population lives, differs significantly from the 25 remaining mu-nicipalities, in terms of social and economic indicators (Table 10.1).

The average population density of the region is 118.5 inhabitants/km^2, with the highest density in Ribeirão Preto city, with 929.9 inhabitants/km^2. By con-trast, at least half of the remaining municipalities have a population density rate lower than 75 inhabitants/km^2. The proportion of urban residents varies from 99.7% in Ribeirão Preto to less than 70% in sparsely populated municipalities.

Table 10.1 Demographic and economic profile* of the municipalities comprising the Ribeirão Preto catchment area, Brazil

	Ribeirão Preto (Main city)	Remaining cities Median (Range)
Population (inhabitants)	604,682	23,862 (1,953–110,074)
Territorial area (km²)	167	347 (111–929)
Population density (inhabitants/km²)	929.8	75.0 (13.2–308.4)
Urban residents (%)	99.7	95.8 (64.6–98.9)
Human Development Index (HDI)	0.800	0.735 (0.686–0.778)
HDI national ranking	40th	897th (145th to 2,282nd)
Per capita gross domestic product (US$)	9,143.20	5,254.80 (2,234.80–20,747.40)
Infant mortality (n/1000 birth)	9.6	11.9 (4.8–52.3)
Illiteracy (%)	3.4	7.4 (5.0–12.2)

*2010 Brazilian Census, https://cidades.ibge.gov.br/; http://www.atlasbrasil.org.br/

The Human Development Index (HDI) of the municipalities ranges from 0.686 to 0.800, with a per capita gross domestic product (GDP) of 3.57[1] times the minimum wage for Ribeirão Preto and 2.83 times the minimum wage for the whole region. Illiteracy varies from 3.4 to 12.2% of the total population, with 7.5 average years of schooling for individuals aged 15 to 64 years. Health data point to a birth rate of 14/1,000 inhabitants, with an average infant mortality rate of 9.9/1,000 live births. Almost all municipalities have adequate urban internal infrastructure, with garbage collection (99.3%), water supply (98.4%), and sanitary sewage (93.9%) (https://www.seade.gov.br).

Historically, the economy of the Ribeirão Preto catchment area has been based on agribusiness, characterized by large monocultures of coffee, in the late nineteenth/early twentieth century, and, more recently, of sugarcane. For several decades, this productive activity has been responsible for an internal seasonal migratory process that occurs every year, mainly through the migration of individuals from the Northeast of Brazil to work in the sugarcane fields.

Mental health services in Ribeirão Preto

The region's health network is hierarchically organized according to the complexity of patients' needs, with services distributed in primary, secondary, and tertiary healthcare, following the principles of the Brazilian Unified Health

---

[1] Minimum wage at the end of 2010 was equivalent to US$306.09.

System (Sistema Único de Saúde, SUS). Ribeirão Preto city is the regional reference for the most complex cases, particularly for the small towns of the region. Access to emergency care is organized through a unified medical regulation system, which directs cases according to their clinical needs and the availability of beds for urgent and emergency care of clinical, traumatic, and psychiatric cases.

Since the 1990s, the mental health network of the Ribeirão Preto catchment area has been operating in a hierarchical and decentralized care model, comprised of community-based mental health services at the local level, with inpatient care when required.

Although with some differences regarding technological and human resources, community-based mental health services are available in all the municipalities of the Ribeirão Preto catchment area. Psychiatric beds for acute patients are available in psychiatric hospitals (160 beds), in psychiatric wards in a general hospital (22 beds), and in an emergency psychiatry unit (8 beds) located in a general emergency hospital.

Patients with a first-episode psychosis can be enrolled in the Psychosis Early Intervention Programme (PEIP) of the Ribeirão Preto Medical School, University of São Paulo, Brazil, comprised of integrated outpatient and inpatient units, managed by a multi-professional staff. The PEIP had been created as a consequence of the STREAM study, aiming to provide qualified care for the individuals identified as incident cases, but has kept its activities even after the end of the STREAM data collection. Since 2013, the programme has admitted around 100 new patients per year (Corrêa-Oliveira et al., 2022).

Patients older than 12 years old, without restriction regarding maximum age, can be referred to the PEIP by general or specialized community-based services. There is also no restriction related to comorbidities, including substance-related problems and other medical conditions.

The PEIP provides a 2-year follow-up period, with weekly to monthly appointments, depending on symptom severity, pharmacological treatment, and a variety of psychosocial interventions focused on the preservation/recovery of global functioning.

The STREAM study

Data collection took place from 1 April 2012 to 31 March 2015. All mental health services in the region, including inpatient and community-based mental health services, were regularly contacted by trained researchers looking for persons aged between 16 and 64 years old, in their first contact with mental health services due to psychotic symptoms not related to other medical conditions or psychoactive substance intoxication or withdrawal. To identify cases that were potentially missed, a leakage study was also carried out in the 12 months following the end of the inclusion period, based on the review of 65,469 medical records of patients attending the mental health services of the catchment area during the 3-year period of the study.

The diagnosis was established by trained researchers using the Structured Clinical Interview (SCID) for Diagnostic and Statistical Manual of Mental Disorders 4th edition (DSM-IV), translated into Portuguese with good psychometric properties (Del-Ben et al., 2005). Patients were classified as having either non-affective (DSM-IV codes 295.xx, 297.1, and 298.8) or affective psychoses (DSM-IV codes 296.04, 296.44, 296.64).

Over the 3-year period, 588 people with first-episode psychosis were identified (Del-Ben et al., 2019). A subsample of individuals with first-episode psychosis (n=218) were included in a case-sibling-control study, for which extensive data on demographic characteristics, social risks, and psychological mechanisms were collected, according to the EU-GEI protocol, plus some potential biological markers collected specifically for the Brazilian study, such as plasma cytokines.

The case-sibling-control study also included 99 patients' siblings without a history of psychotic symptoms, and a representative sample of 318 community-based controls, stratified according to the demographic profile of the local population.

Demographic and clinical features of the incident cases of first-episode psychosis

The majority of the participants were men (62.5%), had reported themselves as having 'white' skin colour (52.4%), were not married (50.7%), were engaged in an occupational activity (61.7%), and had less than nine years of study (62.2%). The median age of illness onset was 29.0 years old (interquartile range: 21.0–39.0), which was lower in men (26.0; 20.0–36.0) than in women (31.0; 24.0–42.0).

The median duration of untreated psychosis (DUP) was 14 weeks (4.0–41.0), which was lower in non-affective psychosis (9.0; 4.0–22.0) than in affective psychosis (21.0; 8.0–59.5). Although the DUP observed in the Brazilian study is comparable with other centres (Cascio et al., 2012), it is higher than observed more recently in some European countries (Jongsma et al., 2018). This discrepancy may be explained by the fact that the implementation of early intervention services is still developing in Brazil. As mentioned before, the first early intervention programme for patients with first-episode psychosis in the Ribeirão Preto catchment area was created during the STREAM study.

Based on the 2015 Brazilian Census, the total population at risk during the 3-year period of the study was estimated as 3,071,862 person-years. The overall incidence rate of first-episode psychosis, adjusted by sex and age (using direct standardization to the world population; https://esa.un.org/unpd/wpp/Downl oad/Standard/Population/), was 19.46 (95% CI=18.71–20.20)/100,000 person-years (Del-Ben et al., 2019). This rate is higher than that observed in São Paulo city (Menezes et al., 2007), 10 years before, and similar to smaller European cities, but clearly lower than the rates observed in some northern European metropolises, confirming the heterogeneity of the incidence of psychosis across the globe.

Similar to previous studies carried out in HICs (Ochoa et al., 2012), the adjusted incidence of first-episode psychosis was higher in young individuals aged 20–24 years old (27.21; 95% CI= 24.83–29.59) and 25–29 years old (25.08; 95% CI=22.68–27.47), and in men (21.21; 95% CI=20.12–22.29) than in women (17.66; 95% CI=16.66–18.67). These data can be seen in Figure 10.1.

Self-reported skin colour

The proportion of people with first-episode psychosis who reported their skin colour as white was lower than the 66.3% reported by the Brazilian Census for the Ribeirão Preto catchment area, suggesting a higher risk of first-episode psychosis among Black or mixed individuals, following findings relating to minority ethnic groups in Europe (Jongsma et al., 2018). The adjusted incidence rate of psychosis among self-reported non-white persons was 19.72 (95% CI= 18.97–20.46), whereas in white individuals was 15.36 (95% CI=14.70–16.02) (Fig. 10.1).

This higher incidence among non-white people is probably related to social adversities since, in general, Black/mixed Brazilians have lower socioeconomic status compared with white Brazilians, as a consequence of the unsolved social and racial inequalities arising from over 350 years of slavery in the country, which was definitively abolished only in 1888.

Population density

The incidence of first-episode psychosis was lower in Ribeirão Preto (17.05; 95% CI=16.03–18.07) than the average incidence in the remaining cities of the region (21.53; 95% CI=20.47–22.59). The incidence rate ratio (IRR=1.27; 95% CI=1.08–1.51) indicated the incidence was around 27% higher among those living in the remaining 25 cities compared with Ribeirão Preto city.

Thus, the main town of the region, the place of residence of 46% of the population at risk, with a population density of 929.8 inhabitants/km^2, had a lower incidence rate than the average incidence of the remaining cities of the region, with

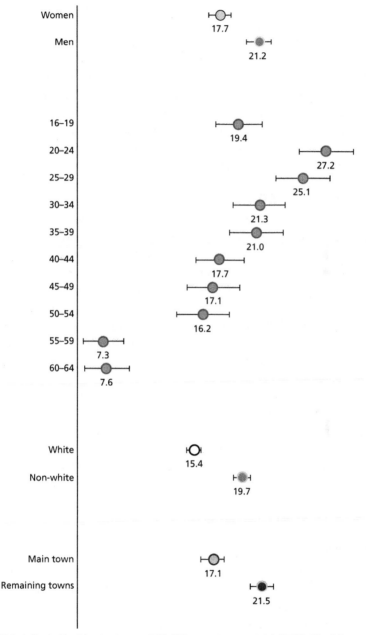

Fig. 10.1 Adjusted incident rates per 100,000 person-year at risk (95% CI) of first-episode psychosis in the Ribeirão Preto Catchment Area, Brazil, by demographic characteristics. Adjusted by sex and age, standardized by the global population.
Source: data from Del-Ben C. M. et al. (2019). Urbanicity and risk of first-episode psychosis: incidence study in Brazil. *Br J Psychiatry*, *215*(6), 726–729.

much lower population densities (median = 75 inhabitants/km^2), as can be seen in Table 10.1. Considering population density as a proxy of urbanicity, these data are in the opposite direction of previous studies that point to an association between urbanicity and the risk of psychosis. Probably these results are due to socioeconomic indicators, which are worse in the remaining cities than in the main town.

Interestingly, a similar pattern was observed in Italy, where a higher incidence of psychosis was associated with lower population density (Jongsma et al., 2018). Moreover, urban residence was not associated with elevated odds of psychotic experiences or the diagnosis of psychosis in an analysis considering data from 42 LMICs (DeVylder et al., 2018).

Internal migration

Migration has been associated with psychosis, and more recently, internal migration has also been implicated as a risk factor for psychosis. The STREAM study may provide some useful information about this, since Ribeirão Preto has increasing rates of internal migration (6.5, in 2000, to 7.6/1,000 inhabitants/year, in 2010). On the other hand, the city of São Paulo, which historically was an attraction pole of migrants, has shown negative rates of internal migration (–5.07, in 2000, to –2.97/1,000 inhabitants-year, in 2010) (http://www.imp.seade.gov.br).

For this purpose, we looked at the two already mentioned Brazilian incidence databases (São Paulo city and Ribeirão Preto catchment area) with their distinct socioeconomic and population profiles, and verified if the place of birth and the time of continuous living in the catchment area where the psychosis started may be a valid predictor of psychosis (Shuhama et al., 2019). Although the continuous time of living in the catchment area may be just a proxy for the effects of migration, our data did not support the association of internal migration as a risk factor for psychosis, neither in São Paulo, nor in Ribeirão Preto (Table 10.2). Possible explanations for these negative results include the language unicity of the country and changes in the migration patterns, involving shorter distances and stability of family and/or social support.

Cannabis use

Several studies point to a relationship between cannabis use and psychosis, suggesting that the greater the use of cannabis, the greater the risk of psychosis. In this context, the EU-GEI consortium assessed the impact of different patterns of cannabis use on the incidence of psychosis (Di Forti et al., 2019). In total, 901 people with psychosis from six countries were included in the study, being 192 (21.3%) from Brazil, residents of the Ribeirão Preto catchment area, and 1,277 individuals without psychosis from the same communities (302 from Brazil/Ribeirão Preto Catchment area).

The study confirmed that daily use of cannabis was associated with a three-fold increase in the risk of developing psychosis, but this association became more pronounced when the participants reported daily use of cannabis with high concentrations of tetrahydrocannabinol (THC).

Specifically, in the Ribeirão Preto catchment area, the use of cannabis with a high concentration of THC was reported by only a small proportion of studied participants (1.5% of population-based controls and 3.6% of patients). On the other hand, daily use of cannabis was observed in 7.4% of controls and 25.0% of patients, indicating a 2.4 times higher risk of occurrence of psychosis among individuals with daily use of cannabis.

The role of cannabis use as a risk factor for psychosis was also confirmed in healthy individuals from the local community. The occurrence of psychotic experiences, measured through the Community Assessment of Psychic Experiences adapted to Brazil (CAPE-33), was more often observed among community-based participants that reported using cannabis more than once a week, in comparison with those reporting no or occasional use of cannabis (Ragazzi et al., 2020).

Childhood trauma

In a subsample of individuals with first-episode psychosis, compared with their unaffected biological siblings and community-based controls, the association between childhood trauma and psychosis that is usually described in wealthy countries (Stanton et al., 2020) was also confirmed in the Ribeirão Preto catchment area (Corsi-Zuelli et al., 2019). At least one type of childhood maltreatment was reported by 43.9% of the patients and 22.7% of the controls, which represents a risk of psychosis 2.7 higher among those with a history of childhood maltreatment compared with those without early trauma. Interestingly, unaffected siblings of people with first-episode psychosis also described a high frequency of childhood trauma (35.1%). The occurrence of early trauma was also associated with psychotic experiences in community-based individuals (Ragazzi et al., 2020).

Biological markers

Although the last few decades have brought a significant advance in the neurobiology of mental disorders, no biological marker has yet been identified with sufficient sensitivity and specificity to be included as a diagnostic criterion, similar to what is observed in other medical conditions. In order to contribute to the search for greater precision in psychiatric diagnosis, we evaluated possible associations between changes in potential peripheral blood markers and psychosis.

Table 10.2 Migration as time living in catchment areas São Paulo (2002–2005) and Ribeirão Preto (2012–2015)—predicting first-episode psychosis in two Brazilian case–control samples

Continuous living (years)	Patients n (%)	Controls n (%)	Unadjusted OR (95% CI)	p	Adjusted* OR (95%CI)	p
São Paulo						
Since birth	72 (36.00)	149 (37.25)	–	–	–	–
At least 11	74 (37.00)	134 (33.50)	1.21 (0.77–1.90)	0.416	1.07 (0.65–1.79)	0.781
6 to 10	27 (13.50)	44 (11.00)	1.27 (0.71–2.27)	0.415	1.11 (0.58–2.12)	0.753
3 to 5	14 (7.00)	41 (10.25)	0.70 (0.35–1.39)	0.304	0.62 (0.30–1.28)	0.193
Up to 2	13 (6.50)	32 (8.00)	0.84 (0.42–1.71)	0.637	0.66 (0.31–1.42)	0.293
Ribeirão Preto						
Since birth	86 (40.38)	141 (44.34)	–	–	–	–
At least 11	56 (26.29)	91 (28.62)	1.01 (0.66–1.55)	0.967	1.07 (0.64–1.78)	0.791
6 to 10	17 (7.98)	25 (7.86)	1.11 (0.57– 2.18)	0.751	1.07 (0.51–2.24)	0.850
3 to 5	20 (9.39)	27 (8.49)	1.21 (0.64–2.30)	0.550	1.13 (0.56–2.26)	0.733
Up to 2	34 (15.96)	34 (10.69)	1.64 (0.95–2.83)	0.076	1.57 (0.86–2.87)	0.145

* Adjusted by sex, age (only Ribeirão Preto), marital status, reported skin colour, and years of education.

Reproduced from Shuhama R (2019) 'From where we came: absence of internal migration effect on psychosis in two case-control Brazilian samples'. *Schizophrenia Research* 212:241–242 with permission from Elsevier.

The initial results of the STREAM project pointed to a reduction in plasma concentrations of N-methyl-D-aspartate (NMDA) receptor subunits in people with first-episode psychosis, in comparison with community controls and unaffected siblings of patients (Loureiro et al., 2018), which is consistent with a dysfunction of the glutamatergic system in the neurobiology of psychoses. Moreover, people with first-episode psychosis showed, in comparison with community-based controls and unaffected siblings, increased plasma concentrations of both pro-inflammatory (IL-6 and TNF-alpha) and anti-inflammatory cytokines (IL-10, TGF-beta), which supports the findings from HICs and extends the evidence for a role of the immune system in people with first-episode psychosis to a LMIC (Corsi-Zuelli et al., 2019).

A desired near future

The preliminary results from the Ribeirão Preto catchment area suggest that some risk factors for psychosis observed in wealthy countries, such as sex, age, ethnicity, cannabis use, and childhood trauma are also present in LMICs. On the other hand, other factors, such as population density and internal migration, may not have the same effects, with a possibly more pronounced effect of socioeconomic adversities in the occurrence of psychosis in LMICs. Further studies focusing on particular environmental characteristics related to social adversities, such as economic and racial discrimination, that may better explain the incidence of psychosis in a socioeconomically deprived context, are needed.

In this context, we believe that special attention should be given to the responsibility of universities, particularly public units, which in Brazil are the centres of science production, to promote the transfer of knowledge to the community, aiming to facilitate access to care and to minimize the impact of the social prejudice related to psychosis.

Finally, other subjects that deserve to be targeted for further studies are quality of patient care, and the improvement of mental health services, such as effective actions to reduce the DUP, and its negative consequences on outcomes (Penttilä et al., 2014). There is an urgent need for more investment in the organization of community mental health services, particularly those focused on the implementation of early identification and intervention protocols for psychoses, aiming to avoid or at least minimize all the individual and social impairments related to untreated psychosis.

References

Cascio, M. T., Cella, M., Preti, A., Meneghelli, A., & Cocchi, A. (2012). Gender and duration of untreated psychosis: a systematic review and meta-analysis. *Early Interv Psychiatry*, 6(2), 115–127.

Charlson, F. J., et al. (2018). Global epidemiology and burden of schizophrenia: findings from the Global Burden of Disease study 2016. *Schizophr Bull*, 44(6), 1195–1203.

Corrêa-Oliveira, G. E., et al. (2022). Early intervention in psychosis in emerging countries: findings from a first-episode psychosis programme in the Ribeirão Preto catchment area, southeastern Brazil. *Early Interv Psychiatry*, 16(7), 800–807.

Corsi-Zuelli, F., et al. (2019). Cytokine profile in first-episode psychosis, unaffected siblings and community-based controls: the effects of familial liability and childhood maltreatment. *Psychol Med*, 50(7), 1139–1147.

Del-Ben, C. M., et al. (2005). Accuracy of psychiatric diagnosis performed under indirect supervision. *Braz J Psychiatry*, 27(1), 58–62.

Del-Ben, C. M., et al. (2019). Urbanicity and risk of first-episode psychosis: incidence study in Brazil. *Br J Psychiatry*, 215(6), 726–729.

DeVylder, J. E., Kelleher, I., Lalane, M., Oh, H., Link, B. G., & Koyanagi, A. (2018). Association of urbanicity with psychosis in low- and middle-income countries. *JAMA Psychiatry*, 75(7), 678–686.

Di Forti, M., et al. (2019). The contribution of cannabis use to variation in the incidence of psychotic disorder across Europe (EU-GEI): a multicentre case-control study. *Lancet Psychiatry*, 6(5), 427–436.

Gayer-Anderson, C., et al. (2020). The EUropean Network of National Schizophrenia Networks Studying Gene–Environment Interactions (EU-GEI): incidence and first-episode case–control programme. *Soc Psychiatry Psychiatr Epidemiol*, 55(5), 645–657.

Jongsma, H. E., et al. (2018). Treated incidence of psychotic disorders in the multinational EU-GEI study. *JAMA Psychiatry*, 75(1), 36–46.

Loureiro, C. M., Shuhama, R., Fachim, H. A., Menezes, P. R., Del-Ben, C. M., & Louzada-Junior, P. (2018). Low plasma concentrations of N-methyl-D-aspartate receptor subunits as a possible biomarker for psychosis. *Schizophr Res*, 202, 55–63.

Menezes, P. R., Scazufca, M., Busatto, G., Coutinho, L. M. S., McGuire, P. K., & Murray, R. M. (2007). Incidence of first-contact psychosis in São Paulo, Brazil. *Br J Psychiatry*, 191(SUPPL. 51), s102–s106.

Ochoa, S., Usall, J., Cobo, J., Labad, X., & Kulkarni, J. (2012). Gender differences in schizophrenia and first-episode psychosis: a comprehensive literature review. *Schizophr Res Treatment*, 2012, 916198.

Penttilä, M., Jääskeläinen, E., Hirvonen, N., Isohanni, M., & Miettunen, J. (2014). Duration of untreated psychosis as predictor of long-term outcome in schizophrenia: systematic review and meta-analysis. *Br J Psychiatry*, 205(2), 88–94.

Ragazzi, T. C. C., et al. (2020). Validation of the Portuguese version of the community assessment of psychic experiences and characterization of psychotic experiences in a Brazilian sample. *Braz J Psychiatry*, 42(4), 389–397.

Shuhama, R., et al. (2019). From where we came: absence of internal migration effect on psychosis in two case-control Brazilian samples. *Schizophr Res*, 212, 241–242.

Stanton, K. J., Denietolis, B., Goodwin, B. J., & Dvir, Y. (2020). Childhood trauma and psychosis: an updated review. *Child Adolesc Psychiatr Clin N Am*, 29(1), 115–129.

11

Trinidad and Tobago

Gerard Hutchinson

Introduction

International interest in the epidemiology of psychosis in Caribbean populations emerged because of the high reported rates of psychotic illness among
first- and second-generation Caribbean migrants to Britain. These rates have
been found to be 4.7 to 5.6 times greater than that in the comparative white
British population in meta-analyses of studies investigating this phenomenon
(Kirkbride et al., 2012; Tortelli et al., 2015).

A significant Caribbean presence in Britain began when approximately 700
passengers who were mostly Jamaican but including nationals of other English-
speaking Caribbean islands arrived in London on the Empire Windrush in June
1948 having sailed from Jamaica. These Caribbeans were at the time British
Commonwealth citizens, and had travelled to Britain seeking work in the
aftermath of the Second World War to help in the rebuilding of Britain (Mead,
2007). Between 1948 and 1970, it is estimated that approximately half a million migrants arrived from the English-speaking Caribbean and in so doing
prompted the establishment of a multicultural Britain (Fryer, 1984). They provided labour in hospitals, transport, postal services, construction, and other
public services. They had families and this led to second and third and subsequent generations of Black Caribbean British nationals who have shifted
the cultural and social landscape in Britain (Phillips, 2001). At the time of the
Windrush, the English-speaking Caribbean countries were still colonies of the
British Empire (Peach, 1991). Unlike their African and Asian counterparts,
English was their first language so they expected to assimilate very easily since
their education and political systems at home were derived from the British colonial rulers (Phillips, 2001).

One unanticipated outcome of their presence was reports of increased rates
of psychotic illness which began to be first documented in the early 1960s in
the psychiatric literature (Harrison et al., 1988; Pinto et al., 2008). One of the
several hypotheses put forward to explain these high rates was that the high
rates might have been a migrant effect and may have been due to high rates in

the Caribbean countries from which these migrants came (Bhugra & Jones, 2001; Sharpley et al., 2001). This led to incidence studies in Jamaica (Hickling & Rodgers-Johnson, 1995), Trinidad (Bhugra et al., 1996), and Barbados (Mahy et al., 1999) which sought to establish the rates of first-episode schizophrenia in these Caribbean countries using similar methodologies to studies in Britain. It was found that, for each of the islands, the incidence rates were consistent with those reported for the white British population from the studies emerging out of Britain.

Since then, other European countries have consistently reported high rates of psychosis among migrants from Africa and the Caribbean, with the closest parallel to Britain being the Netherlands, which still has close ties to its dependencies in the Caribbean (the Dutch Caribbean) and the formerly colonized, now independent Suriname. Increased rates of psychotic illness have also been found among the Caribbean migrants from Suriname who had moved to the Netherlands (Selten et al., 1997; Selten et al., 2005). Because these migrants and their descendants generally experienced more social and economic deprivation than their host counterparts, social disadvantage has come to be accepted as a risk factor for psychosis partially as a result of these consistent migrant findings (Stilo et al., 2017). Socioenvironmental risk factors for psychosis include migration, discrimination, and negative social experiences, which are likely to have a cumulative effect of influencing the onset and course of psychosis in this population (Morgan et al., 2010; Sharpley et al., 2001).

About the Caribbean and Trinidad and Tobago

The Caribbean generally refers to the archipelago of islands that border the Caribbean Sea. It is also a place anchored in a common history of slavery, plantation societies, and colonization. This colonization has given rise to English, Spanish, French and Dutch-speaking islands, and also includes countries Guyana and Belize which geographically are part of South and Central America, respectively. The English-speaking islands and Guyana are also known as the West Indies (Caribbean Atlas, 2013).

Trinidad and Tobago (TT) is an English-speaking twin Caribbean island republic with an atypical Caribbean profile. Its economy is driven by the oil and gas energy industry and therefore is more industrialized than its Caribbean neighbours, for whom tourism is the major income earner. It is categorized as a high-income country (International Monetary Fund, 2017). It is a former British colony but was also held previously by Spanish colonizers and occupied by French settlers before the British took over in 1797. When it became a Crown Colony, it featured the strange arrangement of a French-speaking population living with Spanish laws but run by the British. The Spanish influence remains, with the capital being Port of Spain and the other major city being San Fernando. Many parts of the island retain their Spanish names such as San Juan, Valencia, Santa Cruz, and Diego Martin (Williams, 1962). Geographically, it lies at the southernmost tip of the Caribbean chain and historically it is thought to have separated from the South American continent due to geologic activity. Its closest land mass is Venezuela and therefore also absorbs a very strong Spanish influence (US Library of Congress, 1987).

The population is approximately 1.35 million as of the last census (2011). TT presents an approximately equal ethnic mix of Indian (37.6%) and African (36.3%) descended individuals, with smaller number of Mixed heritage (24.1%), and a range of other ethnicities including White European, Chinese, and Middle Eastern (Central Statistical Office 2013). It is therefore a highly heterogeneous population in terms of ethnicity and culture.

Overview of current evidence

Incidence

The first major study attempting to measure the incidence of schizophrenia in Trinidad was conducted by Bhugra et al. (1996) who found an incidence rate of 2.2/10,000 (22/100,000) for broad schizophrenia and 1.6 (16/100,000) for narrowly defined schizophrenia. In incidence studies in Jamaica and Barbados, the rates reported were 2.1 (21/100,000) and 1.2 (12/100,000), and 3.2 (32/100,000) and 2.8 (28/100,000) for broadly defined and narrowly defined schizophrenia, respectively (Hickling & Rodgers-Johnson, 1995; Mahy et al., 1999). These three studies used the same methodology as a study in London (Bhugra et al., 1997) so that valid comparisons could be made about incidence rates. This methodology utilized the Present State Examination (PSE) and recruited individuals seeking help from mental health services. The rates in the native Caribbean populations were more consistent with those reported for the white British population and significantly lower than those for Caribbeans in London and other UK cities (Sharpley et al., 2001). Compared with cases in Trinidad (Bhugra et al., 1997), Black Caribbean cases in London were more likely to be admitted because of self-neglect, perceived threat, and assault of others. Unemployment, living alone, and separation from parents during childhood were also more common (Mallett et al., 2002). With regard to unemployment, for example, the rate was much higher for the British Black Caribbean population than for the Trinidad sample.

More recently two incidence studies have been completed. Hutchinson and Murray (2006) found a rate of 240/830,000 (28/100,000) for broad schizophrenia.

In a pilot study (INTREPID I) comparing first-contact untreated cases from Ibadan, Nigeria, Chengalpet, India, and East Trinidad, Morgan et al. (2016) reported a rate of 36.5/100,000 in the Trinidad group for broadly defined psychoses inclusive of affective psychoses. This represented untreated cases with a median period of duration of psychosis before detection of 38 weeks. The rates in two other participating centres were 45.9 in Chengalpet, India, and 31.2 in Ibadan, Nigeria. For comparison, the pooled incidence rate in Britain between 1950–2009 was reported to be 31.7 (Kirkbride et al., 2012). In the recently published study of treated incidence in 17 catchment areas and six countries (five in Europe and one in Brazil), the pooled incidence rate was found to be 21.4/100,000 person-years (Jongsma et al., 2018). This suggests that the incidence rate is slightly higher than the international rates and indeed the pooled rate in Britain.

Some other interesting findings have emerged from the INTREPID study as although the incidence rate in Chengalpet was greatest for all psychoses, the age and sex standardized rates for schizophrenia in Ibadan and Trinidad were higher than in India, while the rates of other psychoses were higher in India. This is consistent with what was found among first-time admissions to a psychiatric unit in San Fernando, Trinidad, where those of Indian descent were more likely to have affective presentations, including affective psychoses and alcohol-related problems, while those of African descent were more likely to have non-affective psychosis and cannabis or cocaine use (Hutchinson et al., 2003). The issue of misdiagnosis in Britain as a reason for the marked differential in incidence rates has also been raised (Hickling, 2005). Hickling suggested that racism in the clinical interaction as well as cultural insensitivity contributed to misdiagnosis. This view has been challenged (see Chapter 4). It is also worth noting that racism and social alienation may also express itself in society and in the mental health system as risk factors for the development of severe mental illness in Britain. Timimi (2014) has suggested that the formal diagnostic labels and systems be abolished altogether because they serve to increase stigma and worsen long-term prognosis. In spite of the many social issues in the Caribbean, the onset of serious mental illness in this population is less so when compared with their Caribbean counterparts in Britain.

The limitation in comparing these studies is that the case-finding methods were not the same. For example, in the studies in Jamaica, Trinidad, London, and Barbados (Bhugra et al., 1997; Mahy et al., 1999), only patients who presented to formal mental health services were included. In the INTREPID study (Morgan et al., 2016), patients were additionally identified through traditional and church healers. In Trinidad, it has been found that perceptions of mental illness continue to be influenced by both medical and supernatural illness models, and help is sought from both domains, often simultaneously (Ramkissoon et al., 2017). This may also be a factor influencing incidence measurement, as there may be a population who do not present to services because their beliefs explain psychosis in spiritual and/or supernatural terms and therefore they only seek help from these sources. Ultimately help-seeking is affected by beliefs about causation and the perception of treatment effectiveness (Cohen et al., 2016) and incidence studies depend on help-seeking behaviour, so they become inextricably tied to service access and provision. Cohen et al (2016) also reported that slightly less than half of the INTREPID pilot sample in Trinidad attributed their mental illness onset to spiritual or supernatural causes.

Risk factors

Many risk factors have been identified for psychosis in general and schizophrenia in particular. It is thought psychosis emerges as a consequence of complex processes combining genetic vulnerability with a range of developmental and environmental exposures that eventually culminate in disorder (Davis et al., 2016). These include genes and family history, gender, abnormal neural development, social cognition, maternal and individual nutrition, migrant status, early cannabis use, childhood trauma, and/or isolation and urbanicity (Davis et al., 2016; Heckers, 2009). Migrant status is expressed through ethnic minority status as in the case of Black Caribbeans in England. Urbanicity is the other strongly supported risk factor and both of these may be mediated through adverse social experiences across the developmental life course (Heinz et al., 2013; Radua et al., 2018).

While no large-scale studies have been conducted to conclusively establish the major risk factors for psychosis in Trinidad, the available evidence suggests that young men living in urban environments are most vulnerable. Beyond this, the two greatest risk factors for psychosis in Trinidad seem to be cannabis use and family history (Hutchinson & Murray, 2006). This underscores the need for more detailed research into the factors that contribute to the development of psychotic illness in this population. This is the focus of INTREPID II, which is due to report in 2023. The trend towards decriminalization and legalization of cannabis use is especially relevant to mental health care delivery, particularly for the adolescent and young adult period when cannabis use generally begins or is intensified. The role of family history either as an environmental factor or as a genetic factor also needs to be established as this will be important in the development of preventative interventions and the investigation of gene-environment interactions.

Not enough is known about parental separation and childhood adversity in the context of psychosis and these are areas ripe for further study in Trinidad as risk factors for psychosis. There is an ethnic skew towards people of African descent developing non-affective psychotic illnesses which may be related to cannabis and perhaps cocaine use. East Indians, on the other hand, have more affective disorders and problems with alcohol use (Hutchinson et al., 2003; Hutchinson & Murray, 2006). In Trinidad, high rates of homicide are seen in the African population compared with high rates of suicide in the Indian population (Hutchinson, 2005). Two of the parallel features of homicidal behaviour with psychosis epidemiology are the prominence of men and substance use/abuse (Falk et al., 2014). Social and economic factors have been proffered as reasons for variations in a range of mental health problems such as depression, mania, and substance abuse in Jamaican and Guyanese Caribbean populations, but psychotic illness was not a focus of this study (Lacey et al., 2016).

The issues with substance use may be one of the reasons that young men are particularly vulnerable. Early exposure to cannabis during adolescence (before age 14 years) has been found to increase the risk of developing psychotic symptoms as one grows older in a Trinidadian population (Konings et al., 2008).

Neurodevelopmental factors in schizophrenia related to pregnancy and birth complications have been found to be similar for a Trinidadian sample and their white British counterparts, and lowest for Black Caribbeans in London. This suggests that these complications constitute a baseline risk for schizophrenia in all populations but do not explain the increased risk among Black Caribbeans living in England or indeed differential rates within populations (Bhugra et al., 2003).

Social disadvantage is increased in first presentation psychosis compared with population-based controls. The markers of this disadvantage include long term separation from parents and/or death of parent/s before age 17, living alone, unemployment, and being single with few close friends, all of which are associated with increased risk of psychosis (Stilo et al., 2013). This may be why inferior social status has recently been touted as a likely explanation for findings of increased rates in migrants and ethnic minorities (Van der Ven & Selten, 2018).

In the Trinidadian population, there are high levels of childhood exposure to various forms of abuse, neglect, and exploitation (GOTT-UNICEF, 2012). These may all contribute to an increased risk for psychosis onset. Childhood sexual abuse and neglect, antenatal and postpartum depression in mothers, and experience of and/or exposure to trauma may all be risk factors that can be modified to affect the likelihood of onset of psychotic illness (Bebbington et al., 2011; Varese et al., 2012; Plant et al., 2013). Childhood sexual abuse in particular seems to be highly prevalent (Children's Authority of Trinidad and Tobago, 2016) and recent efforts to address this issue and provide interventions for those affected may positively impact psychosis incidence and prevalence in the decades to come. Violent trauma is also now a consistent risk exposure as rates of homicide and gang-related violence have increased significantly, especially in urban communities (Seepersad, 2016).

Services

Mental health services are sectorized geographically such that each sector has approximately similar base populations. The geographic distribution of residents in Trinidad results in seven sectors, with services in West Trinidad, Port of Spain, North East Trinidad, East, South East, Central, and South Trinidad. Tobago is a separate sector and has a psychiatric unit in its general hospital with attendant outpatient clinics. A mental health team is attached to each sector so that they become familiar with the specific problems that affect individuals living in that sector. The team comprises psychiatrists, community nurses (mental health officers), and a social worker. Outpatient clinics are held in each sector and inpatients are treated in either the main psychiatric hospital (St Ann's Hospital) or in one of the two general hospital units (Maharajh & Parasram, 1999). This model is one that is generally utilized in the English-speaking Caribbean, particularly in the major territories of Jamaica, Barbados, and Trinidad and Tobago, which coincidentally all house campuses of the University of the West Indies.

Most antipsychotic medication is available, with atypical antipsychotics being the drugs of choice. There is still a great deal of stigma associated with mental illness and there has not been a development of advocacy or patient support groups in the country. This is an area that remains to be more fully established and supported.

The Mental Health Act was most recently revised in 2000 and allows for involuntary admissions either through medical referral or a combination of medical and family referral. The mental health officers are also licensed to admit individuals who are behaving in a way suggestive of mental illness in a public place (WHO-AIMS, 2011).

There is generally little formal contact between mental health services and traditional healing or religious healers, but it is generally acknowledged that individuals with mental health problems will sometimes seek out help from these sources. This is related to a belief system that attributes the causation of mental health problems to spiritual or supernatural influence or action (Arthur &Whitley, 2015; Ramkissoon et al., 2017).

A review of the factors affecting the development of mental health services flagged insufficient funding (e.g. in Trinidad and Tobago less than 5% of the health budget is dedicated to mental health), weakness of user and family associations, and a lack of human resources. There is also a need to develop research capacity to interrogate models of care and trial these to determine those that are most culturally appropriate and likely to be effective (Caldas de Almeida, 2013).

A research agenda

Apart from the previously mentioned studies, there have been no major research programmes conducted into the aetiology or course and outcome of psychosis in the English-speaking Caribbean. The two incidence studies (Bhugra et al., 1996; Hickling & Rodgers-Johnson, 1995; Mahy et al., 1999) and the more recent INTREPID research were all funded and supported by British funders and coordinated by the Institute of Psychiatry, Psychology and Neuroscience in London (apart from the Hickling & Rodgers-Johnson study) and largely deemed significant because of the high rates of psychosis among Caribbean descended patients in Britain. What is needed is a research agenda that addresses the needs of the Caribbean and is supported by funding that would assist in the development of research capacity in mental health for the Caribbean region.

Research is not generally seen as a priority investment area for funding in the English-speaking Caribbean, perhaps because of limited resources and other more urgent priorities, though there are signs that this is changing (Hickling et al., 2013; Sharpe & Shafe, 2016). There are several areas in mental health for which more objective information and analysis are needed. There has been no comprehensive national or regional prevalence or incidence study on mental illness, and that is a major priority. The presentation and diagnostic utility of the two major systems, ICD and DSM, need to be assessed in our populations with a determination of the appropriate thresholds for diagnosis that can be applied consistently.

Research is needed that would allow a more detailed determination of risk and protective factors for psychotic illness, including the role of genetics and family history and the relationship with cannabis use. The role of trauma and psycho-social adversity also remains to be fully elucidated in this population. Other social variables such as ethnicity, place of residence, and the role of developmental illnesses and factors related to comorbidity and premature mortality also need to be explored in this population. Other areas such as homelessness and forensic mental health also need to be researched. Intervention research is also required to determine the benefits of early intervention, consistent compliance, and social and family support with regard to symptom control and societal functioning, and the use of indigenous and herbal medicine.

The Ministry of Health has indicated its intention to move towards a more comprehensive community-based model of mental healthcare delivery. Needs assessments, community resources, and attitudes need to be explored to give this initiative its best chance of success.

The costs of mental illness and the relative cost benefits of effective treatments also need to be investigated through research. Surveillance and data-gathering systems need to be researched to ensure that the best and most accurate data is collected in the public health system.

Research is also needed into ways in which collaboration with the operations of the traditional and religious healing sector might be developed. Support for and research into the likely value of user and family support associations and the importance of public advocacy for mental health-related issues are also priorities if stigma and discrimination are to be successfully overcome.

Conclusion

While the rates of psychosis are not far elevated compared with populations in the more developed world, there are some interesting trends that provide food for thought regarding the factors that might determine incidence and prevalence of psychotic illness. There does seem to be an ethnic skew toward a greater risk for non-affective psychosis in those of African origin, with affective psychoses being more common in those of Indian origin. Drug use, particularly cannabis, is a risk factor for psychosis in the Trinidad population. Young urban men of African descent may be the single greatest population group at risk. Attention must therefore be paid to awareness of this risk among parents and children in this age of decriminalization and legalization of recreational marijuana use. Belief systems continue to attribute mental illness to spiritual and supernatural causes and these may contribute to longer periods of untreated psychosis and therefore higher prevalence rates. Research priorities include a large population-based study to determine the population prevalence of mental illness inclusive of psychotic illness and from that determine the risk factors affecting the population that might explain the presence of psychosis in some and its absence in others. There are also no genetic-related research findings to explore the role of this risk factor in the development of psychotic illness in this population. There are also relatively high rates of sociodevelopmental factors such as childhood sexual abuse and parental separation in early life, and this might also contribute to the development of psychosis in those at risk as has been reported elsewhere. Childhood adversities, especially those involving hostility and threat, are now accepted as strong risk factors for the onset of psychotic disorder (Morgan & Gayer-Anderson, 2016).

Exposure to and experiencing of violent trauma is also becoming more commonplace, and this must be addressed as a general mental health need but also specifically in the prevention of long-term psychotic reactions as a response to this trauma (Shavers, 2013; Yousseff, 2010). Violent crime and the fear of these crimes are both risks that need to be addressed in the prevention of mental illness and the promotion of mental health.

There remains an urgent need to rapidly develop research on mental health in Trinidad and Tobago, to inform strategies for prevention, intervention, and service delivery that are rooted in the challenges and needs of Trinidadian society.

References

Arthur, C. M. & Whitley, R. (2015). Head take you. Causal attributions of mental illness in Jamaica. *Transcult Psychiatry, 52*(1), 115–132.

Bebbington, P., et al. (2011). Childhood sexual abuse and psychosis: data from a cross-sectional national psychiatric survey in England. *Br J Psychiatry, 199*(1), 29–37.

Bhugra, D., et al. (1996). First contact incidence rates of schizophrenia in Trinidad and one year follow-up. *Br J Psychiatry, 169*(5), 587–592.

Bhugra, D., Leff, J., Mallett, R., Corridan, B., & Rudge, S. (1997). Incidence and outcome of schizophrenia in whites, African Caribbeans and Asians in London. *Psychol Med, 27*(4), 791–798.

Bhugra, D. & Jones, P. B. (2001). Migration and mental illness. *Adv Psychiatr Treat, 7*, 216–223.

Bhugra, D., et al. (2003). Pregnancy and birth complications in patients with schizophrenia in Trinidad and London. *West Indian Med J, 52*(2), 124–126.

Caldas de Almeida, J. M. (2013). Mental health services development in Latin America and the Caribbean. Achievements, barriers and facilitating factors. *Int Health, 5*(1), 15–18.

Caribbean Atlas Project (2013). Introduction: what is the Caribbean? Caribbean Atlas. Retrieved from http://www.caribbean-atlas.com/en/themes/what-is-the-caribbean/introduction.html

Central Statistical Office (2013). Trinidad and Tobago 2011 Publication and Housing Census Demographic Report. Ministry of Planning and Sustainable Development, Government of the Republic of Trinidad and Tobago.

Children's Authority of Trinidad and Tobago (2016). Annual Report of the Children's Authority of T&T for the period ending 30 September 2015, 31.

Cohen, A., et al (2016). Concepts of madness in diverse settings: a qualitative study from the Intrepid project. *BMC Psychiatry, 16*(1), 388.

Davis, J., et al. (2016). A review of vulnerability and risks for schizophrenia. Beyond the two hit hypothesis. *Neurosci Biobehav Rev, 65*, 185–194.

Falk, O., Wallinius, M., Lundstrom, S., Frisell, T., Anckarsater, N., & Kerekes, N. (2014). The one percent accountable for 63% of violent crime convictions. *Soc Psychiatry Psychiatr Epidemiol, 49*(4), 559–571.

Fryer, P. (1984). *Staying power: the history of black Britain.* London: Pluto Press Ltd.

Government of Trinidad and Tobago (GOTT)—UNICEF (2012). Trinidad and Tobago strategic action for children: GOTT—UNICEF work plan 2013-2016. GOTT—UNICEF. Retrieved from https://docplayer.net/21059703-Trinidad-and-tobago-strate gic-actions-for-children-and-gott-unicef-work-plan-2013-2014-1.html

Harrison, G., Owens, D., Holton, A., Neilson, D., & Boot, D. (1988). A prospective study of severe mental disorder in Afro-Caribbean patients. *Psychol Med*, *18*(3), 643–657.

Heckers, S. (2009). Who is at risk for a psychotic disorder? *Schizophr Bull*, *35* (5), 847–850.

Heinz, A., Deserno, L., & Reininghaus, U. (2013). Urbanicity, social adversity and psychosis. *World Psychiatry*, *12*(3), 187–197.

Hickling, F. W. & Rodgers-Johnson, P. (1995). The incidence of first contact schizophrenia in Jamaica. *Br J Psychiatry*, *167*(2), 193–196.

Hickling, F. W. (2005). The epidemiology of schizophrenia and other mental health disorders in the Caribbean. *Revista Panam Salud*, *18*(4/5), 256–262.

Hickling, F. W., Gibson, R. C., & Hutchinson, G. (2013). Current research on transcultural psychiatry in the Anglophone Caribbean. Epistemological, public policy and epidemiological challenges. *Transcult Psychiatry*, *50*(6), 858–875.

Hutchinson, G., Ramcharan, C., & Ghany, K. (2003). Gender and ethnicity in first admissions to a psychiatric unit in Trinidad. *West Indian Med J*, *52* (4), 300–303.

Hutchinson, G. (2005). Variation of homicidal and suicidal behavior in Trinidad and the associated risk factors. *West Indian Med J*, *54*(5), 319–324

Hutchinson, G. & Murray, R. M. (2006). Risk factors for first episode schizophrenia in Trinidad and Tobago. *Schizophr Res*, *81*, Suppl 1, 238.

International Monetary Fund (2017). Trinidad and Tobago: Selected Issues. International Monetary Fund (IMF), Western Hemisphere Dept, Country Report 17/353. Washington, DC: IMF.

Jongsma, H., et al. (2018). Treated incidence of psychosis in the multinational EU-GEI study. *JAMA Psychiatry*, *75*(1), 36–46.

Kirkbride, J. T., et al. (2012). Incidence of schizophrenia and other psychoses in England 1950-2009: a systematic review and meta-analyses. *PLoS One*, *7*(3), e31660.

Konings, M., Henquet, C., Maharajh, H. D., Hutchinson, G., & Van Os, J. (2008). Early exposure to cannabis and risk for psychosis in young adolescents in Trinidad. *Acta Psychiatr Scand*, *118*(3), 209–213.

Lacey, K. K., Powell Sears, K., Crawford, T. V., Matusko, N., & Jackson, J. S. (2016). Relationship of social and economic factors to mental health problems in a population-based sample of Jamaicans and Guyanese. *BMJ Open*, *6*(12), e012870.

Maharajh, H. D. & Parasram, R. (1999). The practice of psychiatry in Trinidad and Tobago. *Int Rev Psychiatry*, *11*(2–3), 173–183.

Mahy, G. E., Mallett, R., Leff, J., & Bhugra, D. (1999). First-contact incidence rate of schizophrenia in Barbados. *Br J Psychiatry*, *175*, 28–33.

Mallet, R. M., Leff, J., Bhugra, D., Pang, D., Hua Zhao, J. (2002). Social environment, ethnicity and schizophrenia. A case control study. *Soc Psychiatry Psychiatr Epidemiol*, *37*(7), 329–335.

Mead, M. (2007). Empire Windrush. Cultural memory and archival disturbance. *MoveableType*, *3*, 112–128.

Morgan, C., Charalambides, M., Hutchinson, G., & Murray, R. M. (2010). Migration, ethnicity and psychosis: toward a socio-developmental model. *Schizophr Bull*, *36*(4), 655–664.

Morgan, C. & Gayer-Anderson, C. (2016). Childhood adversities and psychosis: evidence, challenges, implications. *World Psychiatry*, *15*, 93–102.

Morgan, C., et al. (2016). The incidence of psychoses in diverse settings, INTREPID (2): a feasibility study in India, Nigeria, and Trinidad. *Psychol Med*, *46*(9), 1923–1933

Peach, C. (1991). *The Caribbean in Europe: contrasting patterns of migration and settlement in Britain, France and the Netherlands*. Research Paper in Ethnic Relations No. 15, Centre for Research into Ethnic Relations. Coventry: University of Warwick.

Phillips, C. (2001). *Pioneers, fifty years of migration to Britain: a new world order*. New York: Vintage.

Pinto, R., Ashworth, M., & Jones, R. (2008). Schizophrenia among black Caribbeans living in the UK: an exploration of the underlying causes of the high incidence rate. *Br J Gen Pract*, *58*(551), 429–434.

Plant, D. T., Pawlby, S., Sharp, D., Zunszain, P. A., & Pariante, C. M. (2013). Prenatal maternal depression is associated with offspring inflammation at 25 years: a prospective longitudinal cohort study. *Transl Psychiatry*, *6*, e936.

Radua, J., et al (2018). What causes psychosis? An umbrella review of risk and protective factors. *World Psychiatry*, *17*(1), 49–66.

Ramkissoon, A. K., Donald, C., & Hutchinson, G. (2017). Supernatural vs medical: responses to mental illness among undergraduate university students in Trinidad. *Int J Soc Psychiatry*, *63*(4), 330–338.

Seepersad, R. (2016). Crime and violence in Trinidad and Tobago. In: Sutton, H. (ed.) *IDB series on crime and violence in the Caribbean.* Inter-American Development Bank. Technical note no. IDB-TN-1062.

Selten, J. P., Slaets, J. P., & Kahn, R. S. (1997). Schizophrenia in Surinamese and Dutch Antillean immigrants to the Netherlands: evidence of an increased incidence. *Psychol Med*, *27*(4), 807–811

Selten, J. P., Zeyl, C., Dwarkasing, R., Lumsden, V., Kahn, R. S., & Van Harten, P. N. (2005). First contact incidence of schizophrenia in Suriname. *Br J Psychiatry*, *186*, 74–75.

Sharpe, J. & Shafe, S. (2016). Mental health in the Caribbean. In Roopnarine, J. L. & Chadee, D. (eds) *Caribbean Psychology: Indigenous contributions to a global discipline.* Washington DC: American Psychological Association, 305–325.

Sharpley, M., Hutchinson, G., McKenzie, K. & Murray, R. (2001). Understanding the excess of psychosis among the African-Caribbean population in England. *Br J Psychiatry*, *178*, Suppl. 40, s60–s68.

Shavers, C. A. (2013). Exposures to violence and trauma among children and adolescents. *Health*, *5*(2), 298–305

Stilo, S. A., et al (2013). Social disadvantage: cause or consequence of impending psychosis. *Schizophr Bull*, *39*(6), 1288–1295.

Stilo, S. A., et al. (2017). Further evidence of a cumulative effect of social disadvantage on risk of psychosis. *Psychol Med*, *47*(5), 913–924.

Timimi, S. (2014). No more psychiatric labels. Why formal psychiatric diagnostic systems should be abolished. *Int J Clin Health Psychol*, *14*(3), 208–215.

Tortelli, A., et al. (2015). Schizophrenia and other psychotic disorders in Caribbean-born migrants and their descendants in England. A systematic review and meta-analysis of incidence rates 1950–2013. *Soc Psychiatry Psychiatr Epidemiol, 50*(7), 1039–1055.

US Library of Congress (1987). *Caribbean islands: country studies.* Meditz, S. A. & Hanratty, D. M. (eds). Washington DC: Library of Congress.

Van der Ven, E. & Selten, J. P. (2018). Migrant and ethnic minority status as risk factors for schizophrenia—new findings. *Curr Opin Psychiatry, 31*(3), 231–236.

Varese, F., et al. (2012). Childhood adversities increase the risk of psychosis: a meta analysis of patient control, prospective and cross-sectional cohort studies. *Schizophr Bull, 38*(4), 661–671.

Williams, E. (1962). *History of the people of Trinidad and Tobago.* London: Andre Deutsch.

World Health Organization—Assessment of Mental Health Systems (WHO-AIMS) (2011). *WHO-AIMS report on mental health systems in the Caribbean region.* Geneva: WHO.

Youseff, V. (2010). The culture of violence in Trinidad and Tobago—a case study. *Caribb Rev Gend Stud, 4*, 1–8.

12

Nigeria

Oye Gureje, Akin Ojagbemi, and
Oluyomi Esan

Introduction

People's behaviour and attitudes towards psychosis and persons with psychosis are shaped in part by their culture, geographical location, religion, and socioeconomic factors. To a large extent, local and cultural perspectives determine the relationships, attitudes, and behaviours that people have with one another and with persons with psychosis. This chapter reviews the local perspective of psychosis in Nigeria with emphasis on recent research programmes on various aspects of psychosis, descriptions of the treatment systems of psychosis, and the cultural contexts shaping the experience of psychosis. The chapter ends with a brief discussion of priorities for future research and service development.

Treatment systems in Nigeria

Nigeria has a population of about 200 million people and more than 250 ethnic groups. It operates a federal system of government comprising 36 federating units and one territory. There are three tiers of government: federal/central, state, and the local government. These oversee the tertiary, secondary, and primary levels of healthcare, respectively. Healthcare provision in Nigeria is a concurrent responsibility of these three tiers of government. The Federal Government, through the Federal Ministry of Health, formulates, disseminates, promotes, implements, monitors, and evaluates health policies of the Federal Government (Federal Ministry of Health Nigeria, 2016). The Federal Government also funds and coordinates the activities of 20 university teaching hospitals, 22 Federal Medical Centers, and 13 specialty hospitals which include the eight neuropsychiatric hospitals spread over the country. The majority of orthodox mental health services are provided by these eight neuropsychiatric hospitals. Their services are complemented by the departments of psychiatry in the teaching hospitals (Federal Ministry of Health Nigeria, 2016). These hospitals and departments of psychiatry can be regarded as tertiary healthcare facilities. The majority of patients seen in these specialist facilities (outpatient or inpatient) tend to have a severe mental disorder, especially psychotic disorders and most commonly, schizophrenia (World Health Organization & Ministry of Health in Nigeria, 2006). State governments fund and manage various general hospitals, which can be regarded as district-level secondary healthcare facilities. A few general hospitals, and private psychiatric facilities, also provide orthodox mental healthcare services. The first tier of the health service is made up of primary healthcare clinics, which are run by local governments. Even though mental healthcare is included in the service provided at this level of the health system (Abdulmalik et al., 2013; Abdulmalik et al., 2014), very few services for psychosis are available at that level.

Complementary and alternative mental healthcare providers (CAPs), made up of traditional and faith healers (TFH), constitute important service providers, especially for persons with severe mental disorders, a situation that is comparable to several other countries in sub-Saharan Africa (Agara et al., 2008; Ensink & Robertson, 1999). In Nigeria, they operate outside of the formal mental health system.

Service provision

Treatment systems for psychosis in Nigeria include services provided by orthodox mental health practitioners and by TFH. Orthodox mental health services include those provided in outpatient, inpatient, and day treatment facilities, community-based psychiatric units, community residential facilities, as well as in forensic and other residential facilities (World Health Organization, 2006). Access to clinical psychologists and other allied mental health providers such as social workers or occupational therapists are mostly available in the specialist neuropsychiatric hospitals and departments of psychiatry within teaching hospitals. The professionals involved in the treatment of psychosis include a diverse group of practitioners, such as general physicians, psychiatrists, psychologists, psychiatric nurses, general nurses, community health extension workers, and community health officers, with the latter two being involved in the provision of care to the few patients who may present at primary care level. This profile of health providers means that there are wide differences in experience, expertise, and knowledge among these various providers with regard to the management of psychosis.

TFH provide for the mental health needs of a substantial proportion of the population in Nigeria. In particular, they are commonly consulted for severe mental health conditions, including psychotic disorders. TFH typically have facilities for both inpatient and outpatient care. In view of their number, their capacity for admission typically far exceeds what is available in the orthodox facilities in the same catchment area. For example, a study that mapped healer and biomedical services in parts of Ghana and Nigeria found that TFH often have between 2- to 10-fold capacity for patient admission compared with conventional mental health facilities (Esan et al., 2019). In essence, even though outside the formal mental health sector, TFH constitute an important part of the de facto mental healthcare system in Nigeria. TFH use a combination of signs, symptoms, and divination to unearth what may be responsible for such psychotic disorders before treatment. The therapeutic measure offered is determined by the perceived cause of mental illness. Depending on the aetiology found, treatment might include fasting, prayer, flogging the patient, the use of herbs, an offering of sacrifices, or a combination of these treatment modalities (Esan et al., 2019).

Specialist mental health facilities are all located in urban areas in the country. Most mental health specialists in active clinical services are therefore based in these urban areas. As a consequence, and since these facilities are few in number, there are large sections of the country, not just the rural areas, that do not have readily accessible specialist mental health services (Esan et al., 2014).

The limited number of orthodox mental health facilities and professionals reflects the generally poor funding of the service. Less than 5% of the health budget of the Federal Government goes to mental health, with over 90% of this going to the provision of services at the neuropsychiatric hospitals (World Health Organization, 2006).

Services in the formal health sector are not free and a national health insurance scheme only provides some services for a small proportion of the population employed in the public service. The most common access to care for persons with psychosis is therefore through out-of-pocket payment. Problems relating to compliance with treatment and lack of access to the most appropriate forms of treatment are directly related to this mode of payment and are therefore common (Adelufosi et al., 2013).

The concept of mental illness

The concept of mental illness among people in sub-Saharan Africa is largely restricted to psychoses and may not be as encompassing as the standard definitions of mental disorders in the Diagnostic and Statistical Manual of Mental Disorders (DSM) or the International Classification of Diseases (ICD; Jegede, 2005). That is, in the language of the lay public in most African communities, 'mental illness' connotes severe mental disorders with features associated with psychosis as the most common point of reference. Consequently, the majority of the general population in Nigeria are not likely to view conditions such as anxiety disorder, moderate depressive disorder, or bodily distress disorder as mental illnesses. In a study conducted in the Yoruba-speaking area of Nigeria to determine the knowledge and attitude of the people towards mental illness, most respondents thought that people with mental illness were 'mentally retarded', were a public nuisance, and were dangerous because of their violent behaviours (Gureje et al., 2005). These beliefs mirror the grossly disorganized behaviour criterion (A4) in DSM-IV where the DSM states that psychosis may manifest in childlike silliness to unpredictable agitation. Another study which examined the portrayal of mental illness in West African films found that cases of psychosis constituted the majority of the scenes in films depicting mental illness (Atilola & Olayiwola, 2013). In a study examining perceptions and beliefs about mental illness among adults in Karfi village, northern Nigeria, the most commonly noted signs or symptoms of mental illness were aggression, destructiveness, talkativeness, and eccentric behaviours (Kabir et al., 2004).

Aetiology of mental illness

There seems to be a shared understanding about the aetiology of mental illness across the major ethnic groups in Nigeria. Studies conducted among the three main ethnic groups (Yoruba, Hausa, and Igbo) suggest that a common belief is that mental illness may be caused by problematic use of drugs and alcohol, brain disease, genetics, possession by evil spirits, traumatic events, and witchcraft (Gureje et al., 2005; Iheanacho et al., 2016; Kabir et al., 2004; Wieschhoff, 1943). The range of possible causal factors endorsed seems to suggest a broad understanding of the aetiology of mental illness as encompassing biological, psychological, and social origins (Cohen et al., 2016). There is a general tendency to set a very low threshold for the link between the use of illicit drugs and severe mental illness, such that the first presumed cause of a psychotic illness, especially if this occurs in a young man, is illicit drug use irrespective of whether any strong evidence exists for such use or not. Thus, in a study conducted in among Hausa/Fulani speakers in northern Nigeria, misuse of illicit drugs ranked highest among the reported causes of mental illness followed by divine punishment and affliction by demons, in that order (Kabir et al., 2004). Studies conducted among the Yorubas and Igbos also showed the same pattern of reported causes (Aina, 2004; Iheanacho et al., 2016; Jegede, 2005; Olugbile et al., 2009).

Attitudes towards people with mental illness

Negative views about people with psychotic illness are widely held in Nigeria (Gureje et al., 2005; Kabir et al., 2004). This manifests in different forms ranging from the fear of holding a conversation with people with mental illness, to an aversion to having friendships with them or any type of close interaction (such as marriage). Men and people who reside in urban areas have a somewhat more tolerant attitude towards people with mental illness in the Yoruba-speaking areas (Gureje et al., 2005).

Epidemiology of psychotic experiences in Nigeria

In the Nigerian Survey of Mental Health and Wellbeing (NSMHWB), a community-based survey of the prevalence, impact, and antecedents of mental disorders, a lifetime prevalence of 2.1% and a 12-month estimate of 1.1% of non-affective psychosis was found among a representative community sample (Gureje et al., 2010). This is high when compared with the lifetime prevalence of other disorders in the same study. For example, the prevalence of alcohol dependence was 0.2%, drug abuse was 1.0% (Gureje et al., 2006), and bipolar disorder was 0.1%. The estimate for psychotic experiences was lower than the estimates in a cross-national analysis of 31,261 respondents from 18 countries which included Nigeria; respondents were asked about lifetime and 12-month prevalence and frequency of six types of psychotic experiences (PE) (two hallucinatory experiences and four delusional experiences). With a lifetime prevalence of 2.2%, Nigeria was among the four countries with the lowest reported prevalence and with a substantially lower estimate than the mean lifetime prevalence of ever having a psychotic experience of 5.8% across the 18 countries (McGrath et al., 2015). However, as in most other countries, hallucinatory experiences were more frequently reported than delusions, 1.7% vs. 1.0%.

In the NSMHWB study, non-affective psychosis was more common among urban dwellers compared with rural dwellers. Persons with non-affective psychosis were at an elevated risk of reporting both lifetime and 12-month comorbid DSM-IV disorders and experiencing impairment in basic and instrumental role functioning. Men had higher lifetime rates than women. Visual hallucinations were the most common PE. Lifetime psychotic experience was more commonly reported by persons who had never been married or those who had separated or divorced (Gureje et al., 2010).

Overviews of recent research programmes on various aspects of psychosis in Nigeria

The Partnership for Mental Health Development in Sub-Saharan Africa (PaM-D)

PaM-D was set up to create an infrastructure to develop mental health research capacity in sub-Saharan Africa, and to improve global mental health science by conducting innovative public health-relevant research in the region (Gureje et al., 2019). This project brought together institutions in six countries in sub-Saharan Africa in an effort to make major improvements in their health systems—Nigeria, South Africa, Ghana, Kenya, Sierra Leone, and Liberia—with researchers from institutions in the United States and the United Kingdom, and in partnership with government departments and non-governmental organizations. The goals of this project included bringing together stakeholders with expertise in global mental health to create a regional centre supporting research capacity building and innovative mental health service development in the region. The project also aimed to develop and implement targeted programmes of training and mentoring that build mental health research capacity for a broad range of mental health professionals.

The research component of PaM-D consisted of a programme entitled the COllaborative Shared care to IMprove Psychosis Outcome (COSIMPO), and its aim was to test the effectiveness and cost-effectiveness of a collaborative shared care programme between TFH and primary healthcare providers (PHCPs) in improving the outcome of psychosis. It had two parts: (1) a series of formative studies, and (2) a randomized controlled trial (RCT). The formative studies were conducted in Nigeria, Ghana, and Kenya.

One of the activities included the mapping of TFH in a defined catchment area in each of the three countries. Information was collected about the number of facilities, their capacity for the admission of patients, the training and experience of the healers, and their common modalities of treatment for psychosis. Another study was conducted to explore the feasibility of collaboration between TFH and PHCPs. The study assessed the willingness of the healers and orthodox primary care providers to work together for the care of persons with psychosis and identify factors that might constitute barriers and facilitators to such collaboration. A final component of the formative studies was a comprehensive exploration of the experience of psychosis and its care among individuals using the services of TFH and their caregivers, as well as how their understanding of the nature of psychosis might facilitate or impede their acceptance of collaborative shared care.

The main findings of these formative studies include the important role that TFH play in the provision of care for persons with psychosis in Nigeria (Esan et al., 2019). In the catchment area studied, admission places available in the facilities of the healers far outstripped those in formal orthodox facilities (Morgan et al., 2016). Healers generally had long years of training, most often as apprentices under a relative, commonly a father. Their treatment practices were eclectic, consisting of the use of herbs, divination, and rituals. These treatment approaches could be classified as those that were potentially helpful (such as herbs), largely with undefined value but otherwise innocuous (such as animal sacrifices), and potentially or clearly harmful (such as shackling, scarification, or prolonged fasting). Healers as well as orthodox primary care providers were well disposed to collaboration even though both groups recognized important differences in their worldviews about the nature of psychosis, its causes, and the most effective ways to care for persons with the condition (van der Watt et al., 2017). There was a general recognition that collaboration could allow for the tapping of their different skills for the overall good of patients. With regard to illness attribution and in consonance with the literature on the subject (van der Watt et al., 2018), persons experiencing psychosis, their caregivers, as well as healers, espoused the supernatural origin of psychosis as one of the most common aetiological explanations and this belief was an important determinant in seeking help from healers who are believed to have approaches that could help address the root cause rather than the superficial features of psychosis. This observation is similar to findings of the same research group in other contexts as well (Cohen et al., 2016). Self-stigma was a common feature among persons with experience of psychosis and it tended to be associated with a higher likelihood of espousing supernatural causation to psychosis (Makanjuola et al., 2016).

Based on the findings of the formative research, a collaborative shared care intervention package that lays out the boundaries and structure of collaboration between TFH and PHCPs was developed and tested in an RCT conducted in Ghana and Nigeria (Gureje et al., 2017). The study represented the first attempt to empirically test, in an RCT design, a formal collaboration between healers and biomedical providers in the delivery of care to patients with psychosis (and indeed with any health condition). The results suggest that, compared with enhanced usual care, a collaborative model of care was more effective in alleviating symptoms of psychosis, improving disability, shortening the length of admission, and improving adjustment to work following admission. The model was also more cost-effective when overall service costs were considered (Gureje et al., 2020).

The INTREPID study

INTREPID is a programme of research designed to develop robust and comparable methods for the study of schizophrenia and other psychoses in diverse settings and to implement these in a three-country study of the epidemiology, phenomenology, aetiology, and outcome of psychoses.

The pilot work (INTREPID I), conducted over 3 years, focused on defined catchment areas in three countries: Chengalpet taluk (near Chennai), India; Ibadan South East and Ona-Ara, Ibadan, Nigeria; and Tunapuna-Piarco,

Trinidad. The main goals of the pilot were to implement and appraise strategies for: (a) identifying and recruiting untreated and first-episode cases of psychosis; (b) identifying and recruiting representative controls; and (c) following cases over time. The study also attempted to validate and assess the feasibility of a core set of instruments and procedures to collect comparable information across diverse settings on psychopathology, biological and social exposures (including social and cultural contexts), and outcome.

Reports from the study indicated the rate of all untreated psychoses in the Nigerian site was 31.2 per 100,000 person-years and further confirmed the importance of TFH in the provision of care to persons with psychosis in the country (Morgan et al., 2015; Morgan et al., 2016). A more definitive programme of work, INTREPID II, to explore incidence, course, antecedents, and correlates of psychosis is currently ongoing.

The clinical outcome study

This prospective longitudinal study, conducted in Ibadan, Nigeria and Cape Town, South Africa investigated the clinical, sociodemographic, and biological and treatment aspects of schizophrenia spectrum disorders. The research was designed to study the symptom expression of schizophrenia in patients experiencing a first episode of the illness, examine the relationships between symptomatic remission and other measures of outcome, identify clinically relevant predictors of treatment outcome, explore the course of the illness, and specifically the evolution of treatment-refractoriness over time. Also, it was designed to explore antipsychotic dose requirements, sensitivity to antipsychotics, and the profile of side effects experienced by patients in the early course of illness, as well as to evaluate how these factors influence the course and outcome of the illness. The findings of the study have been presented in several publications in peer-reviewed journals (Chiliza et al., 2016; Ojagbemi et al., 2015; Ojagbemi et al., 2015). Among the important findings of the study is that a combination of depot antipsychotics with an assertive monitoring programme to promote medication adherence was an effective and safe intervention in the early phases of schizophrenia, a finding with particular relevance for resource-constrained settings where the choice of medications may be limited.

Contextual challenges of psychosis research

Conducting research on psychosis in Nigeria presents several challenges because of the low incidence of psychosis, the sociocultural context in which care is sought or provided, as well as the stigma associated with psychosis. These challenges are further compounded by a generally poor research funding terrain in the country, as in much of sub-Saharan Africa. Thus, methodologically rigorous large-scale studies are few in this area. Other methodological challenges are discussed in more detail below.

The use of small, non-probability samples

Most studies on psychosis in Nigeria and by extension many parts of sub-Saharan Africa have relied on non-probability samples. In particular, many such studies have used convenience samples (e.g. from hospitals, inpatient facilities, clinics, etc.). These non-probability samples may not be representative of the population of psychotic patients in the community. Clinical samples often have the drawbacks of oversampling psychotic patients who are relatively more impaired. In addition, the patients and their caregivers or relatives sampled in such circumstances are those who are more likely to seek orthodox mental health services compared with alternative/complementary healthcare services. Consequently, the level of education, socioeconomic status, and urbanicity may be confounders of the results obtained. These factors limit the generalizability of the findings of such studies.

This challenge is particularly central to the study of psychosis everywhere. The prevalence of psychotic disorders is relatively low; consequently, a large number of people from the population have to be screened to get an adequate number of subjects to provide sufficient power for many studies on psychosis. This would mean mobilizing more resources and funds for such studies.

Sampling, a process in statistics in which a pre-set number of observations are taken from a larger population, is commonly used to generate manageable study samples that may be representative of a larger population. When subpopulations represent only a small proportion of the general population as in the case of psychotic disorders, it presents major challenges for probability sampling. Researchers consequently resort to finding cost-effective and often, less methodologically sound means for obtaining such samples (Kalton, 1993).

Case ascertainment

A problem which stems from using clinical populations is case ascertainment. Many studies on psychosis rely on case note diagnosis. Several glitches may occur in this regard. Diagnostic inconsistencies in patients' case notes can interfere with a researcher's ability to reliably divide patients into diagnostic categories. Patients may have been given two or three different diagnoses within the same case notes. In many teaching hospitals, case note diagnoses have been made by trainees or residents with varying degrees of experience as diagnosticians. This may result in inconsistencies and inaccurate diagnoses (Javier et al., 1997).

Traditional and faith healers

The de facto mental health providers in Nigeria, and many other sub-Saharan African countries, are the traditional and faith healers (Esan et al., 2019; Gureje et al., 2015). Consequently, mental health specialist services are not appropriately placed for the detection of representative samples of incident or untreated cases of psychosis. An approach to solving this methodological problem is to map all TFH in a geographically defined area, using key informants and snowballing approaches to identify cases. The drawback of this method is that the extent to which such a strategy can comprehensively map all providers and identify a sufficient number of key informants in each site is uncertain. Another challenge of this approach is that, except when adequate preliminary efforts have been made to generate trust, the healers may be suspicious of the motives of the researchers. One example of a programme of work where steps were taken to address some of these challenges is INTREPID 1 (Morgan et al., 2015; Morgan et al., 2016).

Response bias

The tendency to give culturally sanctioned or socially desirable responses is also an issue (Laroi et al., 2014). This is particularly so for a condition that is highly stigmatized. Thus, for example in family studies, people are usually reluctant to disclose that another family member outside the index psychotic patient also has a psychotic disorder. Indeed, obtaining third-person information on the occurrence of psychosis requires a lot of sensitivity and experience from the researcher or interviewer in order to ensure that reliable information is obtained.

Priorities for future research and service development

Given the limited nature of the current evidence available on psychotic disorders, especially from sub-Saharan Africa, it is clear that there are large gaps in our knowledge about the profile and features of psychosis in the region. In particular, information about the prevalence of the condition as well as its course and the determinants of that course is needed. We need large-scale studies of representative samples and epidemiological surveys to find the risk factors, causes, and outcomes of psychotic patients in the community as well as those receiving treatment.

Studies are required to explore aetiological factors of psychosis, including genetics and environmental causes. For example, we do not know the extent to which some of the more commonly occurring infections such as malaria predispose to psychoses, including to diagnosable psychotic disorders.

Concerning treatment, we need to study the best ways to increase access to care for persons with psychotic disorders. For example, evidence is needed on how to integrate the treatment of psychosis into primary healthcare and on the most effective and cost-effective ways to implement sustainable rehabilitation for patients with long-term disabilities as a result of psychotic disorders. The controversy about whether the outcome of psychosis may or may not be better in persons with psychosis from these parts of the world (Cohen et al., 2008) will require robustly planned and implemented epidemiological studies, ideally conducted in several sites and by multidisciplinary teams who are able to explore the questions from cultural and sociological as well as clinical angles. Several putative risk factors, such as poverty, migration, pollution, and urban living, are either on the increase in Africa or are undergoing profound changes. Their associations with the risk and course of psychosis are an important and potentially transformative area of research.

References

Abdulmalik, J., et al. (2014). The Mental Health Leadership and Advocacy Program (mhLAP): a pioneering response to the neglect of mental health in Anglophone West Africa. *Int J Ment Health Syst, 8*(1), 5.

Abdulmalik, J., et al. (2013). Country contextualization of the mental health gap action programme intervention guide: a case study from Nigeria. *PLoS Med, 10*(8), e1001501.

Adelufosi, A. O., Ogunwale, A., Adeponle, A. B., & Abayomi, O. (2013). Pattern of attendance and predictors of default among Nigerian outpatients with schizophrenia. *Afr J Psychiatry (Johannesbg), 16*(4), 283–287.

Agara, A. J., Makanjuola, A. B., & Morakinyo, O. (2008). Management of perceived mental health problems by spiritual healers: a Nigerian study. *Afr J Psychiatry (Johannesbg), 11*(2), 113–118.

Aina, O. F. (2004). Mental illness and cultural issues in West African films: implications for orthodox psychiatric practice. *Med Humanit, 30*(1), 23–26.

Atilola, O. & Olayiwola, F. (2013). Frames of mental illness in the Yoruba genre of Nigerian movies: implications for orthodox mental health care. *Transcult Psychiatry, 50*(3), 442–454.

Chiliza, B., et al. (2016). Combining depot antipsychotic with an assertive monitoring programme for treating first-episode schizophrenia in a resource-constrained setting. *Early Interv Psychiatry, 10*(1), 54–62.

Cohen, A., et al. (2016). Concepts of madness in diverse settings: a qualitative study from the INTREPID project. *BMC Psychiatry, 16*(1), 388.

Cohen, A., Patel, V., Thara, R., & Gureje, O. (2008). Questioning an axiom: better prognosis for schizophrenia in the developing world? *Schizophr Bull, 34*(2), 229–244.

Ensink, K. & Robertson, B. (1999). Patient and family experiences of psychiatric services and African indigenous healers. *Transcult Psychiatry, 36*(1), 23–43.

Esan, O., Abdumalik, J., Eaton, J., Kola, L., Fadahunsi, W., & Gureje, O. (2014). Mental health care in anglophone West Africa. *Psychiatr Serv, 65*(9), 1084–1087.

Esan, O., et al. (2019). A survey of traditional and faith healers providing mental health care in three sub-Saharan African countries. *Soc Psychiatry Psychiatr Epidemiol, 54*(3), 395–403.

Federal Ministry of Health Nigeria (2016). Department of Hospital Services. Retrieved from http://www.health.gov.ng/index.php/department/hospital-services

Gureje, O., Lasebikan, V. O., Ephraim-Oluwanuga, O., Olley, B. O., & Kola, L. (2005). Community study of knowledge of and attitude to mental illness in Nigeria. *Br J Psychiatry, 186*, 436–441.

Gureje, O., Lasebikan, V. O., Kola, L., & Makanjuola, V. A. (2006). Lifetime and 12-month prevalence of mental disorders in the Nigerian Survey of Mental Health and Well-Being. *Br J Psychiatry, 188*, 465–471.

Gureje, O., Nortje, G., Makanjuola, V., Oladeji, B., Seedat, S., & Jenkins, R. (2015). The role of global traditional and complementary systems of medicine in treating mental health problems. *Lancet Psychiatry, 2*(2), 168–177.

Gureje, O., Olowosegun, O., Adebayo, K., & Stein, D. J. (2010). The prevalence and profile of non-affective psychosis in the Nigerian Survey of Mental Health and Wellbeing. *World Psychiatry, 9*(1), 50–55.

Gureje, O., et al. (2020). The effect of collaborative care between traditional/faith healers and primary health care workers to improve psychosis outcome in Nigeria and Ghana (COSIMPO)—a randomized controlled trial. *Lancet, 396*(10251), 612–622.

Gureje, O., et al. (2017). COllaborative Shared care to IMprove Psychosis Outcome (COSIMPO): study protocol for a randomized controlled trial. *Trials, 18*(1), 462.

Gureje, O., et al. (2019). Partnership for mental health development in Sub-Saharan Africa (PaM-D): a collaborative initiative for research and capacity building. *Epidemiol Psychiatr Sci, 28*(4), 389–396.

Iheanacho, T., et al. (2016). Attitudes and beliefs about mental illness among church-based lay health workers: experience from a prevention of mother-to-child HIV transmission trial in Nigeria. *Int J Cult Ment Health, 9*(1), 1–13.

Javier, R. A., et al. (1997). Methodological problems encountered in research with psychiatric inpatients: a case example. *Bull Menninger Clin, 61*(4), 520–531.

Jegede, A. (2005). The notion of 'were' in Yoruba conception of mental illness. *Nord J Afr Stud, 14*(1), 117–126.

Kabir, M., Iliyasu, Z., Abubakar, I. S., & Aliyu, M. H. (2004). Perception and beliefs about mental illness among adults in Karfi village, northern Nigeria. *BMC Int Health Hum Rights, 4*(1), 3.

Kalton, G. (1993). *Sampling considerations in research on HIV risk and illness*. New York: Plenum Press.

Laroi, F., et al. (2014). Culture and hallucinations: overview and future directions. *Schizophr Bull, 40 Suppl 4*, S213–220.

Makanjuola, V., et al. (2016). Explanatory model of psychosis: impact on perception of self-stigma by patients in three sub-Saharan African cities. *Soc Psychiatry Psychiatr Epidemiol, 51*(12), 1645–1654.

McGrath, J. J., et al. (2015). Psychotic experiences in the general population: a cross-national analysis based on 31,261 respondents from 18 countries. *JAMA Psychiatry, 72*(7), 697–705.

Morgan, C., et al. (2015). Searching for psychosis: INTREPID (1): systems for detecting untreated and first-episode cases of psychosis in diverse settings. *Soc Psychiatry Psychiatr Epidemiol, 50*(6), 879–893.

Morgan, C., et al. (2016). The incidence of psychoses in diverse settings, INTREPID (2): a feasibility study in India, Nigeria, and Trinidad. *Psychol Med, 46*(9), 1923–1933.

O'Neil, D. (2016, Friday, May 26, 2006.). Human culture: what is culture? Retrieved from https://www2.palomar.edu/anthro/culture/culture_1.htm

Ojagbemi, A., Akpa, O., Esan, O., Emsley, R., & Gureje, O. (2015). The confirmatory factor structure of neurological soft signs in Nigerians with first episode schizophrenia. *Neurosci Lett, 589*, 110–114.

Ojagbemi, A., Esan, O., Emsley, R., & Gureje, O. (2015). Motor sequencing abnormalities are the trait marking neurological soft signs of schizophrenia. *Neurosci Lett, 600*, 226–231.

Olugbile, O., Zachariah, M. P., Kuyinu, A., Coker, A., Ojo, O., & Isichei, B. (2009). Yoruba world view and the nature of psychotic illness. *Afr J Psychiatry (Johannesbg), 12*(2), 149–156.

van der Watt, A. S. J., et al. (2017). Collaboration between biomedical and complementary and alternative care providers: barriers and pathways. *Qual Health Res, 27*(14), 2177–2188.

van der Watt, A. S. J., et al. (2018). The perceived effectiveness of traditional and faith healing in the treatment of mental illness: a systematic review of qualitative studies. *Soc Psychiatry Psychiatr Epidemiol, 53*(6), 555–566.

Wieschhoff, H. (1943). Concepts of abnormality among the Ibo of Nigeria. *J Am Orient Soc, 63*(4), 262–272.

World Health Organization (2006). WHO-AIMS report on mental health system in Nigeria, WHO and Ministry of Health, Ibadan, Nigeria, 2006. Retrieved from https://www.ecoi.net/en/file/local/1076735/1158_1195574650_nigeria-who-aims-report.pdf

13

Ethiopia

Charlotte Hanlon, Alex Cohen,
and Atalay Alem

Introduction

Ethiopia is one of the very few low- and middle-income countries in which there has been sustained research on psychotic disorders. In this chapter, we provide an overview of and introduction to the major studies that have been conducted.

Historical note

The history of psychiatric epidemiology in Ethiopia can be traced to the 1960s and the work of the Dutch psychiatrist Robert Giel and colleagues (Giel, 1999). This early research involved surveys of outpatient and community populations in a city (Jimma) (Dormaar et al., 1974), a small town (Giel & Van Luijk, 1969), a rural village (Giel & van Liujk, 1970), and a religious site in Addis Ababa (Giel et al., 1974). At about the same time, Lars Jacobsson, a Swedish psychiatrist, investigated the prevalence of psychiatric morbidity in a sample of individuals attending the outpatient clinic of a general hospital in western Ethiopia (Jacobsson, 1985). These studies were important for putting mental health on the map in Ethiopia. However, because all the samples were relatively small and not necessarily representative of the contexts in which the surveys were conducted, estimates of prevalence, let alone incidence rates, were not reliable.

In his brief account of the early history of psychiatry (mid-1960s) in Ethiopia, Giel noted the poor conditions for patients in Amanuel Hospital in Addis Ababa but, on the positive side, also noted that psychiatry was introduced into the curriculum of a new medical faculty and provided the basis for Giel's teaching in Haile Selassie I University (Giel, 1999). In the following decades, two Ethiopian psychiatrists, Fikre Workneh and Abdulreshid Abdullahi, returned to the country after having been trained in the United States and Scotland, respectively. Plans for decentralization of mental health services were developed in 1985 at a workshop hosted by the World Health Organization (WHO). This led to the establishment of training programmes for nurses so that they could provide care in Amanuel Hospital and establish psychiatric outpatient clinics in general hospitals throughout the country. The WHO provided additional Ethiopian physicians with training opportunities abroad in psychiatry during the late 1980s and early 1990s.

Epidemiological studies

In the 1990s, Derege Kebede and Atalay Alem conducted an epidemio-logical survey of major mental disorders among a random sample of adults (n=1420) residing in Addis Ababa (Giel, 1999; Kebede & Alem, 1999b). Although the structured measures—including an Amharic version of the WHO Composite International Diagnostic Interview (CIDI)—were ad-ministered by lay data collectors and reliant on self-report, this survey pro-vided first estimates of the one-month prevalence of a range of disorders (Kebede & Alem, 1999c; Kebede & Alem, 1999d), including schizophrenia (0.3%) and bipolar disorder (0.4%); results that were similar to those of studies conducted in other low- and middle-income countries (Kebede & Alem, 1999b). During this same period, Kebede and Alem conducted fur-ther larger surveys (>10,000 people) to investigate levels of mental distress, the use of alcohol, and suicidal behaviour among representative samples of adults in Addis Ababa (Kebede & Alem, 1999e; Kebede & Alem, 1999a; Kebede et al., 1999) and a rural community around Butajira, south-central Ethiopia (Alem et al., 1999b; Alem et al., 1999c; Alem et al., 1999e). Butajira town and surrounding districts were the sites of a demographic surveillance initiative, which provided an important platform for studies of people with severe mental illness (Berhane et al., 1999). In an initial study, Alem inves-tigated how mental disorders were perceived by community key informants using contextualized vignettes capturing seven neuropsychiatric condi-tions (Alem et al., 1999a). Schizophrenia was recognized by informants and perceived to be the most severe condition. Talkativeness, aggression, and strange behaviour were the most commonly perceived manifestations of mental illness, with community responses focusing on religious and traditional healing. Kebede and Alem then initiated the Butajira study of the sociodemographics and the long-term course and outcome of schizo-phrenia, bipolar disorder, and severe depression (Kebede et al., 2003a; Kebede et al., 2004; Kebede et al., 2005a). This study used rigorous commu-nity case-finding methods (Kebede et al., 2003b):

+ 68,378 persons between the ages of 15 and 49 years in the district of Butijira were screened using the Amharic version of the CIDI.

- House-to-house screening was supplemented by key informant identification of 719 people with probable mental illness.
- Combining these approaches, 2,159 individuals were identified as cases with psychosis or affective disorders. Of these, 919 individuals were, based on clinician-confirmed diagnoses using the gold standard WHO Schedules for Clinical Assessment in Neuropsychiatry (Wing et al., 1990), identified at baseline as experiencing schizophrenia, bipolar disorder, or severe depression.
- Of these, 321 were identified as experiencing schizophrenia (Kebede et al., 2003b).

At baseline, women comprised less than 20% of the sample and were younger than men at illness onset, 21.0 vs. 23.8 years, respectively (Kebede et al., 2004). Both of these findings contrasted with estimates from the Global Burden of Disease Study that suggested no clear differences in prevalence by gender and age (Charlson et al., 2018). The marital status of the sample was as follows: less than one-third were married, slightly more than half had never been married, and not quite a fifth were separated, divorced, or widowed (Kebede et al., 2004). Women were more likely to have been divorced or separated (17.7% vs. 10.1% at baseline) (Mayston et al., 2020). This is in sharp contrast to research in India where the percentage married was generally above 70%; twice that seen in Ethiopia (Hopper et al., 2007). In India, no gender differences in proportion married were reported. The findings from Ethiopia also contrast with high-income countries where women may be twice as likely as men to be married. Subsequent qualitative exploration has shed light on the gendered experience of psychosis, with women who develop psychosis seeming to be differentially disadvantaged when it comes to marrying or remaining married (Hailemariam et al., 2019).

One of the objectives of the Butajira study was to examine the course and outcome of schizophrenia. Baseline assessment found that 67.2% (n=216) of participants appeared to have been ill continuously since onset (Kebede et al., 2003b), a finding that was not in agreement with WHO studies that found a better course and outcome among individuals with schizophrenia residing in low- and middle-income countries (Jablensky et al., 1992). Functional outcomes also belied the notion of better outcomes for persons with schizophrenia in LMICs. For example, of the Butajira sample, fewer than half had ever been married and almost half were unemployed, while 7% were homeless and 3.8% had attempted suicide (Kebede et al., 2003b). Only 10% had ever received treatment.

Follow-up of the Butajira cohort, including 40 incident cases identified by a leakage study, revealed a relatively poor clinical course of illness over an average period of 10 years, e.g. more than one-third experienced one or more repeated episodes, almost 20% had been continuously ill, and less than 12% experienced complete remission after a single psychotic episode (Shibre et al., 2015). In addition, 18.2% (n=65) of the cohort had died during the 10 years of follow-up, mostly from infectious diseases; of those who died, nine members of the cohort (2.5%; 13.8% of those who had died) were the result of suicide (Fekadu et al., 2015b). Non-fatal suicidal behaviour was exhibited by 47 (13.1%) individuals in the cohort (Shibre et al., 2014). Members of the cohort had a standardized mortality ratio about three times higher than the general population of Ethiopia. From another perspective, members of the cohort had a life expectancy, on average, of 46.3 years, or about 10 years less than the general population (Fekadu et al., 2015b).

Follow-up of the Butajira cohort produced several other important insights about the lives of individuals with schizophrenia and the individuals who are responsible for their care. For example:

1) During the first 5 years of the project, Shibre et al. (2012) annually assessed the burden of caregiving using the Family Interview Schedule. Burden scores decreased over time and the decrease was associated with relatively longer periods of remission during follow-up. By contrast, higher caregiver burden scores were associated with relatively high scores of assessments of the severity of negative and positive symptoms.

2) Focus group discussion and interviews, primarily among persons with schizophrenia and their caregivers, examined the reasons why some members of the Butajira cohort were non-adherent to medication regimes (Teferra et al., 2013). Some of the reasons for non-adherence (e.g. lack of effectiveness and side effects) were similar to those found in high-income countries. At the same time, two locally relevant reasons for non-adherence were inadequate food supplies to satisfy increased medication-induced appetite stimulation and 'expectations of cure rather than [the] need for continuing care'.

3) Tsigebrhan et al. (2014) found that individuals with severe mental illness (SMI) were more likely to be the perpetrators or victims of violence than individuals without SMI who lived in the same neighbourhoods. Acts of violence by those with SMI were associated with being unmarried, having experienced stressful life events, and being non-responsive to medications. The risk of being a victim of violence was associated with being unemployed, non-adherence to treatment, and having a history of violent acts.

4) Although functional recovery and the clinical course did not differ between men and women, there was evidence of some differences in the outcomes of

women compared with men (Mayston et al., 2020). Women were less likely to report overall life satisfaction (adjusted odds ratio (AOR) = 0.22, 95% CI = 0.09, 0.53) or good quality of spousal relationships (AOR = 0.09, 95% CI = 0.01–1.04). Men were more likely to have comorbid substance use.

The Butajira project has not only led to important evidence on the course and outcome of psychosis in a rural low-income country in sub-Saharan Africa, but it also spearheaded the development of decentralized mental healthcare in the study districts. As part of the project, psychiatric nurses were employed in the local health centre and provided monthly outreach to a more remote centre. Study participants had free access to antipsychotic medication for the full follow-up period of over 10 years. These psychiatric nurses are now employed by the government in the public hospital in the same district.

Although the Butajira project is among the most robust follow-up studies of a cohort of persons with psychosis, its limitations must be noted:

1) Inclusion of all cases: The mix of recent-onset and long-standing cases 'will influence the findings and the inferences that are ultimately to be drawn' (Bromet, 2008). Nonetheless, when findings from the Butajira cohort have been stratified by recent onset (within 1 or 2 years) vs. longer duration, there is no evidence for better outcomes in the more recent-onset cases.

2) Probable underascertainment of women (5:1 ratio of men to women). Recent research suggests that 'sociocultural factors subject women with SMI to higher levels of physical and social isolation compared to men, greatly affecting community health workers' ability to identify and provide care to women with mental illness' (Ghebrehiwet et al., 2020).

3) Limited case-finding in religious healing sites (Kebede et al., 2003b).

4) Limited investigation of salient biological or psychosocial risk factors in this sociocultural setting, including nutrition, physical ill-health, khat chewing, and exposure to traumatic events.

In addition to analyses of the Butajira database, Ethiopian researchers have examined a range of topics and subpopulations concerning psychosis. For example:

◆ An initial epidemiological study conducted in the Borana community, a nomadic group in Southern Ethiopia found no cases of psychosis using the WHO CIDI (Beyero et al., 2004). However, follow-up qualitative research with key informants led to identification of people with confirmed diagnoses of SMI (Shibre et al., 2010). This study found that 'local beliefs, perceptions, and understandings of symptoms of psychosis', posed challenges to case ascertainment. Further qualitative work indicated that causal attributions for SMI included the supernatural, childbirth, seeing blood, war, use of alcohol, malaria, and heredity. Preferred interventions included consultations with healers and 'wise men', prayer, and 'holy water', responses that were consistent with supernatural attributions. Indeed, biomedical interventions were only considered if other treatments were not effective (Teferra & Shibre, 2012).

♦ Among 1691 adult members of an isolated island community (the Zeway Islanders), the prevalence of bipolar disorder was 1.8% but that of psychosis was only 0.06% when using a combination of key informant screening, house-to-house screening using CIDI, and confirmatory diagnostic interviews (using SCAN) (Fekadu et al., 2004; Kebede et al., 2005b).

♦ Fekadu et al. (2014) investigated the needs of a group of 217 homeless adults in Addis Ababa and determined that 89 (41%) could be diagnosed as having psychosis. Furthermore, of those with psychosis, 80–100% of their basic needs were unmet—according to an assessment using an adapted version of the Camberwell Assessment of Needs Short Appraisal Schedule—and almost 30% had a physical disability; only 10% had received medical care, and most were not originally from Addis Ababa and had lived on the streets for two or more years.

♦ Assessment of functional status, as well as the conceptual bases underlying the assessments, are fraught with difficulties (Balaji et al., 2012; Isaac et al., 2007). Habtamu et al. (2015) conducted qualitative research with the aim of gaining in-depth understandings of functioning and disability in people with SMI in rural Ethiopia, as well as informing the development of socioculturally appropriate measures (Habtamu et al., 2016). This research suggests that 'functional impairment in people with [psychosis] is the result of not only symptoms associated with the illness, but also … social, economic and family related causes'. Furthermore, and of particular concern for assessing functional status, engagement in agricultural activities was not adequately captured in a dichotomous (yes/no) category. Rather, agricultural work included tasks with a range of difficulties and 'was not just a matter of going to work in the fields, but that the quality of the work and productivity had to be taken into consideration'.

From epidemiology to intervention

The Programme for Improving Mental Health Care (PRIME, 2011–2019) was the next important psychosis research project in Ethiopia (Lund et al., 2012). It built on the findings of the Butajira study but focused on participatory research to expand access to mental healthcare in the rural district of Sodo, which is about 100 kilometres south of Addis Ababa. The objective of the project was to develop, implement, and scale-up a plan that would coordinate community, facility, and health systems interventions to support the integration of mental health services in primary care settings for individuals with psychosis (Fekadu et al., 2015a). The intervention packages were informed by the contextual needs of people with psychosis (Mall et al., 2015). Formative research carried out 're-source mapping', which demonstrated that although biomedical services were lacking, the district in which the study took place had extensive community resources, e.g. religious organizations, microfinance institutions, funeral asso-ciations, and a large number of community-based health extension workers, that could be used to provide care for individuals with schizophrenia (Selamu et al., 2015). Using trained key informants, people with probable psychosis were identified in the community and referred to primary care for diagnosis and ini-tiation of care by primary care workers trained in the WHO Mental Health Gap Action Programme (WHO, 2008; WHO, 2016). Confirmatory diagnoses of psychotic disorders or bipolar disorder were provided by mental health special-ists using a gold standard semi-structured clinical interview (Baron et al., 2018). PRIME improved on the Butajira psychosis study methodology for case ascer-tainment by including women community-based health extension workers and key informants, leading to a lower men-to-women ratio (42.7% were women). A total of 300 people with psychosis engaged in care, equating to an estimated 80% population coverage (Hailemariam et al., 2020). There was little evidence of case leakage. Probable cases who did not engage (n=63) were more likely to live rurally but were less disabled (Hailemariam et al., 2020). There was limited recruitment in religious healing sites, but the involvement of religious leaders on the community advisory board for PRIME helped to increase awareness.

Key findings at the baseline of PRIME were: lifetime and current access gap for biomedical care were 41.8 and 59.9%, respectively, while the corresponding figures for faith and traditional healing were 15.1 and 45.2% (Fekadu et al., 2019); only 11.3% received minimally adequate biomedical care in the current episode (Fekadu et al., 2019); long duration of untreated psychosis (median 5 years); high rates of restraint (25%) in the preceding 12 months; high exposure to traumatic events (Fekadu et al., 2019; Ng et al., 2019); high lifetime experi-ence of homelessness (36.3%) (Fekadu et al., 2019); relatively low reported dis-crimination (higher in urban residents) (Forthal et al., 2019); higher poverty (Hailemichael et al., 2019a; Hailemichael et al., 2019c) and food insecurity (Tirfessa et al., 2019) compared with population controls.

Over a follow-up period of 12 months, in the 300 people with psychosis who initially engaged with integrated primary mental healthcare, there were reduc-tions in symptom severity, disability, self-reported discrimination, restraint, and suicidality (Hanlon et al., 2019). Household food insecurity was also reduced (Tirfessa et al., 2020). However, 11 people died during the follow-up period, underscoring the need for more proactive attention to physical healthcare. In PRIME, only 29.8% received minimally adequate care over the follow-up period (at least four clinic contacts attended) (Hanlon et al., 2019), with continuous engagement in care undermined by affordability, stigma, and challenges conveying people to care when unwell (Hailemariam et al., 2017).

The PRIME research demonstrated the need for the development of a community-based rehabilitation programme for people with schizophrenia residing in the Sodo district (Asher et al., 2015; Asher et al., 2016). This project, known as RISE (Rehabilitation In people with Schizophrenia in Ethiopia), conducted formative research to ensure that the intervention would be locally valid and feasible. The major formative research findings of RISE included:

- Use of restraints is frequent and is the result of a combination of the lack of treatment options and high levels of family burden due to the need to provide care to ill members (Asher et al., 2017).
- People with schizophrenia have little decision-making authority concerning their treatment. This renders them vulnerable to coercive practices (Souraya et al., 2018).

A pilot study of a community-based intervention demonstrated that increased family support, expanded access to care, and growth in income brought about improved functioning among individuals with schizophrenia (Asher et al., 2018). In a fully powered cluster randomized controlled trial, the RISE programme led to greater improvement in the functioning of people with schizophrenia compared with those who only accessed integrated primary mental healthcare (Asher et al., 2022).

In the neighbouring district, a further randomized controlled trial was conducted to evaluate integrated primary mental healthcare for people with psychosis, the 'TaSCS' trial (Hanlon et al., 2016). The TaSCS trial was nested within the ongoing Buajira project, benefitting from the community-ascertained sample of people with psychosis. In TaSCS, 324 people with psychosis were randomized to continue receiving centralized, psychiatric nurse-led outpatient care, or transfer to their catchment area primary healthcare facility for continuing care delivered by non-specialist health workers trained in the WHO Mental Health Gap Action Programme. After 18 months of follow-up, the clinical and functional outcomes of people with psychosis randomized to primary care were just as good as those who continued to receive care from mental health specialists (Hanlon et al., 2022).

The multi-country Emerging Mental Health Systems in Low- And Middle-Income Countries (EMERALD) programme included Ethiopia and focused on the need to strengthen mental health systems to support expanded access to mental healthcare (Thornicroft & Semrau, 2019). In Sodo district, EMERALD studies at the baseline of PRIME implementation of primary mental healthcare showed that households of people with psychosis when compared with households without an affected person had fewer assets, lower annual income, faced higher levels of catastrophic out-of-pocket healthcare expenditure, and were more likely to have to withdraw children from school or reduce healthcare contacts to save money (Hailemichael et al., 2019a; Hailemichael et al., 2019b). Over the 12-month intervention period, households of a person with psychosis were less likely to access community-based health insurance but did experience a greater increase in income than comparison households (Hailemichael et al., 2022). EMERALD also focused on the involvement of people with psychosis and other mental health conditions in mental health system strengthening. A formative study found that there was a very low experience of involvement at baseline, but interest in greater involvement (Abayneh et al., 2017). This led to the development and implementation of empowerment and training interventions to equip people with mental health conditions to advocate for their rights and be meaningfully involved in improving care. A participatory action research pilot study in Sodo district achieved mobilization of the community to support people with mental health conditions and their caregivers, the establishment of a grassroots representative organization, and reported benefits to participants in terms of social inclusion and connectedness (Abayneh et al., 2020; Abayneh et al., 2022a; Abayneh et al., 2022b).

Future research

In a newly funded research project, SCOPE, there will be an investigation of the association between khat use and psychosis. Khat is an evergreen plant that contains amphetamine-like stimulants (cathinones). Khat chewing is widespread in Ethiopia (Ethiopian Public Health Institute, 2015; Alem et al., 1999d; Alemu et al., 2020) and has been shown to be associated with self-reported psychotic symptoms in community surveys (Ongeri et al., 2019) and with clinical ratings of current psychotic symptoms (Odenwald et al., 2005). There are also plans to evaluate the consequences of traumatic events on the onset of psychosis, to conduct in-depth research on conceptualizations of personal recovery, and how family interaction patterns may influence the course and outcome of psychosis in Ethiopia (Temesgen et al., 2020). Building on these findings, the SCOPE project will develop methods to detect recent-onset psychosis and will design new intervention models that are inclusive of people who are homeless or abandoned, address biopsychosocial needs, mitigate against adverse outcomes, and support recovery.

Conclusion

This chapter presents a brief summary of the research about psychosis that has been conducted in Ethiopia. As important as this research might be, the work in Ethiopia is most distinguished by how it has developed from a focus on epidemiological research to research to inform treatments and interventions, especially for individuals with psychosis. Furthermore, it must be noted that, at first, the research was conducted by a small cadre of Ethiopians who, overtime, encouraged and mentored junior researchers who eventually took on the conduct of the projects and trials. Ethiopia now has a large number of mental health researchers who are carrying out important programmes to improve the lives of individuals with psychosis.

References

Abayneh, S., et al. (2017). Service user involvement in mental health system strengthening in a rural African setting: qualitative study. *BMC Psychiatry*, *17*, 187.

Abayneh, S., Lempp, H., Alem, A., Kohrt, B., Fekadu, A., & Hanlon, C. (2020). Developing a Theory of Change model of service user and caregiver involvement in mental health system strengthening in primary health care in rural Ethiopia. *Int J Mental Health Systems*, *14*, 51.

Abayneh, S., Lempp, H., Kohrt, B. A., Alem, A., & Hanlon, C. (2022a). Using participatory action research to pilot a model of service user and caregiver involvement in mental health system strengthening in Ethiopian primary healthcare: a case study. *Int J Ment Health Syst*, *16*, 33.

Abayneh, S., Lempp, H., Rai, S., Girma, E., Getachew, M., Alem, A., Kohrt, B. A., & Hanlon, C. (2022b). Empowerment training to support service user involvement in mental health system strengthening in rural Ethiopia: a mixed-methods pilot study. *BMC Health Serv Res*, *22*, 880.

Alem, A., Jacobsson, L., Araya, M., Kebede, D., & Kullgren, G. (1999a). How are mental disorders seen and where is help sought in a rural Ethiopian community? A key informant study in Butajira, Ethiopia. *Acta Psychiatr Scand Suppl*, *397*, 40–47.

Alem, A., Kebede, D., Jacobsson, L., & Kullgren, G. (1999b). Suicide attempts among adults in Butajira, Ethiopia. *Acta Psychiatr Scand Suppl*, *397*, 70–76.

Alem, A., Kebede, D., & Kullgren, G. (1999c). The epidemiology of problem drinking in Butajira, Ethiopia. *Acta Psychiatr Scand Suppl*, *397*, 77–83.

Alem, A., Kebede, D., & Kullgren, G. (1999d). The prevalence and socio-demographic correlates of khat chewing in Butajira, Ethiopia. *Acta Psychiatr Scand Suppl*, *397*, 84–91.

Alem, A., Kebede, D., Woldesemiat, G., Jacobsson, L., & Kullgren, G. (1999e). The prevalence and socio-demographic correlates of mental distress in Butajira, Ethiopia. *Acta Psychiatr Scand Suppl*, *397*, 48–55.

Alemu, W. G., Zeleke, T. A., Takele, W. W., & Mekonnen, S. S. (2020). Prevalence and risk factors for khat use among youth students in Ethiopia: systematic review and meta-analysis, 2018. *Ann Gen Psychiatry*, *19*, 16.

Asher, L., et al. (2015). Development of a community-based rehabilitation intervention for people with schizophrenia in Ethiopia. *Plos One*, *10*, e0143572.

Asher, L., et al. (2016). Community-based Rehabilitation Intervention for people with Schizophrenia in Ethiopia (RISE): study protocol for a cluster randomised controlled trial. *Trials*, *17*, 299.

Asher, L., Fekadu, A., Teferra, S., De Silva, M., Pathare, S., & Hanlon, C. (2017). 'I cry every day and night, I have my son tied in chains': physical restraint of people with schizophrenia in community settings in Ethiopia. *Global Health*, *13*, 47.

Asher, L., Hanlon, C., Birhane, R., Habtamu, A., Eaton, J., Weiss, H.A., Patel, V., Fekadu, A., & De Silva, M. (2018) Community-based rehabilitation intervention for people with schizophrenia in Ethiopia (RISE): a 12 month mixed methods pilot study. *BMC Psychiatry*, 18(1):250.

Asher, L., et al. (2022). Community-based rehabilitation intervention for people with schizophrenia in Ethiopia (RISE): results of a 12-month cluster-randomized controlled trial. *Lancet Glob Health*, *10*(4), e530–e542.

Balaji, M., Chatterjee, S., Brennan, B., Rangaswamy, T., Thornicroft, G., & Patel, V. (2012). Outcomes that matter: a qualitative study with persons with schizophrenia and their primary caregivers in India. *Asian J Psychiatr*, *5*, 258–265.

Baron, E. C., et al. (2018). Impact of district mental health care plans on symptom severity and functioning of patients with priority mental health conditions: the Programme for Improving Mental Health Care (PRIME) cohort protocol. *BMC Psychiatry*, *18*, 61.

Berhane, Y., et al. (1999). Establishing an epidemiological field laboratory in rural areas—potentials for public health research and interventions (special issue). *Ethiop J Health Dev*, *13*, 1–47.

Beyero, T., Alem, A., Kebede, D., Shibre, T., Desta, M., & Deyessa, N. (2004). Mental disorders among the Borana semi-nomadic community in Southern Ethiopia. *World Psychiatry*, *3*, 110–114.

Bromet, E. J. (2008). Cross-national comparisons: problems in interpretation when studies are based on prevalent cases. *Schizophr Bull*, *34*, 256–257.

Charlson, F. J., et al. (2018). Global epidemiology and burden of schizophrenia: findings from the global burden of disease study 2016. *Schizophr Bull*, *44*, 1195–1203.

Dormaar, M., Giel, R., & Van Luijk, J. N. (1974). Psychiatric illness in two contrasting Ethiopian outpatient populations. *Soc Psychiatry*, *9*, 155–161.

Ethiopian Public Health Institute (2015). Ethiopia STEPS survey 2015 fact sheet. Addis Ababa, Ethiopia: EPHI. Retrieved from http://www.ephi.gov.et/

Fekadu, A., et al. (2014). Burden of mental disorders and unmet needs among street homeless people in Addis Ababa, Ethiopia. *BMC Med*, *12*, 138.

Fekadu, A., et al. (2015a). Development of a scalable mental healthcare plan for a rural district in Ethiopia. *Br J Psychiatry*, *208*(Suppl 56), s4–s12.

Fekadu, A., et al. (2015b). Excess mortality in severe mental illness: 10-year population-based cohort study in rural Ethiopia. *Br J Psychiatry*, *206*, 289–296.

Fekadu, A., et al. (2019). The psychosis treatment gap and its consequences in rural Ethiopia. *BMC Psychiatry*, *19*, 325.

Fekadu, A., et al. (2004). Bipolar disorder among an isolated island community in Ethiopia. *J Affect Disord*, *80*, 1–10.

Forthal, S., Fekadu, A., Medhin, G., Selamu, M., Thornicroft, G., & Hanlon, C. (2019). Rural vs urban residence and experience of discrimination among people with severe mental illnesses in Ethiopia. *BMC Psychiatry*, *19*, 340.

Ghebrehiwet, S., et al. (2020). Gender-specific experiences of serious mental illness in rural Ethiopia: a qualitative study. *Glob Public Health*, *15*, 185–199.

Giel, R. (1999). The prehistory of psychiatry in Ethiopia. *Acta Psychiatr Scand Suppl*, *397*, 2–4.

Giel, R., Kitaw, Y., Workneh, F., & Mesfin, R. (1974). Ticket to heaven. Psychiatric illness in a religious community in Ethiopia. *Soc Sci Med*, *8*, 549–556.

Giel, R. & Van Luijk, J. N. (1970). Psychiatric morbidity in a rural village in south-western Ethiopia. *Int J Soc Psychiatry*, *16*, 63–71.

Giel, R. & Van Luijk, J. N. (1969). Psychiatric morbidity in a small Ethiopian town. *Br J Psychiatry*, *115*, 149–162.

Habtamu, K., Alem, A., & Hanlon, C. (2015). Conceptualizing and contextualizing functioning in people with severe mental disorders in rural Ethiopia: a qualitative study. *BMC Psychiatry*, *15*, 34.

Habtamu, K., Alem, A., Medhin, G., Fekadu, A., Prince, M., & Hanlon, C. (2016). Development and validation of a contextual measure of functioning for people living with severe mental disorders in rural Africa. *BMC Psychiatry*, *16*, 311.

Hailemariam, M., Fekadu, A., Medhin, G., Prince, M., & Hanlon, C. (2020). Equitable access to mental healthcare integrated in primary care for people with severe mental disorders in rural Ethiopia: a community-based cross-sectional study. *Int J Ment Health Syst*, *13*, 78.

Hailemariam, M., Fekadu, A., Prince, M., & Hanlon, C. (2017). Engaging and staying engaged: a phenomenological study of barriers to equitable access to mental healthcare for people with severe mental disorders in a rural African setting. *Int J Equity Health*, *16*, 156.

Hailemariam, M., et al. (2019). 'He can send her to her parents': the interaction between marriageability, gender and serious mental illness in rural Ethiopia. *BMC Psychiatry*, *19*, 315.

Hailemichael, Y., et al. (2019a). Catastrophic out-of-pocket payments for households of people with severe mental disorder: a comparative study in rural Ethiopia. *Int J Ment Health Syst*, *13*, 39.

Hailemichael, Y., et al. (2019b). Mental health problems and socioeconomic disadvantage: a controlled household study in rural Ethiopia. *Int J Equity Health*, *18*, 121.

Hailemichael, Y., et al. (2019c). Catastrophic health expenditure and impoverishment in households of persons with depression: a cross-sectional, comparative study in rural Ethiopia. *BMC Public Health*, *19*, 930.

Hailemichael, Y., et al. (2022). The effect of expanded access to mental health care on economic status of households with a person with a mental disorder in rural Ethiopia: a controlled before-after study. *Int J Ment Health Syst*, DOI: 10.21203/rs.3.rs-1006902/v1.

Hanlon, C., et al. (2016). Task sharing for the care of severe mental disorders in a low-income country (TaSCS): study protocol for a randomised, controlled, non-inferiority trial. *Trials, 17,* 76.

Hanlon, C., et al. (2022). Efficacy and cost-effectiveness of task-shared care for people with severe mental disorders in Ethiopia (TaSCS): a single-blind, randomised, controlled, phase 3 non-inferiority trial. *Lancet Psychiatry, 9,* 59–71.

Hanlon, C., et al. (2019). Impact of integrated district level mental health care on clinical and social outcomes of people with severe mental illness in rural Ethiopia: an intervention cohort study. *Epidemiol Psychiatr Sci, 29,* e45.

Hopper, K., Harrison, G., Janca, A., & Sartorius, N. (eds) 2007. *Recovery from schizophrenia: an international perspective.* Oxford: Oxford University Press.

Isaac, M., Chand, P., & Murthy, P. (2007). Schizophrenia outcome measures in the wider international community. *Br J Psychiatry Suppl, 50,* s71–7.

Jablensky, A., et al. (1992). Schizophrenia: manifestations, incidence and course in different cultures. A World Health Organization ten-country study. *Psychol Med Monogr Suppl, 20,* 1–97.

Jacobsson, L. (1985). Psychiatric morbidity and psychosocial background in an outpatient population of a general hospital in western Ethiopia. *Acta Psychiatr Scand, 71,* 417–26.

Kebede, D. & Alem, A. (1999a). The epidemiology of alcohol dependence and problem drinking in Addis Ababa, Ethiopia. *Acta Psychiatr Scand Suppl, 397,* 30–34.

Kebede, D. & Alem, A. (1999b). Major mental disorders in Addis Ababa, Ethiopia. I. Schizophrenia, schizoaffective and cognitive disorders. *Acta Psychiatr Scand, 100,* 11–17.

Kebede, D. & Alem, A. (1999c). Major mental disorders in Addis Ababa, Ethiopia. II. Affective disorders. *Acta Psychiatr Scand, 100,* 18–23.

Kebede, D. & Alem, A. (1999d). Major mental disorders in Addis Ababa, Ethiopia. III. Neurotic and somatoform disorders. *Acta Psychiatr Scand, 100,* 24–29.

Kebede, D. & Alem, A. (1999e). Suicide attempts and ideation among adults in Addis Ababa, Ethiopia. *Acta Psychiatr Scand Suppl, 397,* 35–39.

Kebede, D., Alem, A., Deyassa, N., Shibre, T., Negash, A., & Beyero, T. (2003a). Socio-demographic correlates of depressive disorder in Butajira, rural Ethiopia. *Cent Afr J Med, 49,* 78–83.

Kebede, D., Alem, A., & Rashid, E. (1999). The prevalence and socio-demographic correlates of mental distress in Addis Ababa, Ethiopia. *Acta Psychiatr Scand Suppl, 397,* 5–10.

Kebede, D., Alem, A., Shibre, T., Negash, A., Deyassa, N., & Beyero, T. (2004). The sociodemographic correlates of schizophrenia in Butajira, rural Ethiopia. *Schizophr Res, 69,* 133–141.

Kebede, D., Alem, A., Shibre, T., Negash, A., Deyassa, N., & Beyero, T. (2005a). Socio-demographic correlates of bipolar disorder in Butajira, rural Ethiopia. *East Afr Med J, 82,* 34–39.

Kebede, D., et al. (2003b). Onset and clinical course of schizophrenia in Butajira-Ethiopia—a community-based study. *Soc Psychiatry Psychiatr Epidemiol, 38,* 625–631.

Kebede, D., Fekadu, A., Alem, A., Beyero, T., Shibire, T., & Deyessa, N. (2005b). The distribution of mental disorders among an isolated island community in southern Ethiopia. *Ethiop Med J, 43,* 71–77.

Lund, C., et al. (2012). PRIME: a programme to reduce the treatment gap for mental disorders in five low- and middle-income countries. *PLoS Med, 9,* e1001359.

Mall, S., et al. (2015). 'Restoring the person's life': a qualitative study to inform development of care for people with severe mental disorders in rural Ethiopia. *Epidemiol Psychiatr Sci, 26*(1), 43–52.

Mayston, R., et al. (2020). The effect of gender on the long-term course and outcome of schizophrenia in rural Ethiopia: a population-based cohort. *Soc Psychiatry Psychiatr Epidemiol, 55,* 1581–1591.

Messias, E. L., Chen, C.-Y., & Eaton, W. W. (2007). Epidemiology of schizophrenia: review of findings and myths. *Psychiatr Clin North Am, 30,* 323–338.

NG, L. C., Medhin, G., Hanlon, C., & Fekadu, A. (2019). Trauma exposure, depression, suicidal ideation, and alcohol use in people with severe mental disorder in Ethiopia. *Soc Psychiatry Psychiatr Epidemiol, 54,* 835–842.

Odenwald, M., et al. (2005). Khat use as risk factor for psychotic disorders: a cross-sectional and case-control study in Somalia. *BMC Med, 3,* 5.

Ongeri, L., et al. (2019). Khat use and psychotic symptoms in a rural Khat growing population in Kenya: a household survey. *BMC Psychiatry, 19,* 137.

Selamu, M., et al. (2015). Beyond the biomedical: community resources for mental health care in rural Ethiopia. *PLoS One, 10,* e0126666.

Shibre, T., et al. (2014). Suicide and suicide attempts in people with severe mental disorders in Butajira, Ethiopia: 10-year follow-up of a population-based cohort. *BMC Psychiatry, 14,* 150.

Shibre, T., et al. (2015). Long-term clinical course and outcome of schizophrenia in rural Ethiopia: 10-year follow-up of a population-based cohort. *Schizophr Res, 161,* 414–420.

Shibre, T., et al. (2012). Predictors of carer-burden in schizophrenia: a five-year follow-up study in Butajira, Ethiopia. *Ethiop Med J, 50,* 125–133.

Shibre, T., Teferra, S., Morgan, C., & Alem, A. (2010). Exploring the apparent absence of psychosis amongst the Borana pastoralist community of Southern Ethiopia. A mixed method follow-up study. *World Psychiatry, 9,* 98–102.

Souraya, S., Hanlon, C., & Asher, L. (2018). Involvement of people with schizophrenia in decision-making in rural Ethiopia: a qualitative study. *Global Health, 14,* 85.

Teferra, S., Hanlon, C., Beyero, T., Jacobsson, L., & Shibre, T. (2013). Perspectives on reasons for non-adherence to medication in persons with schizophrenia in Ethiopia: a qualitative study of patients, caregivers and health workers. *BMC Psychiatry, 13,* 168.

Teferra, S. & Shibre, T. (2012). Perceived causes of severe mental disturbance and preferred interventions by the Borana semi-nomadic population in southern Ethiopia: a qualitative study. *BMC Psychiatry, 12,* 79.

Temesgen, W. A., Chien, W. T., Valimaki, M. A., & Bressington, D. (2020). Predictors of subjective recovery from recent-onset psychosis in a developing country: a mixed-methods study. *Soc Psychiatry Psychiatr Epidemiol, 55*(9), 1187–1199.

Thornicroft, G. & Semrau, M. (2019). Health system strengthening for mental health in low—and middle-income countries: introduction to the Emerald programme. *BJPsych Open*, 5, e66.

Tirfessa, K., Lund, C., Medhin, G., Hailemichael, Y., Fekadu, A., & Hanlon, C. (2019). Food insecurity among people with severe mental disorder in a rural Ethiopian setting: a comparative, population-based study. *Epidemiol Psychiatr Sci*, 28, 397–407.

Tirfessa, K., et al. (2020). Impact of integrated mental healthcare on food insecurity of households of people with severe mental illness in a rural African district: a community-based, controlled before-after study. *Trop Med Int Health*, 25, 414–423.

Tsigebrhan, R., Shibre, T., Medhin, G., Fekadu, A., & Hanlon, C. (2014). Violence and violent victimisation in people with severe mental illness in a rural low-income country setting: a comparative cross-sectional community study. *Schizophr Res*, 152, 275–282.

Wing, J., et al. (1990). SCAN: schedules for clinical assessment in neuropsychiatry. *Arch Gen Psychiatry*, 47, 589–593.

World Health Organization (2008). *Mental Health Gap Action Programme (mhGAP): scaling up care for mental, neurological, and substance use disorders.* Geneva: WHO.

World Health Organization (2016). *Mental Health Gap Action Programme Intervention Guide (mhGAP-IG) for mental, neurological and substance use disorders in non-specialized health settings, version 2.0.* Geneva: WHO.

14

KwaZulu-Natal, South Africa

Jonathan K. Burns and Bonginkosi Chiliza

Introduction

In this chapter, we provide an overview of services for and research on psychotic disorders in KwaZulu-Natal (KZN), South Africa. KwaZulu-Natal (KZN) is the second largest province in South Africa with a population of 11.1 million of which 35% are under 15 years of age (Stats SA, 2016). It is diverse, ethnically and religiously. The ethnic proportions are as follows: Black African 87%, Asian/Indian 7.9%, white 3.9%, and 'coloured' (mixed ancestry) 1.2%. Over 68% of the adult population have never married. 71.1% affiliate with Christianity, 7.4% with Traditional African Religion, 4% with Hinduism, and 1.7% with Islam. Further, the average household size is 3.8 persons, 47% of households are headed by women, and 17% are headed by children aged 19 and younger. In terms of highest educational achievement in adults aged 20 and over, 16.6% have had no education at all, 6.7% primary only, 70.9% secondary only, and 5.8% tertiary only.

Context and risks for psychosis

KZN is a region beset with major economic and social challenges, many of which have been identified as significant risk factors for psychosis. These include high rates of poverty, inequality, unemployment, internal displacement and migration, HIV/AIDS, substance misuse, and exposure to violence, especially childhood sexual abuse. Poverty rates are high with 42.5% of people 'living in poverty'. Eighteen per cent (18%) of dwellings are traditional and 9% are informal, 39% do not have a flush/chemical toilet, 11% have no electricity, and 19% have no access to safe drinking water. Only 9% of households have access to the internet. The unemployment rate in adults aged 25–34 years is 36%. Migration is relatively low in KZN, with 5.3% of the population born outside of South Africa. The majority of immigrants (78%) are from other countries on the African continent. However, as is the case for all of South Africa, this region has a long history of rural-to-urban migration ('migrant labour'), driven by economic and political factors closely tied up with the country's history of racial discrimination legislated inequality. This has led to large numbers of people in the rural areas living in poverty with limited economic and social activities.

South Africa is at the epicentre of the HIV pandemic with 20% of all people living with HIV globally and 20% of all new infections being in the country. KwaZulu-Natal is the province with the highest number of people living with HIV, with 27% (2.1 million out of the 7.9 million people nationally) of the country's total. This represents an overall population prevalence of 19%, with the highest prevalence in women aged 35–39 years (66.4%) and men aged 40–44 years (59.6%) (Kharsany et al., 2018).

Crime rates are very high in KZN with 2019 figures being: murder rate 39.1 per 100,000 population; rape rate 68.5 per 100,000; and aggravated robbery rate 198 per 100,000 (Crimestats, 2019). Particularly grim is the fact that over 40% of reported rape cases in South Africa are of children, with the recent Optimus study reporting that 37% of boys and 34% of girls had experienced some form of sexual abuse (Artz et al., 2018). Finally, cannabis use in adolescence is relatively high with a recent high school survey reporting 11% lifetime prevalence of cannabis use (Dlamini et al., 2015).

One might speculate, based on this profile of risk, that KZN is likely to have incident rates of psychosis that approximate (or even exceed) the higher end of the range of reported rates globally. But a significant caveat to this speculation is the fact that almost all the evidence we have on environmental risk for psychosis has been generated in countries of the Global North. A key research priority is to determine whether the same risk relationships exist in regions of the Global South; and if so, then to determine the strength of such relationships.

Services for psychosis in KZN

In KZN, biomedical mental health services are few, under-resourced, and understaffed and mainly located in large urban centres. There are 27 general psychiatrists working in the public health sector in the province (0.24 per 100,000 population). Subspecialists are even rarer, with only three child and adolescent psychiatrists and three forensic psychiatrists. Acute inpatient beds are located in specialist psychiatric hospitals, in psychiatric units within some regional general hospitals, and in general medical wards within local district hospitals (staffed by non-specialist doctors and nurses). It is estimated that the province has approximately 25% of the number of acute beds required to meet national norms (Burns, 2010), while an audit of 2010/2011 admission data showed that only 19.8% of expected psychiatric admissions (predicted from modelling) actually took place (Burns, 2014). Community mental health services are similarly inadequate and modelling revealed that in the same year only 21% of expected ambulatory visits for mental healthcare took place in the province (Burns, 2014). Thus, in line with observations made in other regions of the Global South, the overall treatment gap for people with mental disorders in KZN is approximately 80%. A recent study attempted to cost the expenditure of public mental healthcare (Docrat et al., 2019). They found that KZN spends about 5.5% of the total healthcare budget on mental health, with the majority of the costs going towards inpatient care for people with psychosis.

Specific mental health services for psychosis are generally unavailable and there are no early intervention services in the province. In Durban, there is a specialist clinic at the main teaching hospital for patients with first-episode psychosis who are full-time students or in full-time employment. The multidisciplinary specialist clinic focuses on preserving and improving functioning of the patients.

Efforts to develop community mental health services in KZN were arguably hindered by the misguided implementation of a national policy of integration of mental health into primary care. In the early 2000s, decisions were taken to dismantle 'stand-alone' community mental health teams and redeploy staff to primary care facilities in an attempt to integrate mental health services into primary healthcare. The effects of this policy decision were catastrophic, with most areas of the province lacking mental health professionals in the community and large numbers of hospitalized patients finding little or no support post-discharge (Hlongwa & Sibiya, 2019). The result has been a 'revolving door' pattern of discharge and subsequent early readmission for patients with severe mental disorders in the region (Tomita & Moodley, 2016).

In terms of treatments available for people with psychosis, most patients have access to typical antipsychotics such as haloperidol and chlorpromazine, while atypical antipsychotics are generally only available at psychiatric hospitals and units in urban centres. In general, access to long-acting injectable antipsychotics is limited to typical agents such as fluphenazine decanoate. Clozapine is available for individuals with treatment-resistant schizophrenia, but in practice only prescribed at urban psychiatric facilities where psychiatrists are available. The situation is different in the private sector (an estimated 15% of the population have medical insurance and can access private care), where a wide range of novel antipsychotics including long-acting injectables are available.

Some of the larger cities in KZN have mental health charities and non-governmental organizations that provide some community-based care including a few residential facilities for people with severe mental disorders such as schizophrenia. For example, Pietermaritzburg Mental Health Society provides some services to that city, although a significant proportion of the people they support have intellectual disabilities rather than mental disorders.

An important source of support and care in KZN for people with mental health problems including psychosis is traditional health practitioners (THPs). Officially recognized by the South African government in 2007 with the passing of the Traditional Health Practitioners Act, THPs play a very significant role in South African society. There are an estimated 25,000 THPs in KZN and these include diviners, herbalists, faith healers, and traditional birth attendants (Gqaleni et al., 2007). The widespread availability of THPs in areas where health and especially mental health services are scarce (or absent), together with the fact that approximately 70% of the population are thought to consult THPs, means that THPs constitute a vital community-based resource for people with health problems. A systematic review found that approximately half of the individuals seeking biomedical healthcare for mental disorders in Africa choose traditional and religious healers as their first care provider (Burns & Tomita, 2015). In a hospitalized first-episode sample in KZN, 39% had first consulted a THP (notably only 19% had consulted a psychiatrist), while approximately half attributed their symptoms to spiritual causes (Burns et al., 2010b). Thus, it is clear that in this setting, where biomedical mental health services are limited and often inaccessible, THPs constitute an important source of care for people with mental health problems including psychosis.

Current evidence on psychosis from KZN

Incidence of psychosis

There have been no large-scale epidemiological studies of psychosis in KZN and thus the evidence base for prevalence and incidence is thin. It is reasonable to speculate that incidence rates of psychosis are likely to be at the high end of the range of rates reported globally. This is because, as elaborated earlier, there are several significant population-wide risk factors in the province, namely: high levels of poverty, the HIV/AIDS pandemic, high levels of interpersonal violence and trauma including early childhood abuse, and widespread cannabis use.

There have been two small studies in discrete regions that provide some indication of likely incidence rates. The first was based on a review of clinical records of hospitalized patients with first-episode psychosis from a specific catchment region (Burns & Esterhuizen, 2008). All new cases (n, 160) aged 15–49 from the Municipality of Umgungundlovu (population-at-risk approximately 500,000) admitted to Town Hill Hospital, the psychiatric referral centre for the region, were included, which gave a treated incidence rate for this region of 31.5 per 100,000. The second was a Fogarty-funded pilot study, the INCET Study, which was designed to establish methods for a subsequent incidence study of psychosis in a rural region of KZN called Vulindlela (Veling et al., 2019). This region is contained within the Umgungundlovu Municipality. Using an innovative case-detection strategy at the community level where THPs were trained and referred clients they suspected may have psychosis, 44 individuals with incident psychosis (DSM-IV criteria) were detected over 6 months. With a population-at-risk of 170,000 for Vulindlela, this gave an incidence rate for this area of 51.8 per 100,000. Assuming that both a treated incidence rate (hospitalized) and a community-based rate (based only on THP referrals) underestimate the actual incidence of psychosis, it is reasonable to speculate that incidence rates in this region of KZN are well above the global mean incidence rate from a recent meta-analysis (Jongsma et al., 2019) of 26.6 per 100,000 and may approximate rates at the upper end of the range (80–90 per 100,000).

Outcome of psychosis

Contrary to findings from World Health Organization studies in the 1980s and 1990s that outcome of schizophrenia is better in the Global South, there is a relatively large evidence base that has subsequently accumulated suggesting that this may not be the case. In KwaZulu-Natal, clinicians have for a long time had the opinion, based solely on anecdotal experience with their patients, that most individuals with psychosis have a high rate of relapse, have persistent distressing symptoms, experience marked social and occupational decline, and are subject to significant social rejection and stigma. The only empirical data available to substantiate this view comes from a follow-up study of the 160 hospitalized patients with first-episode psychosis identified through record review and alluded to earlier (Burns, unpublished data). Contact details were available for 115 of these individuals and, 3 years after hospitalization, a community psychiatric nurse attempted to trace them using these details as well as via local community clinics. Of the 52 individuals traced, 8 (15%) had died, 55% were being followed up and were taking treatment, 19% had seen a psychiatrist during the 3-year period, and 40% had been readmitted at least once. Fifty per cent (50%) were still symptomatic in that they were regularly experiencing at least one positive psychotic symptom, auditory hallucinations (40%) and paranoid delusions (38%) being the most common. Twelve per cent (12%) were currently suicidal, 14% were using cannabis daily, 30% were physically unwell, and 35% volunteered problems with the side effects of their psychiatric medication. Functional outcomes were also poor with 80% unemployed (general population norm 45%), greater household crowding (compared with the general population), and lower individual and household income (compared with the general population).

Metabolic syndrome and psychosis

In the Global North, metabolic syndrome is a well-established comorbidity in people with psychosis and, while antipsychotic medications are responsible for a proportion of the increased rates in this population, there is some suggestive evidence that individuals with schizophrenia and bipolar disorder may have an inherent increased risk associated independently with these illnesses. Importantly, rates of metabolic syndrome are high in the Black South African population, with rates especially high in women and with increasing age (Motala et al., 2011). In KwaZulu-Natal, Saloojee et al. (2016) found no difference in prevalence of metabolic syndrome in 276 patients with psychotic disorders (schizophrenia, bipolar disorder, and schizoaffective disorder) compared with matched controls. However, patients did have higher waist circumference and lower HDL cholesterol than controls. Also, in women and in those aged 55 and over, patients differed from controls in terms of prevalence of metabolic syndrome (Saloojee et al., 2016; Saloojee et al., 2017). In 67 antipsychotic-naïve first-episode psychosis patients, Saloojee et al. (2018) reported no difference in metabolic syndrome compared with controls and a low incidence of metabolic syndrome after 1 year of antipsychotic treatment. However, at 1 year patients had increased waist circumference. The conclusion from this work is that it may be that, in a context where the 'baseline' population prevalence of metabolic syndrome is high, individuals with psychosis are not at a particularly greater risk. Also, it is possible that antipsychotic-related metabolic side effects are mitigated by race and ethnicity. Clearly, further research in diverse populations is needed to test this hypothesis.

Cannabis use and psychosis

Cannabis is widely used in KwaZulu-Natal, and its use and impact have been investigated in several studies in the province. In an inpatient sample of adults (n, 54) with first-episode psychosis (FEP), 35% of patients reported current cannabis use and this was associated with shorter duration of untreated psychosis (Burns et al., 2010a). A separate study at the same psychiatric hospital enrolled 87 adults with psychotic disorders and reported a lifetime prevalence of cannabis use of 49% and current use of 43% (Davis et al., 2016). Higher proportions of lifetime cannabis use (61.4%) were reported in 70 adolescents admitted with psychosis (Paruk et al., 2009); while a similar proportion (56%) of lifetime use was reported in 45 adolescents with FEP (Paruk et al., 2015). In the latter study, adolescents with FEP were more likely to currently use cannabis (37.8%) than adolescent controls with non-psychotic mental disorders (15.6%) (Paruk et al., 2018).

Causal attributions and help-seeking

As discussed earlier in this chapter, THPs are an important source of support and care for many people in KZN, including those with mental illness. THPs are available and accessible in people's communities and they address questions about why an individual has become ill at this time and in this way, and provide a spiritual framework and explanation that meets these needs (Burns & Tomita, 2015). A large proportion of individuals with FEP attribute their symptoms to spiritual circumstances such as having failed to observe a certain traditional ritual, having been bewitched, or being called by the ancestors to undergo training as a THP (Burns et al., 2010b). These beliefs about symptoms lead individuals and their families to consult THPs rather than biomedical health providers who will not address these issues. Research in KZN has shown that help-seeking behaviours and pathways to care for people with psychosis are very complex and often lead to delays in engaging biomedical mental health services with consequent long durations of psychosis (Burns et al., 2010b; Burns & Tomita, 2015; Labys et al., 2016; Tomita et al., 2015). Individuals and their families often move back and forwards between different types of providers and sometimes consult more than one type simultaneously (e.g. hospital doctor and THP). While generally protective against poor mental health, good neighbourhood social capital has also been shown to delay biomedical treatment-seeking in those with FEP in this context (Burns & Kirkbride, 2012).

Selected case studies of psychosis research in KZN

INCET Study

Funded by NIMH/Fogarty, the INCET Study set out to pilot and establish methods for a subsequent epidemiological study of psychosis in rural KZN. The site and main pilot have been described earlier, but in addition to this pilot, important preparatory work was conducted to engage with local traditional leadership, THPs, and other community stakeholders and potential gatekeepers. Also, research instruments were adapted, translated, and piloted. An effective strategy for case detection in the community was developed involving referrals from THPs, and the basis was laid for an incidence study of psychosis in the region (Veling et al., 2019).

PSYMAP-ZN Study

'PSYchosis MAPping in KwaZulu-Natal' is a 3-year project funded by the Medical Research Council (MRC) (UK) and MRC (South Africa) and is a collaboration between the Universities of KwaZulu-Natal and Exeter, UK. It commenced in July 2019 and has several objectives: (1) Mapping the catchment area (Msunduzi Municipality, population 500,000) to identify all potential biomedical and informal providers/gatekeepers for cases; (2) To detect all incident/untreated cases of psychosis within the catchment area over a period of 2 years (expect approximately 300 cases); (3) To recruit into a case-control study 240 FEP cases with matched controls and family/caregivers; (4) Conduct baseline assessments for diagnosis, symptoms, function, quality of life, childhood trauma, substance use, HIV status and cognition, and undertake qualitative work on pathways to care and help-seeking; (5) Spatial epidemiological methods using GIS to map the distribution of cases across the catchment area in relation to various area-level risk factors and to map help-seeking pathways. In addition, this study used methods aligned with the INTREPID II programme so that results will be comparable with those from Nigeria, India, and Trinidad. Further funding will be sought for PSYMAP-ZN to support longitudinal follow-up of the cohort and add-on studies such as genomics.

Amathwasa Study

The Amathwasa Study, developed in parallel to the INCET Study, investigated psychosis and psychotic-like symptoms in the amathwasa, or apprentice THPs, in the Vulindlela community. In Zulu traditional culture, an individual may become acutely unwell with various somatic and psychological symptoms and this illness (ukuthwasa) may be interpreted by a THP as a 'calling' from the ancestors to enter training and become a THP. Some of the features of this illness would be regarded as psychotic or psychotic-like within a psychiatric framework. In the Amathwasa Study, extensive ethnographic and qualitative work was carried out to understand this condition and the process of 'healing' into which the person enters as an apprentice THP (or uthwasa) (Van der Zeijst et al., 2021a). In addition, 48 amathwasa (all early in their apprenticeships) were recruited through THPs in Vulindlela and were assessed with the CAPE to measure symptoms and the SCAN to assign a DSM-V diagnosis. Seventeen per cent (17%) met criteria for a psychotic disorder (15% unspecified psychotic disorder; 2% depressive disorder with psychotic features) and 6% for depressive disorder without psychosis; 54% had subthreshold persistent hallucinations without distress and dysfunction; and 23% had no diagnosis (Van der Zeijst et al., 2021b). A 3-year follow-up has also been conducted with these individuals, but not reported at the time of writing. What is very interesting from this work is the fact that almost all amathwasa appear to improve remarkably during their apprenticeship period—in terms of symptoms and function. Most go on to respected and often lucrative occupations as THPs, while retaining some experiences such as auditory hallucinations (as they communicate with the ancestors as the basis for their practice). Speculatively, the amathwasa training experience may act as an indigenous 'natural intervention' that promotes recovery from psychotic illness/psychotic experiences and reintegration into society in a high-status role.

HIV psychosis study

The HIV first-episode psychosis (FEP) study will recruit and follow-up HIV infected (120) and non-infected (120) patients presenting with a FEP in Durban over 12 months. The study aims to determine and compare the prevalence of risk factors (such as family history, substance use, and trauma), clinical presentation (psychotic, mood, and cognitive symptoms), and outcomes (symptoms, quality of life, viral load) at 3, 6, and 12 months in HIV-infected and HIV-non-infected patients with FEP. In addition, in the HIV-infected FEP patients, clinical presentation will be analysed for correlations with clinical markers of HIV disease such as duration of HIV infection, CD4 count, viral load, CSF, and neuroimaging where available. The project will recruit adults, 18–45 years, presenting with FEP as defined by DSM-V criteria for a primary psychotic illness. Participants will be assessed at baseline, 3, 6, and 12 months and treated using a standardized treatment protocol. This will be the first longitudinal study to compare the two groups in a sub-Saharan African setting, in the antiretroviral era. The study is particularly important in an environment with a high HIV infection burden and limited mental healthcare resources, and where many people with a first episode of psychosis are HIV positive (Mashaphu & Mkize, 2007).

A research agenda for priority research on psychosis in KZN

This chapter has briefly sketched the current service and research landscape for psychoses in a province in South Africa. There are several important research studies that shed—or promise to shed—light on psychoses in a setting characterized by a high prevalence of risks for psychosis. Looking forward, several priority research areas on psychosis in KZN are indicated:

+ Obtaining good representative epidemiological evidence on prevalence, incidence, risk factors for, and course and outcome of psychosis in this context.
+ Understanding the relationship between HIV and psychosis including its impact on the epidemiology of psychosis, clinical phenomenology, and diagnosis, as well as treatment strategies.
+ The genetics and epigenetics of psychosis in this African context.

- Physical health in people with psychosis in KZN, a region where non-communicable diseases are on the rise as sub-Saharan Africa 'goes through the epidemiological transition'.

- The development and testing of better mental health services for people with psychosis, including collaboration between biomedical and other providers (such as THPs) to improve early detection and long-term outcome.

- The development of innovative approaches to render good care in a resource-scarce setting (e.g. through task-shifting), including the development and testing of culturally adapted therapeutic interventions (especially those that can be delivered in community settings).

- Effective and acceptable strategies to reduce stigma and improve the integration of people with psychosis into meaningful social and occupational roles.

References

Artz, L., Ward, C. L., Leoschut, L., Kassanjee, R., & Burton, P. (2018). The prevalence of child sexual abuse in South Africa: the Optimus Study South Africa. *SAMJ*, *108*(10), 791–792.

Burns, J. K. (2010). Mental health services funding and development in KwaZulu-Natal Province: a tale of inequity and neglect. *S Afr Med J*, *100*, 662–666.

Burns, J. K. (2014). The burden of mental disorders in KwaZulu-Natal: mapping the treatment gap. *S Afr J Psychiatry*, *20*(1), 6–10.

Burns, J. K. & Esterhuizen, T. (2008). Poverty, inequality and the treated incidence of first-episode psychosis—an ecological study from South Africa. *Soc Psychiatry Psychiatr Epidemiol*, *43*(4), 331–335.

Burns, J. K., Jhazbhay, K., & Emsley, R. A. (2010a). Cannabis predicts shorter duration of untreated psychosis and low negative symptoms in first-episode psychosis: a South African study. *Afr J Psychiatry*, *13*(5), 395–399.

Burns, J. K., Jhazbhay, K., & Emsley, R. A. (2010b). Causal attributions, pathway to care and first-episode psychosis: a South African perspective. *Int J Soc Psychiatry*, *57*(5), 538–545.

Burns, J. K. & Kirkbride, J. B. (2012). Social capital, pathway to care and duration of untreated psychosis: findings from a low and middle income country context. *S Afr J Psychiatr*, *18*(4), 163–170.

Burns, J. K. & Tomita, M. A. (2015). Traditional and religious healers in the pathway to care for people with mental disorders in Africa: a systematic review and meta-analysis. *Soc Psychiatry Psychiatr Epidemiol*, *50*(6), 867–877.

Crimestats (2019). Provinces by crime. Retrieved from https://www.crimestatssa.com/provincesbycrime.php

Davis G, et al. (2016). Substance use and duration of untreated psychosis in KwaZulu-Natal, South Africa. *S Afr J Psychiatr*, *22*(1), a852.

Dlamini, S., Jinabhai, N., Esterhuizen, T., Friedland, G., & Taylor, M. (2015). Prevalence and correlates of cannabis use amongst Kwazulu-Natal high school students. *Int J Epidemiol*, *44*(Suppl 1), i83–i184.

Docrat, S., Besada, D., Cleary, S., Daviaud, E., & Lund, C. (2019). Mental health system costs, resources and constraints in South Africa: a national survey. *Health Policy Plan*, *34*(9), 706–719.

Gqaleni, N., Moodley, I., Kruger, H., Ntuli, A., & McLeod, H. (2007). Traditional and complementary medicine: health care delivery. In Harrison, S., Bhana, R., & Ntuli, A. (eds) *South African health review*. Durban: Health Systems Trust, 175–185.

Hlongwa, E. N. & Sibiya, M. N. (2019). Challenges affecting the implementation of the policy on integration of mental health care into primary healthcare in KwaZulu-Natal province. *Curationis*, *42*(1), e1–e9.

Jongsma, H. E., et al. (2019). International incidence of psychotic disorders, 2002–17: a systematic review and meta-analysis. *Lancet Public Health*, *4*(5), e229–e244. ISSN 2468-2667. https://doi.org/10.1016/S2468-2667(19)30056-8

Kharsany, A. B. M., et al. (2018). Community-based HIV prevalence in KwaZulu-Natal, South Africa: results of a cross-sectional household survey. *Lancet HIV*, *5*(8), e427–e437.

Labys, C. A., Susser, E. S., & Burns, J. K. (2016). Psychosis and help-seeking behavior in rural KwaZulu Natal: unearthing local insights. *Int J Ment Health Syst*, *10*, 57.

Mashaphu, S. & Mkize, D. L. (2007). HIV seropositivity in first-episode psychosis. *S Afr J Psychiatr*, *13*, 90–94.

Motala, A. A., Esterhuizen, T., Pirie, F. J., & Omar, M. A. (2011). The prevalence of metabolic syndrome and determination of the optimal waist circumference cutoff points in a rural South African community. *Diabetes Care*, *34*(4), 1032–1037.

Paruk, S., Ramlall, S., & Burns, J. K. (2009). Adolescent onset psychosis: a 2-year retrospective study of adolescents admitted to a general psychiatric unit in Durban. *S Afr J Psychiatr*, *15*(4), 86–92.

Paruk, S., Jhazbhay, K., Singh, K., Sartorius, B., & Burns, J. K. (2015). Clinical correlates of first-episode early onset psychosis in KwaZulu-Natal, South Africa. *J Child Adolesc Ment Health*, *27*(2), 103–111.

Paruk, S., Jhazbhay, K., Singh, K., Sartorius, B., & Burns, J. K. (2018). A comparative study of socio-demographic and substance use correlates in early-onset psychosis. *Early Interv Psychiatry*, *12*(3), 339–347.

Saloojee, S., Burns, J. K., & Motala, A. (2016). Metabolic syndrome in South African patients with severe mental illness: prevalence and associated risk factors. *PLOS One*, *11*(2), e0149209.

Saloojee, S., Burns, J. K., & Motala, A. (2017). High risk of metabolic syndrome among black South African women with severe mental illness. *S Afr J Psychiatr*, *23*, a1089.

Saloojee, S., Burns, J. K., & Motala, A. A. (2018). Metabolic syndrome in antipsychotic naïve African patients with severe mental illness in usual care. *Early Interv Psychiatry*, *2*(6), 1137–1143.

Tomita, A., et al. (2015). Duration of untreated psychosis and the pathway to care in KwaZulu-Natal, South Africa. *J Nerv Ment Dis*, *203*(3), 222–225.

Tomita, A. & Moodley, Y. (2016). The revolving door of mental, neurological, and substance use disorders re-hospitalization in rural KwaZulu-Natal Province, South Africa. *Afri Health Sci*, *16*(3), 817–821.

Van der Zeijst, M. C. E., et al. (2021a). Ancestral calling and traditional health practitioner training as an intervention in mental illness: an ethnographic study from rural KwaZulu-Natal, South Africa. *Transcult Psychiatry*, *58*(4), 471–485.

Van der Zeijst, M. C. E., et al. (2021b). Psychopathology among apprentice traditional health practitioners: a quantitative study from rural KwaZulu-Natal, South Africa. *Transcult Psychiatry*, *58*(4), 486–498.

Veling, W., et al. (2019). Identification of patients with recent-onset psychosis in KwaZulu Natal, South Africa: a pilot study with traditional health practitioners and diagnostic instruments. *Soc Psychiatry Psychiatr Epidemiol*, *54*, 303–312.

15

Central and Eastern Europe

Dzmitry Krupchanka, Petr Winkler, Arunas Germanavičius, Jan Pfeiffer, Cyril Höschl, Oksana Plevachuk, and Orest Suvalo

Introduction

Central and Eastern Europe (CEE) is a region of Europe combining countries of the former Soviet Union (Belarus, Estonia, Latvia, Lithuania, Moldova, Russia, Ukraine) and countries of the former Eastern bloc (Albania, Bosnia-Herzegovina, Bulgaria, Croatia, Czech Republic, Hungary, Kosovo, Macedonia, Montenegro, Poland, Romania, Serbia, Slovakia, Slovenia). The total population of the region is more than 323 million, of which about 180 million are in the Russian Federation (UN, 2015). The countries of CEE have many historical commonalities, and many challenges and barriers to the development of appropriate mental healthcare (MHC) are shared. However, there are also substantial differences related to diverse economic performance, sociopolitical contexts, and dissimilar development after the collapse of communism. To illustrate the commonalities, we begin with a brief overview of mental healthcare in the region; to illustrate differences, we describe in more detail the specific situations in Ukraine, Lithuania, and the Czech Republic (Czechia).

During the second half of the twentieth century, psychiatry in CEE was influenced by constraints imposed on it by the Soviet Union (Bloch, 1978; Höschl et al., 2012; Scheffler et al., 2008). The only officially acceptable scientific discourse was materialism and, in relation to the mind and behaviour, physiology of learning as proposed by I. P. Pavlov. Psychiatry in the USSR was systematically involved in the political repression of opponents of the regime (van Voren, 2010). Social problems were regarded as leftovers of capitalism that were to be solved spontaneously as a consequence of the progress of communism. Sociology, as well as a majority of the social sciences, were considered 'bourgeois quasi-sciences', and were de facto prohibited. Psychiatric research was primarily biologically oriented, mental health promotion was marginalized, spirituality was taboo, and those who had a severe mental disorder, such as psychosis, were confined in large psychiatric institutions.

Physical and ideological boundaries were dissolved by revolutions in 1989–1991, which led to the collapse of the USSR. Paternalistic, command-style regimes that had prevailed in the political, social, and economic spheres for the preceding 40 years changed completely. Deinstitutionalization and de-stigmatization became major concerns in mental healthcare (MHC). However, despite some progress towards de-hospitalization in all countries of CEE (Füredi et al., 2006; Mundt et al., 2012), the development of community services has been limited (Semrau et al., 2011) and without sufficient political support (Höschl et al., 2012).

An analysis of the development of MHC for people with severe mental illnesses in CEE countries between 1989–1991 to 2016 demonstrated that, in most countries, deinstitutionalization has been proposed but not implemented, psychiatric hospitals consume most of the financial and human resources, decision-making is not driven by evidence, and stigma seems to be high across the region (Winkler et al., 2017). On the other hand, there is increased attention to human rights and user involvement. However, this progress has not been equal across the region, and disparities across countries have widened with time. Generally speaking, MHC in the region remains underfunded with poor intersectional cooperation, e.g. social and psychological approaches are somewhat underdeveloped and community services are available only to a few of those who need them (Dlouhy, 2014). Mental health research can play an important role in supporting reforms, but it remains rather scarce in the region (Evans-Lacko et al., 2014; Forsman et al., 2014; Füredi et al., 2006). Despite these broad similarities, there are considerable differences among individual countries, which are illustrated in the following case studies.

Case studies from three Central and Eastern European countries

Ukraine

Ukraine is a lower-middle-income country with a population of 44.6 million, located in Central-Eastern Europe (World Bank, 2018). It is the second largest country in Europe by area. Health expenditure per capita in 2017 was 177 US dollars (https://apps.who.int/nha/database/ViewData/Indicators/en).

Sociopolitical and historical context

During the twentieth century, the population of Ukraine was exposed to a large number of traumatic events. In addition to two world wars and the great famine of Holodomor between 1932 and 1933, there was the Holocaust against the Jewish population, the deportation of Ukrainians to Siberia, and the expulsion of the Crimean Tatars to other parts of the Soviet Union. Psychiatry was used for political purposes, when approximately one-third of the political prisoners were locked up in psychiatric hospitals (Ougrin et al., 2006; van Voren 2010). Major human rights violations influenced people's behaviour, attitude, and self-esteem.[1] The nuclear explosion in Chornobyl in 1986 led to the displacement of 350,000 people, with negative consequences for the mental and physical health of millions.

After the collapse of the Soviet Union and the declaration of independence in 1991, Ukraine went through the 'Orange Revolution' in 2004 and the 'Revolution of Dignity' in 2013–2014. The last revolution was ended by the occupation of Crimea and part of the Eastern regions of Luhans'k and Donetsk by the Russian military in 2014. In February 2022, while this book was in development, Russia invaded Ukraine and the full scale invasion with huge traumatization and consequences to mental health is still ongoing. The number of people in need of humanitarian aid and protection increased from approximately 3 million people at the start of the year to nearly 18 million a few months later (https://www.unocha.org/ukraine). Approximately 8 million people have been registered as refugees from Ukraine across Europe (https://data.unhcr.org/en/situations/ukraine). At the end of January 2023 there were more than 5 million people registered as internally displaced persons in Ukraine (https://data.unhcr.org/en/documents/details/98705).

The full scale invasion with the horrors of war, rocket attacks on civilian infrastructure, medical institutions, including psychiatric hospitals and care homes, coupled with social and health consequences have dramatically influenced mental health and well-being in Ukraine.

Structure of services

Since its independence, Ukraine has continued to operate a centralized model of healthcare. Legislative procedures for the provision of mental healthcare are outlined in the Ukrainian 'Law on Psychiatric Care', approved in 2000 with amendments made in 2018. In 2009, Ukraine ratified the Convention on the

---

[1] Human rights—Ukraine and the Soviet Union: hearing and markup before the Committee on Foreign Affairs and its Subcommittee on Human Rights and International Organizations, House of Representatives, Ninety-seventh Congress, First Session, on H. Con. Res. 111, H. Res. 152, H. Res. 193, 28 July, 30 July, and 17 September 1981. U.S. Government Printing Office, 1982.

Rights of Persons with Disabilities (CRPD) but legal reforms to bring the law in line with the CRPD are still needed.[2]

The Ukrainian mental health system comprises psychiatric and narcological (substance use) hospitals, psychiatric, and addiction departments in general hospitals, a network of psychoneurological dispensaries, polyclinics with psychiatrists or narcologists on staff, and psychiatric facilities that work under the jurisdiction of other governmental departments. In 2015 there were 86 psychiatric beds per 100,000 population (reduced from 2013 when there were 99 per 100,000).[3] Alongside services overseen by the Ministry of Health, long-term care for patients with neurological disorders, mental disorders, and intellectual disabilities is provided in care homes (145 social care homes, known as 'psychoneurological internats', with around 60,000 residents) that are under the authority of the Ministry of Social Policy.[4]

According to a World Bank report from 2017, the government spent about 2.5% of its total health budget on mental health services, and 89% of this is used to finance large inpatient psychiatric hospitals, usually located in larger cities (Weissbecker et al., 2017). Psychiatric hospitals were funded according to the number of beds provided until April 2020 when the second wave of reforms of healthcare financing was introduced and payment began to operate through the National Health Service of Ukraine.

Challenges in terms of services for people with severe mental illnesses such as psychotic disorders include a large institutionalized psychiatric system, alongside public stigma and low awareness of mental health. Social services for people with mental disorders are limited or absent in the communities. Although community-based mental health services are formally available in outpatient offices and dispensaries and in day-stay departments in psychiatric clinics or dispensaries, these community-based services are mostly located in large cities and are not efficiently organized in terms of evidence based rehabilitation and service provision. Many of these services function as dispensaries (i.e. focusing on a specific illness or sphere, such as narcology or psycho-neurology), and are not always well integrated with other services within communities. The

---

[2] CRPD/C/UKR/CO/1 GE.15-16704(E) Committee on the Rights of Persons with Disabilities Concluding observations: https://tbinternet.ohchr.org/_layouts/15/treatyb odyexternal/Download.aspx?symbolno=CRPD/C/UKR/CO/1&Lang=En

[3] Психічне здоров'я населення України Аналітично-статистичний довідник за 2013–2015 р. Київ 2016: https://ipz.org.ua/wp-content/uploads/2018/01/MH-report-for_INTE RNET_All_ua.pd

[4] Review of social care homes and the development of a plan of action. February 2017. D. Juodkaitė et al.: https://www.gip-global.org/files/final-eng-report-internats-2.pdf

delivery of mental healthcare in primary care is also very limited (Weissbecker et al., 2017) and the accessibility of services is hampered by high out-of-pocket (informal) payments. This noted, since 2022, the Ministry of Healthcare, with international partners, has actively promoted mhGAP trainings for primary health care and the National Health Service of Ukraine created a new service package according to which PHC services staff trained in mhGAP receive funds from the state. Also, online courses on mhGAP for primary health workers are freely available.

In 2014, the Ministry of Health of Ukraine developed the National Strategy on Health Reform 2015–2020 to improve access to healthcare and the quality of services and to mitigate financial risks for the population (Weissbecker et al., 2017). In 2017, the Parliament of Ukraine adopted a law to launch single purchaser of health services (the National Health Service of Ukraine, NHSU), thus transforming the country's approach to financing healthcare providers, which was subsequently established in 2018. These financing changes were implemented for the primary care sector from 2018, and came into force for specialist and secondary care in April 2020. However, the financing reforms for specialized care have had mixed results and have been criticized for some of their unintended consequences, such as discharging people who have been institutionalized in hospitals for many years into communities where services are not developed.

Alongside these reforms, at the end of 2017 the government of Ukraine adopted a Concept Note on Mental Health,[5] in which a number of key directions were outlined for reforming the mental health system in order to better meet the needs of its population. Among these proposals were awareness raising, reducing discrimination and human rights violations, developing professional capabilities, increasing accessibility of care, decentralizing the mental health system, and transitioning towards greater provision of services within the community, prevention strategies, and empowerment of primary care. The action plan for implementing the Concept Note was adopted at October 2021.

At the beginning of full scale Russian invasion, the Ukrainian mental healthcare system had remained largely unchanged since Ukrainian independence in 1991 (Quirke et al., 2020). After February 2022, some mental health institutions were attacked and occupied; some patients were evacuated to the more safe places in the country. The quality of inpatient psychiatric facilities need to be improved; care has a mostly biomedical focus with few non-medical

5   Ministry of Health of Ukraine. Concept note of the state targeted mental health program in Ukraine lasting until 2030 [Internet]. Cabinet of Ministers of Ukraine; 2017 Dec: (https://zakon.rada.gov.ua/laws/show/1215-2021-%D1%80#Text)

services. Social care homes act largely as centres to provide indefinite care and treatment for people with higher levels of psychosocial disabilities, rather than seeking to rehabilitate and integrate these persons into the community. There are also high levels of stigma associated with both common and severe mental disorders, creating significant challenges in ensuring access to diagnosis and appropriate treatment. This said, prior to the Russian invasion, there were indicators of change. In 2021, with the support of the WHO, the Ministry of Healthcare launched Community Mental Health Teams (CMHTs) (https://www.who.int/news-room/feature-stories/detail/mental-health-in-ukraine--how-community-mental-health-teams-are-providing-care-amidst-the-ongoing-war). Further, since the invasion, there is increasing understanding of mental health needs and the first lady, Olena Zelenska, began the National Programme on Mental Health and Psychosocial Support (https://www.president.gov.ua/en/news/olena-zelenska-rozpovila-yak-vtilyuyetsya-iniciativa-zi-stvo-80109).

Research

Research on psychotic disorders in Ukraine is limited, which means there is next to no evidence base to inform public health strategies and service development. There are some regional reports that provide estimates of incidence (e.g. around 15 per 100,000 between 2014 and 2017) and lifetime prevalence (e.g. around 0.4%),[6] but the quality of the research that underpins these and therefore the validity of the estimates is hard to judge. Most recent studies of mental health in Ukraine have focused on common mental disorders, substance use, and trauma among internally displaced persons or soldiers, without particular attention to psychosis (e.g. Roberts et al., 2019). Most of the very small number of studies of psychosis conducted in Ukraine concern clinical characteristics of psychosis, psychopharmacological interventions, and strategies for the rehabilitation of patients after a psychotic episode (e.g. Mruh et al., 2020; Rakhman et al., 2019; Maruta et al., 2018; Boiko et al., 2017; Mudrenko et al., 2017; Markova et al., 2014; Yuryeva et al., 2010). The collective monograph 'Early intervention in Psychosis (new diagnostic and therapeutic paradigms)', edited by P. Voloshyn and N. Maruta, contains the results of research conducted by the Ukrainian scientists, devoted to the problems of treatment of the primary psychotic episode (Kharkiv, 2019).

---

[6] Психічне здоров'я населення України Аналітично-статистичний довідник за 2013–2015 р. Київ 2016 https://ipz.org.ua/wp-content/uploads/2018/01/MH-report-for_INTERNET_All_ua.pdf

Czech Republic (Czechia)

The Czech Republic is a landlocked country with roughly 10.5 million inhabitants. Economically it is one of the most developed countries in the region. According to the World Bank, its GDP per capita at purchasing power parity was USD37,370 in 2018. About 4.14% of the total healthcare budget was spent on mental health in 2015 (USD 52.1 per capita), out of which 55.7% was allocated to psychiatric hospitals (Broulikova et al., 2019). Affecting approximately 104,000 people, the economic burden of psychosis was estimated to be USD1.4 billion in 2010 (Ehler et al., 2013).

Policy and service reform

In the Czech Republic, the development of community care started after the fall of communism in 1989. Several NGOs were then established by enthusiasts who made use of special governmental funds dedicated to the development of community alternatives to institutional care for people with disabilities. In 1994, the framework of the programme entitled 'MATRA' supported by the Dutch government triggered further development and cooperation between Czech and Dutch providers of community services. Assertive community treatment and other individually oriented community services were piloted and implemented but have never reached country-wide coverage. Czech community care providers have been financially dependent on successful grant proposals and, as a consequence, uncertain employment for personnel and irregular services for clients have become features of the community mental health system in the Czech Republic (Höschl et al., 2012).

Despite several attempts, the locus of care has not yet shifted from large psychiatric hospitals to community-based services. The policy changed in 2013, when the Czech Ministry of Health published a document entitled The Strategy for Mental Health Care Reform, which sought to increase the quality of life of people with mental illnesses through deinstitutionalization, decreasing stigma, and supporting evidence-based mental healthcare development in the Czech Republic. The Strategy for Mental Health Care Reform resulted in 10 three- to five-year-long implementation projects that started in 2017–2018. Three of these projects are dedicated to the development of a network of 30 recovery-oriented 'Community Mental Health Centers'. One project focuses on developing, piloting, and evaluating three teams providing early detection and early intervention services for people with psychosis. Another project sought to develop, pilot, and evaluate community mental health teams for: (a) people with dual diagnosis (comorbid severe mental illnesses and substance abuse); (b) those with forensic issues; (c) children and adolescents with mental health problems; (d) older age people with mental health problems; and (e) people treated by outpatient psychiatrists. Yet another project aims for the deinstitutionalization of psychiatric hospitals and for improving adherence to CRPD.

There have been several recent developments in the provision of mental healthcare. Seventeen community mental health centres (CMHC) have been established across the country. These are innovative services based on multidisciplinary teams, which include both healthcare and social workers. Another 12 CMHCs started to operate in 2020–2021. Over 1,600 long-term patients with severe mental illnesses were discharged from psychiatric institutions. The QualityRights toolkit was used to assess the quality of care in all but one of Czech psychiatric hospitals—based on the results of this assessment and in collaboration with the World Health Organization (WHO), the work has started to improve the situation in Czech psychiatric hospitals (Winkler et al., 2020). There is also a nationwide evidence-based de-stigmatization programme running in all regions of the Czech Republic. A system for evidence-based decision-making and monitoring of the quality and performance of the Czech mental healthcare system has also been developed; and financing of healthcare services was adjusted to prioritize acute inpatient care and community care over long-term hospitalizations. Recently, the Governmental Council for Mental Health was established, and the Czech government has already approved the National Mental Health Action Plan 2020–2030, which covers all target groups and which includes also promotion, prevention, early intervention, and a focus on human rights. In addition, a National Suicide Prevention Action Plan and a National Action Plan for Alzheimer's Disease and other Dementias were developed and, while the former was already approved by the government, the latter is currently being reviewed by relevant stakeholders. There are many more ongoing activities related to mental healthcare reform, and it is not possible to list them all within this chapter.

The development of a single mental health act has been discussed within the context of other reforms. Currently the rights of people with mental health problems are covered by general legislation, which includes legislation related to both human rights and the provision of MHC. Compulsory treatment is regulated by law, but it is a common practice that patients agree with the treatment soon after being involuntarily admitted. The use of coercive measures is also an issue, e.g. the EUNOMIA (an international study focused on the use of coercive measures in psychiatry in 12 European countries) project reported restraint measures were used in 46% of patients involuntarily hospitalized in Prague's inpatient facilities (Kališová et al., 2014). This extensive use of restraint measures might be associated with understaffed services (Kališová et al., 2014). Patient and family organizations exist and are becoming more influential due to their inclusion in the recent reform processes. Peer workers are also getting more and more recognition as professionals in outpatient social services.

Structure of services

MHC in the Czech Republic is concentrated in 18 psychiatric hospitals, which consume about 56% of the MHC budget. These hospitals have over 500 beds on average, and the two largest accommodate over a thousand beds. There were an additional 1,200 beds in 26 psychiatric wards of general hospitals in 2017 (IHIS, 2018).

Outpatient private psychiatrists oversee the care of the vast majority of patients with psychosis who receive some form of treatment. In 2017, 51,564 patients with psychosis were getting treatment from private psychiatrists (IHIS, 2018). There are about 60 recovery-oriented community mental health teams. These are unevenly distributed around the country and operate on a regional level. These teams are currently being transformed into the CMHC as described earlier. The majority of patients with psychosis are not in their operational scope and so many receive only general social services with no particular focus on the needs of this population. Access to rehabilitation, employment, multi-disciplinary teams, and other services are, therefore, available only to a fraction of patients with psychosis.

Standardized and validated instruments are not used for the diagnosis of people with mental health problems. Diagnosis is made by psychiatrists according to the tenth revision of the International Classification of Disease (ICD-10) codes, which need to be strictly adhered to (Winkler et al., 2015a). Patients may enter or leave care at almost any time. Patients may be admitted to a psychiatric hospital as well as to any other inpatient facility without any previous referral. The absence of a clear system of referrals makes the system somewhat complicated. When a patient is discharged from inpatient care, his or her outpatient psychiatrist is contacted and the patient is formally handed over to him or her. However, there is no follow-up or feedback, and a patient may simply make no appearance there. However, this practice has been changing because of the reforms detailed earlier and the effort is being made to make sure that each patient is offered assistance from a community mental health team or community mental health centre before his or her discharge.

Research: register, health service, and survey data

The Czech Republic maintains a national register of inpatient hospitalizations, including those for psychiatric disorders. The register is based on Protocols of Discharges (for details see Krupchanka et al., 2018) which must be filled in for every patient at the end of a hospital stay. We have analysed data from this register and looked at the discharges for psychosis (defined as F2x in ICD-10) between 1998 and 2012. There were between 110 and 120 discharges for psychosis per 100,000 population every year, giving a total of 47,052 hospitalizations for 21,538 individuals with psychosis, of which 2,042 (9.5%) were long-term patients, i.e. in hospital for more than a year. Two hundred and sixty (260) patients were in hospital for more than 20 years (Winkler et al., 2015b). This partly explains the excessively long average duration of treatment for psychosis which was 115 days in 2012 (IHIS, 2013). Overall, nearly one-fifth of all inpatient hospitalizations in 2013 were because of psychosis (IHIS, 2014).

Outpatient medical treatment is reported and registered much less rigorously. Only aggregate data are available, and these are based on annual reports filled in by each of the outpatient care providers. In 2013 there were 873 psychiatric outpatient facilities, and the annual report was delivered by 803 (92%) of them. The number of patients treated for psychosis in all outpatient facilities has been slowly but steadily rising in the last 20 years; in the 15 years between 2002 and 2017, there was an increase from 40,110 to 51,564 patients (IHIS, 2003; IHIS, 2018). This increase cannot be explained by population growth, but other factors such as increased willingness to seek help, increased incidence, or increased longevity might have played a role. Outpatient social services are not reported and registered on a national level, which makes it difficult to estimate how many patients receive such services.

A population survey to estimate the prevalence of mental disorders, including psychosis, was last conducted in November 2017. This research used the Mini-International Neuropsychiatric Interview as a screening measure and was conducted on a representative sample of the Czech non-institutionalized adult population (Winkler et al., 2018). This research suggested that 1.5% of people experienced a psychotic disorder in a given year, and that those who experienced psychotic disorders had a considerably higher disability (Median WHODAS rating = 22; IQR = 16–29) than the general population with no mental disorder (Median WHODAS rating = 12; IQR = 12–17) (Formánek et al., 2019). This survey was repeated twice during the COVID-19 pandemic in order to assess changes in the prevalence of current mental disorders in the country (Winkler et al., 2020).

In the Czech Republic, there is a lack of social science research on mental health because of the dominance of biological psychiatry. Although some research in psychiatric epidemiology was pursued prior to 1989, research in health services has been rare; research into stigma and discrimination, user-led or user-collaborative research, and mental health economics research has been basically non-existent. This is now changing with the establishment, in 2015, of the National Institute of Mental Health and a reasonably large Department of Public Mental Health.

Republic of Lithuania

The Republic of Lithuania is an upper-middle-income country (GDP $16,506.9 per capita) with a population of three million. Health expenditure per capita is $966 (WHO, 2014), of which 7% goes to MHC (WHO, 2005). Psychoses affect around 32,300 people, with an estimated cost to the economy of €232 million (Gustavsson et al., 2011).

Socio-political and historical contexts

During the period 1918–1940, Lithuania was an independent Baltic state with relatively underdeveloped psychiatric services. The university psychiatric clinic was based in the temporary capital city of Kaunas and was led by Professor Juozas Blazys. His interests were broad and, in 1938, he published a book about the history of culture and ideas of tolerance. At the same time, the National Brain Research Institute in Vilnius (led by Professor Maksymilian Rose) applied modern neuro-histological methods (Santiago Ramón y Cajal) and treatments. This served as a basis for young neuropsychiatric researchers who emigrated before the Second World War (WW2) to Canadian and North American institutes of psychiatry and neurology (e.g. Jerzy Olszewsky, Igor Klatzo). Electroconvulsive therapy (ECT) for the treatment of psychosis was introduced in Vilnius by Dr Antanas Smalstys in 1940, just a couple of years after it was discovered by Bini and Cerletti. After WW2, Smalstys was accused by the Russian KGB of using ECT to torture psychiatric patients and Soviet army captives and he was sentenced to 25 years in Siberia.

Suicide rates rose dramatically during the Soviet period: from 5–7 per 100,000 before WW2 to about 45 per 100,000 in the period 1994–1996 (Haghighat, 1997). This may be explained by many factors, including transgenerational trauma during the Soviet period (genocide and deportations, partisan resistance, oppression by KGB, forced collectivization, and atheization, etc.), current neoliberal and rapid societal and economic changes with massive psychosocial strain, cycles of violence, self-harming behaviours (such as drinking, smoking, reckless driving, and alcohol-related deaths), and lack of social support (Gailienė & Kazlauskas, 2005; Rutz, 2004). Since a peak in 1994–1996, the suicide rate has dropped to 26.1 per 100,000 (https://apps.who.int/gho/data/node.sdg.3-4-data?lang=en) but it remains among the highest in Europe.

Stigma in psychiatry and society toward and among people with psychosis has deep roots in Lithuania. Being a political instrument during the Nazi occupation (Felder, 2013), psychiatry remained a tool of power during the Soviet occupation of Lithuania after the Second World War. Since the Soviet regime used psychiatry and psychiatric diagnoses (so-called sluggish schizophrenia) as tools to control dissidents (Kowalewski, 1979; van Voren, 2009), stigma remains deeply rooted in society. An international study on stigma and schizophrenia (INDIGO) has shown that, due to stigma, a majority of people with schizophrenia stop applying for jobs, continuing their education, seeing friends, and seeking social interactions (Thornicroft et al., 2009).

There are several user organizations that represent people with psychosis; however, there is no single umbrella organization. Some users' organizations receive municipal or state small grants for targeted activities, but they do not have an impact on policies or clinical practice in psychiatry. The psychological burden of carers for people with psychosis has negative impacts on families, which have never had their own organization. In part, this is due to deep stigma. A study of 51 relatives of people with a first episode of psychosis found this period to be the most difficult and overwhelming experience in their lives, which is not currently addressed by services (Povilaitienė, 2011).

Structure of services

After the Soviet collapse, Lithuania inherited a highly centralized and inefficient system of psychiatric care. Changes were brought by making psychiatry more open and efficient.

Since 1992, ICD-10 has been used and all MHC services for psychoses (F2x of ICD-10) have been provided free of charge and paid for by the national health insurance company ('Sick Fund'). Access to reimbursed cost for medications is based on the ICD diagnosis and is not equal for different categories. It results in a skewed statistic, as psychiatrists are made to diagnose conditions allowing better access to medications for patients (best reimbursement options are for people with schizoaffective disorder [F25.xx] compared with other psychoses). There is also a lack of modern and validated diagnostic tools and psychometric scales.

Since 1997, outpatient MHC has expanded across all geographic regions of Lithuania and is now provided in 108 primary MHC centres (Pūras et al., 2004). This care is specialized and provided by multidisciplinary teams. However, in practice service gaps, especially for people with psychosis, result in direct referrals to psychiatric hospitals. For instance, a study followed-up a sample of people with psychosis after being discharged from two psychiatric hospitals and found that half of the sample who lived in the capital city Vilnius were readmitted; of these, a majority by-passed primary MHC and, instead, were referred directly by emergency services, carers, or themselves (Germanavičius et al., 2004).

The prevailing treatment for people with psychosis (medications, ECT) is based on a biological model of psychosis. The use of ECT is increasing each year (Lookene et al., 2014). Psychotherapies for people with psychosis are used very rarely, because many psychiatrists believe that it could be harmful during acute psychosis and because psychological therapies are inadequately covered from the national 'sick fund' (€12 per hour in 2015). It does not correspond to market prices (€20–50 per hour) and very few psychotherapists agree to take patients not privately funded. The number of specialists providing cognitive-behavioural therapy is very low: about 20, compared with 250–300 psycho-dynamic therapists.

In 1995, social rehabilitation for people with psychosis was established in Siauliai psychiatric hospital under the leadership of Dr Eugenijus Mikaliunas. In 2001 the first community-based centre for psychosocial rehabilitation was established in Vilnius ('Vilniaus Psichosocialinės reabilitacijos centras', www.protnamis.lt). This programme provides multidisciplinary services using the CARE model (Wilken & Hollander, 2005) and is partially paid for by international donors (Open Society Fund) and partly by the municipality. Vocational rehabilitation services and job support models for out-patients with disability due to psychosis have been developed and now provide services for about 250 patients yearly. Since 2016, the national 'sick fund' has reimbursed the cost of psychosocial rehabilitation services (hospital and outpatient) but, compared with inpatient cost coverage, it is less than 5%.

Residential services for people with psychosis are not included in coverage from the health budget and are only partly covered by social budgets (state or municipal). In the old Soviet model, a majority of homeless people with psychosis, or those whose relatives refused to live with them, were transferred to so-called psychoneurological pensions (23 institutions for adults, housing up to 6,000 people with a mix of psychiatric diagnoses), usually located in remote areas, and without the possibility of living in the community (Germanavičius et al., 2006). In this institutional model, human rights abuses are documented (Germanavičius et al., 2005). Only recently, the Lithuanian government recognized this as a problem and drafted a reform plan (Pūras et al., 2013). Since 2013, EU Structural Funds have been used to improve services: 5 crisis units in psychiatric and general hospitals were renovated and some acute wards and 27 new daycare centres opened.

Forensic psychiatric care is highly centralized and is provided in the Rokiskis psychiatric hospital. The majority (69.5%) of patients treated there are people with psychosis (F2x.xx of ICD-10) (Sileikaite et al., 2016).

Research

There are two universities (Lithuanian University of Health Sciences (Kaunas), Vilnius University) and one psychiatric institution (Republican Vilnius Hospital) that are conducting and coordinating research focused on psychosis.

Between 2003–2015, these three institutions published 40 out of 58 international publications on psychosis. The impact of the other six institutions producing research in this field has been far less.

Work on psychoses is one of the major priorities for research and includes the following topics:

- Studies on psychosis biomarkers and thyroid pathology (Bunevicius et al., 2014)
- Human rights in psychiatry (Germanavičius et al., 2005, 2006)
- Stigma and schizophrenia, antistigma campains (Germanavičius et al., 2005, 2006)
- Patients and relatives of first-episode psychosis (Povilaitienė et al., 2011)
- Empowerment of users and carers (Germanavičius et al., 2005, 2006)
- Forensic psychiatric services and people with psychosis (Sileikaite et al., 2016)

Between 2003–2015 in Lithuania there were several international research projects (acronyms EUNOMIA, INDIGO, EMILIA, HELPS, ITHACA, COST) focused on psychoses and people with severe mental illness, a further indication of the extent to which this is a research priority in the country.

Conclusions

In this chapter, we have presented the current state and development of mental healthcare for, and research related to, people with psychosis in three CEE countries (Ukraine, Czech Republic, and Republic of Lithuania). We've addressed the sociopolitical and historical context, structure of services, and—where possible—described available epidemiological data and outlined the main directions of research activity.

Similar historical influences shaped the MHC landscape in the region before 1990. After the collapse of the Soviet Union, each country had to substantially reconsider its system of MHC. In Ukraine, services remain centralized and efforts to shift care into the community are still in the process of being conceptualized and established. In the Czech Republic, multiple attempts at reform have been undertaken with limited effect, but the process is now gaining momentum with the publication of 'Strategy of MHC Reform' and work on its implementation. In Lithuania, outpatient care has expanded across the country, but there are a number of gaps including the continued dominance of a biological model of treatment, unequal distribution of community care services, poor access to psychotherapy, rehabilitation and assertive community treatment, and reported human rights abuses of people with psychosis. Service user movements do not exist in Ukraine, have limited impact on policies and clinical practice in Lithuania, but, by contrast, are becoming more and more involved in Czech reforms and provision of care. Mental health policy is still unclear in Ukraine, whereas in Czech Republic and Lithuania explicit plans exist, although their implementation has yet to happen. Research on psychoses needs to be strengthened in all three countries in order to enable evidence-based MHC development. Lithuania seems to be the most active in this regard, and there are a number of promising initiatives recently started in the Czech Republic. Additional attention is necessary to strengthen research and international collaborations in Ukraine.

This chapter illustrates that despite similar historical influences and a number of shared challenges, there are remarkable differences in the current state of the art in CEE. These need to be taken into account when specifying priorities for future development.

A set of recommendations common for the whole region, however, can be formulated. The priorities include:

(1) increased and evidence-based allocation of resources to MHC

(2) continuing the shift of care into the community

(3) development of properly planned policies with clearly stated roles, responsibilities, resources, SMART targets, and with comprehensive involvement of stakeholders

(4) strengthening the voices, empowerment, and inclusion of service users in MHC development

(5) addressing stigma and discrimination

(6) strengthening leadership and human resources, and building research capacity

(7) promoting international collaboration within and beyond the region in order to stimulate the transfer of knowledge

(8) scaling-up of best practices to improve MHC for people with psychosis and other mental illnesses

References

Bloch, S. (1978). Psychiatry as ideology in the USSR. *J Med Ethics*, *4*, 126–131.

Boiko, D. I., Zhyvotovska, L. V., Sonnik, G. T., & Skrypnikov, A. M. (2017). Clinical and psychopathological characteristics of the autoagressive behavior in patients with the first psychotic episode with considering circadian rhythms. *Wiad Lek*, *70*(3 pt 2), 553–557.

Broulikova, H. M., Dlouhy, M., & Winkler, P. (2019). Expenditures on mental health care in the Czech Republic in 2015. *Psychiatr Q*, *91*(1), 113–125.

Bunevicius, R., Steibliene, V., & Prange, A. J. (2014). Thyroid axis function after in-patient treatment of acute psychosis with antipsychotics: a naturalistic study. *BMC Psychiatry*, *14*, 1–9.

Dlouhy, M. (2014). Mental health policy in Eastern Europe: a comparative analysis of seven mental health systems. *BMC Health Serv Res*, 14–42.

Ehler, E., Bednařík, J., Höschl, C., Winkler, P., Suchý, M., & Pátá, M. (2013). Náklady na poruchy mozku v české republice *[Cost of brain disorders in the Czech Republic]. Čes Slov Neurol*, 76, 109, 282–291.

Evans-Lacko S, et al. (2014). The state of the art in European research on reducing social exclusion and stigma related to mental health: a systematic mapping of the literature. *Eur Psychiatry*, 29, 381–389.

Felder, B. M. (2013). 'Euthanasia', human experiments, and psychiatry in Nazi-occupied Lithuania, 1941–1944. *Holocaust Genocide Stud*, 27, 242–273.

Formánek, T., Kagström, A., Cermakova, P., Csémy, L., Mladá, K., & Winkler, P. (2019). Prevalence of mental disorders and associated disability: results from the cross-sectional CZEch mental health Study (CZEMS). *Eur Psychiatry*, 60, 1–6.

Forsman, A. K., Ventus, D. B. J., Van Der Feltz-Cornelis, C. M., & Wahlbeck, K. (2014). Public mental health research in Europe: a systematic mapping for the roamer project. *Eur J Public Health*, 24, 955–960.

Füredi, J., et al. (2006). Psychiatry in selected countries of Central and Eastern Europe: an overview of the current situation. *Acta Psychiatr Scand*, 114, 223–231.

Gailienė, D. & Kazlauskas, E. (2005). Fifty years on: The long-term psychological effects of soviet repression in Lithuania. In Gailienė, D. (ed.) *The psychology of extreme traumatisation: the aftermath of political repression*. Vilnius, Lithuania: Akreta, 67–107.

Germanavičius, A., et al. (2004). *[Analysis of treatment and rehabilitation of persons affected with schizophrenia spectrum disorders in Vilnius]. Psichikos ligų klinika ir gydymas: mokslinės praktinės konferencijos darbų rinkinys. Vilniaus universiteto Psichiatrijos klinika*. Vilnius: Presvika.

Germanavičius, A., Mališauskaitė, L., Povilaitis, R., Pūras, D., Rimšaitė, E., & Šakalienė, D. (2005). Human rights monitoring in residential institutions for mentally disabled and psychiatric hospitals: monitoring report. In Mickevičius, H., Šakalienė, D., & Vyšniauskas, R. (eds) *Vilnius, Lithuania: Human Rights Monitoring Institute; Global Initiative on Psychiatry; Lithuanian Welfare Society for Persons with Mental Disability 'Viltis'*. Vilnius: Vilnius Center for Psychosocial Rehabilitation, 1–34.

Germanavicius, A., Rimsaite, E., Pilt, E., Puras, D., Juodkaite, D., & Leimane, I. (2006). *Human rights in mental health care in Baltic countries. In Mercer E & Rimsaite E (eds.)*. Latvia: Mental Disability Advocacy Center.

Golubeva, N., Naudts, K., Gibbs, A., Evsegneev, R., & Holubeu, S. (2006). Psychiatry in the republic of Belarus. *Int Psychiatry*, 3, 11–13.

Gustavsson, A., et al. (2011). Cost of disorders of the brain in Europe 2010. *Eur Neuropsychopharmacol*, 21, 718–779.

Haghighat, R. (1997). Psychiatry in Lithuania: the highest rate of suicide in the world. *The Psychiatrist*, 21, 716–719.

Höschl, C., Winkler, P., & Pec, O. (2012). The state of psychiatry in the Czech Republic. *Int Rev Psychiatry*, 24, 278–285.

IHIS (2003). *[Psychiatric care 2013]*. Prague: Institute for Health Information and Statistics, Czech Republic.

IHIS (2013). *[Psychiatric care 2012]*. Prague: Institute for Health Information and Statistics, Czech Republic.

IHIS (2014). *[Psychiatric care 2013]*. Prague: Institute for Health Information and Statistics, Czech Republic.

IHIS (2018). *[Psychiatric care 2013]*. Prague: Institute for Health Information and Statistics, Czech Republic.

Kališová, L., et al. (2014) Do patient and ward-related characteristics influence the use of coercive measures? Results from the EUNOMIA international study. *Soc Psychiatry Psychiatr Epidemiol, 49*(10), 1619–1629.

Kowalewski, D. (1979). Dissent in the Baltic republics: characteristics and consequences. *J Balt Stud, 10,* 309–319.

Krupchanka, D., Mladá, K., Winkler, P., Khazaal, Y., & Albanese, E. (2018). Mortality in people with mental disorders in the Czech Republic: a nationwide, register-based cohort study. *Lancet Public Health, 3*(6), e289–e295.

Lookene, M., Kisuro, A., Maciulis, V., Banaitis, V., Ungvari, G. S., & Gazdag, G. (2014). Use of electroconvulsive therapy in the Baltic states. *World J Biol Psychiatry, 15,* 419–424.

Melik-Pashayan, A. E. & Mironova, E. V. (2013). [Experience of stigmatization of schizophrenic patients in republic of Armenia and Republic of Belarus]. *Psychiatry and Psychopharmacotherapy, 3,* 68–72.

Motejl, O. (2008). *[Report from a visit of an institution: psychiatric hospital opava]. Sp. Zn.: 7/ 2008/nz/ls.* BRNO: Public Defender of Rights.

Mruh, O., Rymsha, S., & Mruh, V. (2020). Evaluation of the efficacy of atypical antipsychotic drugs and psychotherapy in patients with paranoid schizophrenia based on the duration of remission. *Georgian Med News,* (**302**), 86–92.

Mudrenko, I., Potapov, A., Sotnikov, D., Kolenko, O., & Kmyta, A. (2017). [Psychotherapeutic interventions in patients with auto-aggressive behavior during the first psychotic episode]. *Georgian Med News,* (**270**), 81–88.

Mundt, A. P., et al. (2012). Changes in the provision of institutionalized mental health care in post-communist countries. *PloS One, 7,* e38490–e38490.

Ougrin, D., Gluzman, S., & Dratcu, L. (2006) Psychiatry in post-communist Ukraine: dismantling the past, paving the way for the future. *The Psychiatrist, 30,* 456–459.

Pishel, V. Y., Ilnytska, T. Y., Drevitska, O. O., & Polyvyana, M. Y. (2019). Prevalence and structure of psychotic disorders in participants of military action. *Arch Psychiatry, 25*(2), 117–118.

Povilaitienė, I. (2011). *Relatives of the first episode psychosis patients: the relationship between appraisal of illness situation, social support, and psychological distress over time.* PhD, Vilnius University.

Pūras, D., Germanavičius, A., Povilaitis, R., Veniute, M., & Jasilionis, D. (2004). Lithuania mental health country profile. *Int Rev Psychiatry, 16,* 117–125.

Pūras, D., Sumskiene, E., & Adomaityte-Subaciene, I. (2013). Challenges of prolonged transition from totalitarian system to liberal democracy. *J Soc Policy Soc Work Transition, 1,* 1–24.

Quirke, E., Suvalo, O., Sukhovii, O., & Zöllner, Y. (2020). Transitioning to community-based mental health service delivery: opportunities for Ukraine. *J Mark Access Health Policy, 8*(1), 1843288.

Roberts, B., et al. (2019). Mental health care utilisation among internally displaced per-sons in Ukraine: results from a nation-wide survey. *Epidemiol Psychiatr Sci*, *28*(1), 100–111.

Rutz, W. (2004). Suicidal behaviour: comments, advancements, challenges. A European perspective. *World Psychiatry*, *3*, 161–162.

Scheffler, R., Potucek, M., & Univerzita, K. (2008). *Mental health care reform in the Czech and Slovak republics, 1989 to the present.* Prague: Karolinum.

Semrau, M., Barley, E. A., Law, A., & Thornicroft, G. (2011). Lessons learned in developing community mental health care in Europe. *World Psychiatry*, *10*, 217–225.

Sileikaite, A., Germanavičius, A., & Cesniene, I. (2016). The relationships of clinical, socio-demographic and criminal factors in a sample of forensic psychiatric patients. In **Frangou, S., Gorwood, P., & Heun, R.** (eds) *24th European Congress of Psychiatry.* Madrid, Spain: Elsevier Masson SAS, 47–51.

Thornicroft, G., Brohan, E., Rose, D., Sartorius, N., & Leese, M. (2009). Global pattern of experienced and anticipated discrimination against people with schizophrenia: a cross-sectional survey. *Lancet*, *373*, 408–415.

UN (2015). *World population prospects: the 2015 revision: key findings and advance tables.* New York: United Nations.

Van Voren, R. (2009). *On dissidents and madness from the Soviet Union of Leonid Brezhnev to the 'Soviet Union' of Vladimir Putin.* New York: Rodopi.

Van Voren, R. (2010). Political abuse of psychiatry—an historical overview. *Schizophr Bull*, *36*, 33–35.

Voloshina, P. V. & Maruty, N. O. (eds) (2019). *Early intervention in psychosis (new diagnostic and therapeutic paradigms).* Kharkiv: Strokov D.V.

Weissbecker, I., et al. (2017). *Mental health in transition: assessment and guidance for strengthening integration of mental health into primary health care and community-based service platforms in Ukraine (English).* Washington (DC): World Bank Group.

WHO (2005). *Mental health atlas 2005.* World Health Organization.

WHO (2014). *Mental health atlas—2014 country profiles.* Geneva: World Health Organization.

Wilken, J. P. & Hollander, D. D. (2005). *Rehabilitation and recovery: a comprehensive approach.* Amsterdam: SWP.

Winkler, P., Formánek, T., Mladá, K., & Cermakova, P. (2018). The CZEch Mental health Study (CZEMS): study rationale, design, and methods. *Int J Methods Psychiatr Res*, *27*(3), e1728.

Winkler, P., Formánek, T., Mladá, K., Kagstrom, A., Mohrova, Z., Mohr, P., & Csemy, L. (2020). Increase in prevalence of current mental disorders in the context of COVID-19: analysis of repeated nationwide cross-sectional surveys. *Epidemiol Psychiatr Sci*, *29*, e173.

Winkler, P., et al. (2020). Adherence to the convention on the rights of people with disabilities in Czech psychiatric hospitals: a nationwide evaluation study. *Health Hum Rights*, *22*(1), 21.

Winkler, P., Horáček, J., Weissová, A., Šustr, M., & Brunovský, M. (2015a). Physical comorbidities in depression co-occurring with anxiety: a cross-sectional study in the Czech primary care system. *Int J Environ Res Public Health*, *12*, 15728–15738.

Winkler, P., Mladá, K., Krupchanka, D., Agius, M., Kar-Ray, M., & Höschl, C. (2015b). Long-term inpatients with psychoses discharged from Czech mental hospitals in 2006–2011 5th Biennial Cambridge & Bedford International Conference on Mental Health 11th–14th September 2015. University of Cambridge, UK. Retrieved from http://www.bcmhr-cu.org/sites/default/files/Abstracts For Conference 20150908.pdf

Winkler, P., et al. (2017). A blind spot on the global mental health map: a scoping review of 25 years' development of mental health care for people with severe mental illnesses in central and eastern Europe. *Lancet Psychiatry*, 4(8), 634–642.

16

Chennai, India

Rangaswamy Thara, Sujit John,
Ramachandran Padmavati, Greeshma
Mohan, and Vijaya Raghavan

Introduction

This chapter provides a snapshot of research on psychotic disorders conducted at the Schizophrenia Research Foundation (SCARF) in Chennai, India over the last three decades. The Schizophrenia Research Foundation (SCARF) is a non-governmental organization in Chennai in South India. Since 1984, SCARF has been committed to providing care and rehabilitation for persons with severe mental disorders, as well as conducting quality research in collaboration with the World Health Organization and other international and national academic and research centres (www.scarfindia.org). In collaboration with many national and international academic and research institutions, an array of studies covering a broad range of topics has been conducted. This includes studies on phenomenology, epidemiology, genetics, course and outcome, community-based interventions, stigma, and the role of work in the lives of persons with schizophrenia. In summarizing this work, we reflect on the highs and lows of research in low-and-middle-income countries and the challenges encountered in conducting community research in low-resource settings. We conclude with a section on priorities for future research and programme development in the Indian context.

Epidemiology

In the latter half of the 1980s, SCARF along with the Department of Psychiatry, Government General Hospital, conducted a large survey in urban Chennai sponsored by the Indian Council of Medical Research. A door-to-door survey of a population of 100,000 identified persons with psychotic disorders. The prevalence of schizophrenia, corrected for age at risk (15–45 years), was 3.87 per 1,000 of the population. It was significant that nearly one-third of these patients had remained untreated for an average duration of 10 years despite having three mental health services in the vicinity. The incidence rate was 35 per 100,000 years (Padmavati et al., 1988; Rajkumar et al., 1993).

Working in the slum areas of Chennai (formerly Madras), one of the authors (RT) developed a community support programme for persons with chronic severe mental illness (SMI). The common elements of the programme were case management with social and vocational rehabilitation offered at SCARF, educational and awareness programmes for families and local communities, income generation, and training in basic skills. This was recognized by the World Bank as one of the innovative slum-based programmes (Thara, 1992).

Coping with schizophrenia

When it was widely believed that persons with schizophrenia in India were unable to perceive early signs of relapse, our pilot study of 30 individuals with longstanding schizophrenia (mean duration of illness around 7 years) revealed that all but four were able to perceive early indicators. Disturbed sleep, slowness, underactivity, and confusion were the common indicators of relapse, according to them. Having a dialogue with oneself, talking to a close relative or friend, seeking psychiatric help, and engaging in some work seemed to be the commonly used coping strategies (Kumar et al., 1989).

Stigma

Stigma is a major factor that influences help-seeking as well as social integration of people with schizophrenia. A study of outpatients at SCARF reported fear of rejection by family and neighbours and the need to conceal facts from others as some of the more stigmatizing factors (Thara & Srinivasan, 2000). Indian families believe marriage to be a cure for mental illnesses, nondisclosure of which is not uncommon at the time of marriage. The Madras Longitudinal Study (MLS) found that 70% of young adults with a diagnosis of schizophrenia went on to marry in the following 10 years and all these were arranged by families with varying extents of disclosure about the disorder (Thara & Srinivasan, 1997). Finding jobs is tough and non-disclosure in job applications is again not uncommon (Loganathan & Murthy, 2011; Padmavati, 2014). Direct discrimination against individuals with schizophrenia is evidenced by the fear of rejection and the need to hide facts (Padmavati, 2014; Thara & Srinivasan, 2000).

A later study (Koschorke et al., 2014) nested in the COmmunity-based Intervention for People with Schizophrenia and their Caregivers in India (COPSI study) (Chatterjee et al., 2014) explored the experiences of stigma and discrimination in three Indian sites using a mixed methods approach. In-depth interviews with people with schizophrenia and caregivers (36 each) were carried out and analysed using thematic analysis. Experiences of negative discrimination were reported less commonly than more internalized forms of stigma experience such as a sense of alienation. Experiences of discrimination were associated with higher positive and lower negative symptoms of schizophrenia, higher caregiver knowledge about symptomatology, and younger age of the patients. Qualitative findings highlight three key domains influencing the themes of 'negative reactions' and 'negative views and feelings about the self', i.e. 'others finding out', 'behaviours and manifestations of the illness', and 'reduced ability to meet role expectations'. It was postulated by the authors that the ability to meet role expectations in marriage, work, and socially acceptable behaviours seemed to matter most (Koschorke et al., 2014).

Interventions

SCARF has piloted several community-based interventions in the rural area of Chengelpet, a district located to the south of the city of Chennai, ranging from community outreach clinics to trialling a task-shifting approach using lay health workers to deliver community-based mental healthcare.

Thiruporur community mental health programme

In 1989, a community-based mental health programme was initiated in the town of Thiruporur, about 45 km directly south of Chennai, with funding support from the International Development Research Centre, Canada (Thara et al., 2008). We decided to piggyback on an ongoing Red Cross community-based rehabilitation (CBR) programme for the physically disabled and trained 40 of their volunteers and community level workers.

The specific aims of the programme initiated were: (a) to increase awareness about mental disorders and their treatments; (b) to integrate a mental health component in the existing healthcare infrastructure by training primary care personnel; and (c) to develop CBR strategies that would be run by a network of trained lay volunteers. We believed that these personnel trained in detecting individuals with mental health problems would also ensure continued availability of mental health services and facilitate gradual withdrawal of the service of SCARF. Towards this end, SCARF ran a monthly mental health clinic in the community and trained 68 multipurpose workers in mental health. An active liaison was also established with the traditional faith healing centres in that area (Hanumanthapuram temple and the Kovalam Dargha) to motivate healers to refer cases to the SCARF clinic in Thiruporur. Over a period of five years, 637 patients were registered, two-thirds of whom were diagnosed with psychotic disorders.

Further, a citizens' group was created, which comprised stakeholders from the community, and was tasked with the responsibility of creating awareness, encouraging help-seeking, organizing mental health clinics, and involving the community in general in the rehabilitation of the patients. The members of the group also created a small fund, tapping local fiscal resources for the implementation of the above activities.

We exited from the area in 1999 since the funding stopped. At that time, we were treating 185 persons with psychotic disorders and we had referred them to available mental healthcare facilities. Six years later, in 2005, we conducted a follow-up of these 185 patients and assessed their clinical status and level of use of the various community services that we had established under the programme (Thara et al., 2008). Sadly, the referral service had been used by only 15% of the patients. Multiple factors such as limited access and associated expenses entailed in seeking treatment and termination of the mental health services provided by the primary health centre (PHC), determined this low level of help-seeking. The citizens' group was also functional for only a year as it had conflicting priorities.

It was clear that while it is feasible to start a wide spectrum of mental health and related social and economic activities in a rural area, community involvement and better motivation on the part of primary care physicians are necessary for their sustainability.

COmmunity-based Intervention for People with Schizophrenia and their Caregivers in India (COPSI)

In order to test the effectiveness of a community-based intervention for people with schizophrenia and their caregivers, a randomized controlled trial was conducted across three sites in India, with the Chengelpet taluk being one of the sites; the others were in Goa and Satara (Maharashtra) (Chatterjee et al., 2014). While the combined data from all the sites reported that the intervention was only modestly more effective than facility-based care, especially for reducing disability and symptoms of psychosis, the results from Chengelpet showed a definite improvement in both symptoms and disability. Reduction in PANSS scores was significant ($p=0.003$), and so was disability ($p=0.01$), but this was not the case in the other two more urban sites. We postulate that, because the intervention in Chengelpet was largely on never treated subjects, it may be a lack of exposure to prior intervention that could account for better outcomes. COPSI also clearly demonstrated that the delivery of services by lay health workers was acceptable to the community at large and that task shifting as a strategy was feasible.

Tele-psychiatry

Following our experience with tele-psychiatry during the tsunami in December 2004, SCARF launched a mobile tele-psychiatry programme in 2010. This was done in the district of Pudukkottai in Tamil Nadu and the programme involved the use of a mobile unit and fixed lines for tele-consultations.

The mobile unit was a bus that was custom-built with a consultation room and a pharmacy. The psychiatrist in Chennai (~450 km from Pudukkottai) carried out a detailed mental state examination through flat-screen televisions and state-of-the-art, high-resolution cameras using a wireless internet connection. The nurse on the bus dispensed the medicine prescribed. This programme, which catered only to persons with severe mental disorders, has treated close to 3,600 persons over a period of 8 years. Apart from medication, counselling and help with employment were also offered by the trained community-level workers in those areas. The TV screen on the bus was used to project short films and messages on mental health during the evenings. This programme is one of SCARF's flagship innovative community-based interventions (Thara & John, 2013).

Explanatory models

Cultural beliefs about mental illness and cultural idioms of distress have long evoked the interest of anthropologists, sociologists, and psychiatrists. In the 1990s, we looked at understanding a rural community's perceptions and explanatory models of mental disorders (Thara et al., 1998). Focus group discussions and in-depth interviews were undertaken using a topic guide to elicit information on signs, causes, reactions, and quest for treatment. The respondents were village leaders, community respondents (who had no relatives with mental illness), and family members of persons with a serious mental disorder who were treated at religious healing centres.

This study found that even a predominantly impoverished and illiterate rural population was able to describe in detail behavioural concomitants of mental illnesses. Altered behaviours were associated with psychoses, depression, and hysteria, as it was known then. Violence was easily identified and clearly associated with psychotic disorders. Many abnormal behaviours were believed to be caused by possession by spirits, devils, curses of the gods, etc., and appeared to determine treatment-seeking patterns, leading many to prefer religious and traditional modes of therapy.

Another study, conducted more than half a decade later, examined the reasons mentally ill patients and their families in India choose to seek help from a religious site (Padmavati et al., 2005). In-depth interviews at religious sites sought explanations for the illness and found them to be largely based on culturally accepted reasons such as evil spirits, planetary positions, or sins of the past life. While the choice of source of help was largely based on the explanations for the illness, there were other factors that influenced this decision, such as advice from religious leaders, priests, astrologers, faith healers, or elders in the family. It is interesting to note that the choice of the place of worship often went beyond the boundaries of religious faith. Irrespective of their religion by birth, patients and families went to temples, dargahs, or churches for a 'cure'. Hindus were seen to visit a Muslim dargah for treatment. A Christian or a Muslim would visit a temple in the hope of a 'cure'. In almost all the centres, ritualistic behaviour patterns were observed.

Research from about 10 years later (Cohen et al., 2016) reported similar findings, i.e. that help-seeking did not always match the religious beliefs of families. Furthermore, while initial responses to mental illness were largely congruent with cultural beliefs, later responses were often more pragmatic and involved consideration of, for example, relative effectiveness and costs of treatments, such that—at later points—families might seek care with biomedical practitioners. This later research also found that families had a broad array of causal attributions, e.g. thinking too much, shock, and head injuries.

Course and outcome

While we have completed a few studies on course and outcome, the MLS has had the longest period of follow-up of persons with first-episode schizophrenia and is one of the few of its kind from low- and middle-income countries.

The original MLS cohort was 90 first-episode patients who met ICD-9 and Feighner criteria for schizophrenia and who were attending the psychiatry outpatient department of the Government General Hospital attached to the Madras Medical College in Chennai, India. From year 10, follow-up was conducted from SCARF (previous follow-ups were conducted by staff at the government general hospital, who later moved to SCARF). Follow-up data at years 10, 20, and 25 have been published (Eaton et al., 1995; Thara et al., 1994; Thara, 2004; Thara, 2012). Clinical and demographic details were recorded every year for the first five years and then at years 10, 20, 25, and 35 after inclusion. At inclusion and follow-up, the ninth edition of the present state examination (PSE) and the psychiatric and personal history schedule (PPHS) were administered to elicit demographic and clinical data. While all attempts were made to ensure regular contact during the first 10 years, the absence of adequate funding thereafter made it difficult to ensure this in the subsequent years (Table 16.1). Table 16.2 illustrates the follow-up rates and clinical status of the cohort at each

Table 16.1 Details of follow-up (Madras Longitudinal Study)

Variable	10 yrs. n (%)	20 yrs. n (%)	25 yrs. n (%)	35 yrs. n (%)
Followed up	76 (84.4)	61 (67.0)	47 (51.0)	30 (33.0)
Drop-out	5 (5.5)	13 (14.4)	18 (20.0)	28 (31.1)
Deaths	9 (10.0)	16 (17.7)	25 (27.7)	32 (35.6)
Suicides	4 (44.4)	7 (43.8)	7 (28.0)	7 (21.9)

of the follow-up periods. At the final follow-up, we found that one-third of the sample could be located, with mortality accounting for another third. A third of these deaths were by suicide. The average age at death was 39.4 years. Marital status and mortality appeared to be related. Half of those who died were single, and another 22% were either separated or divorced. Only 28% were married at the time of death. This requires additional research to determine if marriage is indeed a protective factor in terms of caregiving.

In an interesting paper, Eaton and Thara studied symptom patterns at 10 years (Eaton et al., 1995). The clusters of positive and negative symptoms seemed to be independent, both cross-sectionally and longitudinally. Symptoms in one month were highly predictive of the same the next month.

Further, an analysis at 10 years revealed that marital rates of persons with schizophrenia in India were quite high compared with Western countries. While more men tended to remain single, more women were either separated from their husbands or divorced. Continuous illness or multiple relapses seemed to reduce the prospects of getting married (Thara & Srinivasan, 1997).

Finally, at the end of 10 years, we explored the work and occupational functioning of both men and women in the follow-up sample. A comprehensive evaluation of work functioning of 40 men over a period of 10 years was done. Over 50% had a good occupational outcome, while 4 of 40 never held a job during

Table 16.2 Clinical status at follow-up (Madras Longitudinal Study)

	10 yrs. n (%)	20 yrs. n (%)	25 yrs. n (%)	35 yrs. n (%)
Cohort	76 (84)	61 (68)	47 (52)	30 (33)
Remission	13 (17)	5 (8)	11 (23)	7 (23)
Relapses	58 (76)	51 (84)	31 (66)	19 (63)
Continuous illness	5 (7)	5 (8)	5 (11)	4 (13)
On treatment	53 (70)	32 (52)	27 (57)	15 (50)

the entire period. The employment rate was higher than that seen in developed countries (Srinivasan & Thara, 1997). On similar lines, the long-term home-making functioning of women was also studied using items from the PPHS. The 10-year work outcome was good in 67% of 36 women and poor in the rest. These figures were comparable to the rates seen in men (Srinivasan & Thara, 1999).

Abnormal movements in never treated psychoses

In collaboration with Dr Robin McCreadie of the Crichton Royal Hospital, Dumfries, Scotland, SCARF initiated a series of studies on abnormal move-ments in never treated persons with schizophrenia. Movement disorders were examined in persons aged 50 plus in several settings in Chennai, i.e. outpatient, inpatient, and daycare facilities of SCARF, centres for senior citizens, and a rural community. All subjects fulfilled DSM-IV criteria for schizophrenia. Of the 308 included, it was found that there was no difference in the prevalence and se-verity of abnormal movements in treated and untreated subjects. However, ab-normal movements were much more evident than what was seen in controls. This was a landmark study demonstrating dyskinesias in untreated individuals with schizophrenia (McCreadie et al., 1996). When a subgroup of 37 of these pa-tients were examined for abnormal movements after 18 months, we found that 24% had dyskinesia on both occasions and 33% on one. It seemed that spontan-eous dyskinesia and parkinsonism fluctuate over time (McCreadie et al., 2002).

Another significant piece of work related to this was the use of MRI to com-pare brain volumes in three groups: persons with schizophrenia with and without dyskinesia and non-psychotic matched controls, all from a rural com-munity. The findings suggest that never treated patients with dyskinesia may have striatal pathology and may indeed represent a subgroup of persons with schizophrenia (McCreadie et al., 2002).

INTREPID (International Research Programme on Psychoses in Diverse Settings)

INTREPID is a multi-country programme of research on several aspects of psychoses, including phenomenology, onset, course and outcome, and physical health. The first phase of INTREPID was designed to implement and evaluate methods for identifying, assessing, and following up cases of untreated psych-osis and controls in three sites: Chengalpet (near Chennai), India; Ibadan South East and Ona Ara, Nigeria; and Tunapuna-Piarco, Trinidad (Morgan et al., 2015). The specific sites were chosen to ensure they contained a mix of urban and rural areas. The purpose of this phase was to ensure a comparable set of procedures and methods across the sites that could be implemented in a substantive programme to address questions about the distribution, onset, and course and outcome of psychoses in several countries in the Global South. This substantive programme, INTREPID II, is ongoing.

From data collected as part of the initial phase of INTREPID, we found that rates of all untreated psychoses in Chengelpet taluk were 45.9 (per 100,000 person-years) and roughly half the cases received a diagnosis of schizophrenia (ICD-10). When analyses were restricted to cases with a short duration (i.e. onset within the preceding 2 years), the rate was 15.5 per 100,000 person-years. Further, the duration of psychosis (inclusive of all cases) was close to 5 years (median 4.83 years). The average age of onset was 33.8 years. Overall, there were more women (56.2%) than men with psychoses but when schizophrenia cases alone were considered men outnumbered women (43.2%). Being a rural and remote community, 90% of the cases were identified through non-providers (i.e. key informants and local residents) in the community rather than from the formal mental health service providers who were few and far between.

Further, as part of INTREPID I, we completed a study of help-seeking and be-liefs. In this, almost all the identified patients on the site had first been taken to a faith healer by their families. They received this treatment for varying lengths of time and tended to shift to allopathic care when there was no improvement in the patient's condition (Cohen et al., 2016). About 20% of the identified sample had never received allopathic care, while 27% had discontinued treat-ment. Ninety per cent (90%) of those who discontinued treatment were cur-rently symptomatic. Only 53% of the identified subjects at the time of the study were receiving treatment. The average length of time that was taken prior to an allopathic consultation (excluding the never treated) was 3.2 years (SD 5.1) with the maximum length being 23 years. A significant proportion also sought concurrent magico-religious care.

INTREPID II was initiated in the same sites in 2018 with the primary object-ives of determining the variability—in incidence, presentation, outcome, and impact—of psychotic disorders in diverse countries of the Global South. The two-year course and outcome, help-seeking patterns, and the co-occurrence of physical health problems will also be determined.

Scales and instruments

We have also developed several instruments to be used with our population. These include:

· The Family Burden Scale (BAS): Since almost all persons with a serious mental disorder in India live with their families, we developed a tool to measure both objective and subjective burdens. This was done in collaboration with WHO SEARO, has 40 items, and has been used extensively by researchers in India (Thara et al., 1998).

· The SCARF social functioning index (SSFI): This measures social functioning, which is a critical outcome measure in persons with a serious mental disorder. It has four sections: self-concern, occupational role, role in the family, and other social roles (Padmavati et al., 1995).

Genetic studies

We have completed several studies of the genetics of schizophrenia. For example, in collaboration with the University of Queensland, Australia, we undertook a large community-based genome-wide association study (GWAS) to understand the genetic loci and functional associations among patients with schizophrenia from South India. GWAS was done for 3,092 participants including patients with schizophrenia, their family members, and unaffected controls. A novel association was observed between schizophrenia and chromosome 8q24.3 locus (rs10866912, allele A). This locus directly modifies the abundance of the nicotinate phosphoribosyl transferase gene (*NAPRT1*, a key enzyme for niacin metabolism) transcript in the brain cortex. These findings imply that *NAPRT1* is a novel susceptibility gene for schizophrenia and its relationship with niacin metabolism might have implications for the treatment of schizophrenia (Periyasamy et al., 2019).

First episode psychosis (FEP) programme at SCARF

SCARF and the Prevention and Early Intervention Program for Psychosis (PEPP) at Douglas Hospital, Montreal, collaborated for over a decade on a series of research initiatives on FEP. Developed collaboratively, these studies examined differences in multiple outcome domains (functional, subjective, and clinical) across sites using mixed methods (Iyer et al., 2010). Both centres followed similar early intervention service (EIS) protocols for serving young persons with FEP. These included the use of second-generation antipsychotic medications at the lowest effective doses, case management, family psychoeducation and individual family intervention, emotional support to patients and families, and an overall recovery orientation. Over two years, positive and negative symptoms improved in both sites. However, the improvement was greater in Montreal for positive symptoms and greater in Chennai for negative symptoms (Malla et al., 2020). Not unexpectedly, family support was higher for Chennai patients.

Study on hallucinations

In a multisite study on auditory hallucinations (Luhrmann et al., 2015), people with schizophrenia in three different countries were compared. There were prominent differences in the kinds of voices that people appeared to experience. The voices were described as intrusive, unreal (California sample), largely useful and guiding (Chennai, India), and morally good and causally powerful (Ghana). The researchers proposed a social kindling hypothesis stating that people with serious psychotic disorder pay selective attention to a constant stream of many different auditory and quasi-auditory events because of different cultural invitations, implying variations in ways of thinking about minds, persons, spirits, and so forth.

Challenges faced

Many challenges have been confronted in delivering the research programmes sketched in this chapter. To note just a few.

Conducting research in low-resource settings with large populations spread over vast geographical areas comes with many expected challenges, chiefly logistics. Low levels of literacy, with high poverty in the local population, creates its own set of unique challenges in terms of access to the population, obtaining informed consent, and so on. It takes great tact and effort to establish liaisons with the local community leaders to gain their cooperation for community-based research work.

The almost complete lack of availability of any form of records also poses a challenge, leaving researchers dependent entirely on the ability of the subject and family to recall events and dates, even for something as basic as their date of birth. (This is however now slowly changing with national ID cards being issued by the government.)

Translation of study instruments into the local language and the applicability of some of the items is also a challenge.

Some of the specific challenges encountered within the context of the INTREPID epidemiological study are that, despite the best efforts to extend case-finding, there are factors within and outside the formal healthcare system which hinder this process. We lack access to some of the private hospitals and practitioners in the area who also do not maintain good case records, and the lack of specified catchment-based services allows for persons to seek help from anywhere they wish to, even to go to hospitals in Chennai. Religious practitioners and healers located within churches or temples also deliver treatment and their willingness to share information is varied.

During the COPSI trial, a major challenge was to get families from a largely patriarchal society to accept young women as advisors. Caste considerations in rural communities in Tamil Nadu run deep and there were instances when upper-caste families were reluctant to permit lower-caste women to enter their homes to provide the trial interventions.

International collaborations

It has been a unique experience for us at SCARF to have collaborated with many international researchers. A wealth of data from genetics to anthropology has been generated using rigorous research designs and methodologies. This would not have been possible without the great cooperation we had from patients and families, and the commitment and competence of our rural health workers who formed an integral part of our research teams. There was no room on either side for patronization and condescension. To quote McCreadie, one of our long-term collaborators, 'I have found my research activities in India one of the most satisfying in my psychiatric career . . . What you need is a good idea, money and most of all a clear understanding that the project is carried out by equals' (Thara & McCreadie, 1999).

Priorities for future research and service development

Research in India on various aspects of psychosis needs to be prioritized in order to better understand the aetiology of the disorders including genetic and social determinants and the role of medical, psychological, and psychosocial interventions. With a large part of the country being rural, it is important that this research translates itself to cost-effective and feasible programmes for the rural poor, many of whom live with a mental illness and remain untreated for decades and become progressively disabled. Since stigma and poor awareness of mental health conditions prevent help-seeking, we need to develop—using rigorous methods—programmes that will address both these variables. Community engagement and participation in mental healthcare also needs to be fostered. In the absence of formal mental healthcare services in many parts of the country, the community can play a critical role in the social and economic care of these persons.

Finally, it is equally important to build capacity for research in many academic settings and have a system of incentives that will promote well-planned, scientific research, particularly among early career mental health professionals.

References

Chatterjee, S., et al. (2014). Effectiveness of a community-based intervention for people with schizophrenia and their caregivers in India (COPSI): a randomised controlled trial. *Lancet, 383*(9926), 1385–1394.

Cohen, A., et al. (2016). Concepts of madness in diverse settings: a qualitative study from the INTREPID project. *BMC Psychiatry*, *16*(1), 388

Eaton, W. W., Thara, R., Federman, B., Melton, B., & Liang, K. Y. (1995). Structure and course of positive and negative symptoms in schizophrenia. *Arch Gen Psychiatry*, *52*(2), 127–134.

Iyer, S. N., Mangala, R., Thara, R., & Malla, A. K. (2010). Preliminary findings from a study of first-episode psychosis in Montreal, Canada and Chennai, India: comparison of outcomes. *Schizophr Res*, *121*(1–3), 227–233.

Koschorke, M., et al. (2014). Experiences of stigma and discrimination of people with schizophrenia in India. *Soc Sci Med*, *123*, 149–159.

Kumar, S., Thara, R., & Rajkumar, S. (1989). Coping with symptoms of relapse in schizophrenia. *Eur Arch Psychiatr Neurol Sci*, *239*(3), 213–215.

Loganathan, S. & Murthy, R. S. (2011). Living with schizophrenia in India: gender perspectives. *Transcult Psychiatry*, *48*(5), 569–584.

Luhrmann, T. M., Padmavati, R., Tharoor, H., & Osei, A. (2015). Differences in voice-hearing experiences of people with psychosis in the USA, India and Ghana: interview-based study. *Br J Psychiatry*, *206*(1), 41–44.

Malla, A., et al. (2020). Comparison of clinical outcomes following 2 years of treatment of first-episode psychosis in urban early intervention services in Canada and India. *Br J Psychiatry*, *217*(3), 514–520.

McCreadie, R. G., et al. (1996). Abnormal movements in never-medicated Indian patients with schizophrenia. *Br J Psychiatry*, *168*(2), 221–226.

McCreadie, R. G., Padmavati, R., Thara, R., & Srinivasan, T. N. (2002). Spontaneous dyskinesia and parkinsonism in never-medicated, chronically ill patients with schizophrenia: 18-month follow-up. *Br J Psychiatry*, *181*(2), 135–137.

McCreadie, R. G., Thara, R., Padmavati, R., Srinivasan, T. N., & Jaipurkar, S. D. (2002). Structural brain differences between never-treated patients with schizophrenia, with and without dyskinesia, and normal control subjects: a magnetic resonance imaging study. *Arch Gen Psychiatry*, *59*(4), 332–336.

Morgan, C., et al. (2015). Searching for psychosis: INTREPID (1): systems for detecting untreated and first-episode cases of psychosis in diverse settings. *Soc Psychiatry Psychiatr Epidemiol*, *50*(6), 879–893.

Padmavati, R., Thara, R., & Corin, E. (2005). A qualitative study of religious practices by chronic mentally ill and their caregivers in South India. *Int J Soc Psychiatry*, *51*(2), 139–149.

Padmavati, R., Thara, R., Srinivasan, L., & Kumar, S. (1995). Scarf social functioning index. *Indian J Psychiatry*, *37*(4), 161–164.

Padmavati, R., Rajkumar, S., Kumar, N., Manoharan, A., & Kamath, S. (1988). Prevalence of schizophrenia in an urban community in Madras. *Indian J Psychiatry*, *30*(3), 233.

Padmavati, R. (2014). Stigmatization and exclusion. In Okpaku, S. O. (ed.) *Essentials of global mental health*. Cambridge: Cambridge University Press, 85–92.

Periyasami, S., et al. (2019). Association of schizophrenia risk with disordered niacin metabolism in an Indian genome-wide association study. *JAMA Psychiatry*, *76*(10), 1026–1034.

Rajkumar, S. R. P. R. T. M. S. M., Padmavathi, R., Thara, R., & Menon, M. S. (1993). Incidence of schizophrenia in an urban community in Madras. *Indian J Psychiatry*, *35*(1), 18.

Srinivasan, T. N. & Thara, R. (1997). How do men with schizophrenia fare at work? A follow-up study from India. *Schizophr Res, 25*(2), 149–154.

Srinivasan, T. N. & Thara, R. (1999). The long-term home-making functioning of women with schizophrenia. *Schizophr Res, 35*(1), 97–98.

Thara, R. (2012). Twenty-five years of schizophrenia: the Madras longitudinal study. *Indian J Psychiatry, 54*(2), 134.

Thara, R., Padmavati, R., Aynkran, J. R., & John, S. (2008). Community mental health in India: a rethink. *Int J Mental Health Systems, 2*(11), 1–7.

Thara, R. & John, S. (2013). Mobile telepsychiatry in India. *World Psychiatry, 12*(1), 84.

Thara, R. (1992). An attempt at the development of community-based support systems in the urban slums of Madras, India. *Psychosoc Rehabil J, 16*(1), 155.

Thara, R., Henrietta, M., Joseph, A., Rajkumar, S., & Eaton, W. W. (1994). Ten-year course of schizophrenia—the Madras longitudinal study. *Acta Psychiatr Scand, 90*(5), 329–336.

Thara, R. & Srinivasan, T. N. (1997). Marriage and gender in schizophrenia. *Indian J Psychiatry, 39*(1), 64.

Thara, R. & Srinivasan, T. N. (1997). Outcome of marriage in schizophrenia. *Soc Psychiatry Psychiatr Epidemiol, 32*(7), 416–420.

Thara, R., Islam, A., & Padmavati, R. (1998). Beliefs about mental illness: a study of a rural South-Indian community. *Int J Mental Health, 27*(3), 70–85.

Thara, R. & McCreadie, R. G. (1999). Research in India: success through collaboration. *Adv Psychiatr Treat, 55555*, 221–224.

Thara, R. & Srinivasan, T. N. (2000). How stigmatising is schizophrenia in India?. *Int J Soc Psychiatry, 46*(2), 135–141.

Thara, R. (2004). Twenty-year course of schizophrenia: the Madras longitudinal study. *Can J Psychiatry, 49*(8), 564–569.

Thara, R., Padmavati, R., Aynkran, J. R., & John, S. (2008). Community mental health in India: a rethink. *Int J Ment Health Syst, 2*(1), 11.

17

Hong Kong

Christy Lai Ming Hui, Wing Chung Chang,
Sherry Kit Wa Chan, Edwin Ho Ming Lee,
and Eric Yu Hai Chen

Introduction

In this chapter, we provide an overview of services for and research on psychotic disorders in Hong Kong. Hong Kong is one of the most densely populated cities in the world, accommodating a population of over seven million. The majority of the population is Han Chinese (95%) and the primary language is Cantonese. The city has an overall gender ratio of 876 men to 1,000 women (Population Census Office, 2012), with the preponderance of women also reflected in the population with psychosis (Chen et al., 2005a; Chen et al., 2010). Another distinctive feature of the city is that a majority of the population lives with their family due to factors such as sky-rocketing property prices and traditional Chinese culture. Thus, only 17% of the population lives in single-person households, a rate lower than in the UK (29%; Office of National Statistics, 2013), the US (28%; United States Census Bureau, 2015), and Australia (24%; Australian Bureau of Statistics, 2011).

Overview of services

A government-subsidized public healthcare system is in place in Hong Kong. Local psychiatric care depends heavily on this system and is complemented by rather costly private services. At the time of writing, the psychiatrist-to-people ratio is 4.5:100,000, but only 330 serve the public sector (Cheung, 2016). In total, there are also 1,880 psychiatric nurses (of which 133 are community nurses), and 197 medical social workers serving approximately 150,000 psychiatric patients (Tang et al., 2010). According to territory-wide surveys, approximately 2.5% of the Chinese adult population has a lifetime psychotic disorder (Chang et al., 2017a) and 13.3% of the general Hong Kong population reports having a common mental disorder (CMD; Lam et al., 2015). Evidently, the demand for psychiatric services in Hong Kong is high. While government funding and resources are available to support service provision, they are both of limited supply. In addition to the overflow of demand on the public psychiatric services, the system also struggles to manage formidable social obstacles such as stigma (Lee et al., 2005; 2006; Chan et al., 2016) and the defects in service quality that stem from the unmanageable demand.

In Hong Kong, access to public psychiatric outpatient services requires a referral from a primary care practitioner. Before the implementation of the early intervention programme for psychotic disorders, patients would need to wait for months, or even over a year, for the first consultation. Thus, the duration of untreated psychosis (DUP) was long, averaging 513 days (Chen et al., 2005b). In many cases, patients would make their first contact with psychiatric services during a crisis (e.g. at risk of self-harm or violence) and through attendance in accident and emergency departments or admission to hospital. After gaining access to the public psychiatric system, stabilized patients are then managed in busy general psychiatric outpatient clinics in which the service volume is high. As a result of demands on the service, multiple aspects of it are inadequate, restricting the quality of care received by patients, e.g. consultation times at clinics average 5.6 minutes, follow-ups are infrequent, and the provision of non-pharmacological interventions is limited (Hui et al., 2008), to name a few.

As mentioned, strong social obstacles also add to the constraints on psychiatric services. Whereas stigma for mental illnesses presents a major barrier to help-seeking universally, the phenomenon is of particular significance in Chinese populations, compared with Western cohorts (Knifton et al., 2010). Regardless of improved mental health literacy over the years, a phone-interview study indicates that the level of stigma towards psychosis has not changed in Hong Kong (Chan et al., 2016). Marked stigma and discrimination against individuals with psychotic disorders continue to hinder help-seeking behaviour as well as treatment adherence (Chung & Wong, 2004). In consideration of the pressure faced by public psychiatric services and the lack of specialized care provision, early intervention services for psychosis in Hong Kong were initiated in 2001.

Early intervention for psychoses in Hong Kong

Noting the above mentioned challenges and more, increased efforts were focused on developing early intervention programmes for psychosis over the past two decades in Hong Kong. In 2001, the first territory-wide public service, Early Assessment Service for Young people with psychosis (EASY), was launched by the Hospital Authority (Chen, 2004). It is one of the first early intervention services for psychosis launched in Asia. EASY utilizes prodromal monitoring, case management, and phase-specific interventions for psychosis patients. Upon a formal diagnosis, the service would provide a two-year programme for first-episode psychosis (FEP) patients aged 15–25 years. The programme incorporates outcome evaluation studies, public awareness campaigns, and professional training. Following the establishment of EASY, the Asian Network of Early Psychosis (ANEP) was launched in 2003. The ANEP is an informal network for relevant professionals to promote early intervention and to facilitate knowledge exchange and research on psychosis in Asia.

On top of reinforcing regional communication, the Early Psychosis Foundation (EPISO, www.episo.org), a local independent charitable organization, was founded in 2007. EPISO provides a platform intended to make knowledge about psychosis more accessible, raise awareness of the disorder, and promote existing intervention services.

In 2009, the University of Hong Kong hosted another early intervention project, the Jockey Club Early Psychosis (JCEP) project, providing five-year early intervention for FEP patients aged 26 years old or above (Hui et al., 2014), in an attempt to address the service gap left by EASY at the time. Following evaluation of EASY's services along with the increased need for psychiatric care indicated by JCEP's operations, EASY has undergone a major extension. In 2011, its services were extended to provide three-year early intervention for FEP patients aged 15–64 years in all seven local hospital clusters

To complement the service provision, professional training and caregiver support programmes were developed. A postgraduate programme in psychosis studies was launched in 2011, with the aim of providing professional training in early psychosis to students from various sectors, including social work and nursing. In addition to educating future professionals, the Department of Psychiatry in the University of Hong Kong also launched an internet-based psychosis education programme for caregivers (iPEP, www.ipep.hk) in 2014 (Chan et al., 2016). The interactive website is designed for patients with psychosis and their families, to access up-to-date information to facilitate understanding and care provision for patients.

For better understanding of the early intervention services in Hong Kong, the two major early intervention programmes for psychosis patients, EASY and JCEP, are discussed in-depth in the following sections.

EASY: first local early intervention programme for psychoses

EASY, the government-funded territory-wide initiative founded by the hospital authority, was implemented in 2001 and has undergone two phases of service extension since then. The programme originally targeted FEP patients aged 15–25 years in four hospital clusters in the city. In view of the increasing psychiatric needs of the local population, as indicated by JCEP, the government has since granted increased funding to extend EASY's catchment area to all seven hospital clusters and expanded the target age range to include patients up to 64 years old. It excludes patients who have significant medical illnesses, moderate to severe intelligence deficiency, or substance-induced psychotic episodes.

The programme aims were to: 1) create an easily accessible channel for patients to reduce treatment delay; 2) achieve the best possible clinical outcome during the critical period by providing phase-specific care tailored to the needs of FEP patients; and 3) establish a high-quality data-driven phase-specific intervention model through developing a team of professionals. A steering committee was formed to lead the programme and to develop a management protocol, the Psychological Intervention Programmes in Early Psychosis (PIPE; So et al., 2013), specifically for EASY.

A multidisciplinary intervention team works with community collaborators to serve each of the catchment areas, covering the entire territory. At present, each of the intervention teams consist of two to three psychiatrists, three key workers who are usually psychiatric nurses, one social worker, and half to one clinical psychologist. Specific working groups were also formed during programme development to deal with issues such as media events, training, and research.

Public awareness campaigns

A working group consisting of experienced clinicians and experts from the public affairs division of the Hospital Authority was formed to organize public education programmes that target the social obstacles to the use of services. A major element of the public awareness campaign was the term 'psychosis', which has no proper equivalent in Chinese (Chiu et al., 2010). Prior to this campaign, people who exhibited psychotic symptoms would be referred to as having 'split-personality', which could in fact refer to a different diagnosis, i.e. dissociative identity disorder. In hopes of ameliorating stigma and enhancing understanding of psychosis, a more accurate and informative Chinese term, 'Si Jue Shi Diao/思覺失調', was adopted. The word literally means dysregulation ('Shi Diao/失調') in thinking ('Si/思') and perception ('Jue/覺'), which depicts the conditions of psychosis more accurately and imparts a suggestion of reversibility. The new term was used widely in the campaigns that covered television, radio, printed, and online media, exhibitions, and talks. The new term has been found to be well-adopted by the public through a study of the news coverage of the term over 10 years (Chan et al., 2017). There were also intensive education campaigns to inform the public about psychotic symptoms.

Access to services

Taking into account the long waiting time in the public psychiatric system, EASY aims to set up an easily accessible channel for service contact to encourage early help-seeking. The open and direct system accepts referrals from a wide range of sources, e.g. community programmes, NGOs, schools, as well as within the healthcare system, and can be done through a telephone hotline, email, and walk-ins. These methods lowered the entry barriers to services and encouraged help-seeking in non-stigmatizing community settings such as NGOs and general hospitals.

A two-staged assessment system is adopted. Stage one is an initial telephone screening carried out by case managers, usually clinically experienced psychiatric nurses, to determine whether the individual is a potential client for the service. Ideally, an informant, who is usually the primary caregiver of the potential client, would also take part in the preliminary screening. Eligible cases then enter stage two of the assessment system, where clinicians conduct a diagnostic assessment for them within one week.

Phase-specific intervention

Phase-specific intervention is the key intervention component of EASY. It includes case management, intensive medical follow-up, and enhanced rehabilitation services, all tailored to each patient's phase of illness. For individuals with an at-risk mental state (ARMS) or those who present prodromal symptoms, their ARMS status would be confirmed using the comprehensive assessment of the ARMS (CAARMS; Yung, 2003) before formal enrolment and treatment reception in EASY (Chen et al., 2013). Cases with ARMS or prodrome would then be provided with case management and regular follow-up appointments with a clinician. For patients whose initial contact with EASY coincides with the acute phase of psychosis, they would usually be prescribed a second-generation antipsychotic as first-line treatment, to ameliorate positive symptoms. Additionally, if this is their initial contact with the service, case managers would also begin to establish therapeutic alliances with patients and their families. Following the acute phase of illness, intensive care and case management are continued during the maintenance phase. Beyond sustaining remission from positive symptoms, which is primarily handled by maintenance medication, EASY also recognizes the need to promote an all-rounded recovery. In this respect, case managers would then actively encourage and guide patients in evaluating their recovery progress, with a particular focus on independent living, symptom control, social networks, and employment. Collaborating NGOs would arrange community-based rehabilitation programmes and vocational training for FEP patients in remission. Additionally, specific interventions such as occupational therapy and cognitive-behavioural therapy (CBT) are also available for patients if needed. These interventions follow a strict protocol, with regular reviews by multidisciplinary teams, to regulate the quality and consistency of their delivery.

The Psychological Intervention Programmes in Early Psychosis (PIPE; So et al., 2013) is the protocol designed and developed for EASY. PIPE encompasses three main modules of psychological interventions: (1) enhancement of psychological adjustment to early psychosis via in-depth engagement, extensive psychoeducation, medication adherence, stress management, and relapse prevention; (2) application of psychotherapy to address psychiatric comorbidity; and (3) application of CBT for treatment-resistant psychotic symptoms. Case managers adhere to a standardized PIPE-I module when delivering interventions to patients and their families. Patients who present with more complex needs such as persisting residual symptoms and depressive symptoms would be referred to clinical psychologists, who would then intervene according to PIPE-II and -III.

Outcome evaluation

Since the launch of EASY, there has been an annual average of 3,000 hotline enquiries, 1,000 diagnostic assessments, and 600 new cases admitted into the programme. The median response time between referral and diagnostic assessment has averaged five days (Wong et al., 2012), as opposed to the 16- to 64-week wait at public psychiatric clinics (Hospital Authority, 2019). Even with high caseloads per case manager (1:80–100), EASY was found to be effective in improving the outcome of FEP patients (refer to section 'Review of selected research programmes on psychoses in Hong Kong').

In addition to the success of the programme in improving patient outcomes, cost-effectiveness also constitutes a crucial aspect of EASY's sustainability. Analyses were conducted to compare the direct cost of early intervention and standard care over 24 months and revealed that EASY reduced hospital admissions and improved clinical symptoms, while reducing inpatient costs, accident and emergency department service needs, community psychiatric nurse services, and medical social worker attendances (Wong et al., 2011).

JCEP: specialized early intervention programme for adult-onset psychosis

With funding from the Hong Kong Jockey Club Charities Trust, the University of Hong Kong introduced an early intervention service for adult FEP patients in 2009 to fill the service gap back then. The JCEP targets patients with an FEP onset after the age of 25 and those who were not covered by EASY (Hui et al., 2014). In addition to addressing the age gap that EASY failed to accommodate for, JCEP also tailors its services to differentiate between patients with early—and late-onset. This is in view of earlier literature which has suggested differences in illness symptomatology and treatment response between the two groups (Harris & Jeste, 1988; Pearlson et al., 1989). Much like EASY, JCEP also integrates research, services, and education.

JCEP's case management approach

The JCEP provides specialized and individualized case management in addition to community-based group programmes for more than 1,000 FEP patients aged 26–55, who were otherwise receiving only infrequent and brief outpatient contacts.

Under JCEP, each patient is assigned a case manager who personally engages with the patient and who plans and evaluates the initial years of the intervention. To ensure service quality, the case-per-case manager ratio was set at 1:80. Case managers would engage and track clients' progress in outpatient settings. They would also contact clients by phone, carry out community visits, and work alongside NGO partners at community bases to facilitate treatment. These interventions are designed based on comprehensive assessments of each patient. Case managers generate life charts, which summarize all relevant retrospective (past) and prospective (present) data regarding major life events, illness trajectory, and treatment methodologies, of each patient. The use of life charts then enables case managers to construct the most appropriate treatment plan to tackle the disorder. Different psychosocial treatments are applied depending on individuals' needs. The life coach approach specifically for psychosis patients was pioneered in JCEP as a way to facilitate functional recovery.

Depending on the needs and preferences of the patients, they may be referred to two local NGO partners, Caritas Hong Kong (Social Work Services) and the Mental Health Association of Hong Kong, for participation in a variety of group programmes. These include psychoeducation, coping skills, family work, vocational training, communication skills, relapse prevention, and physical activities. These interventions are carried out in non-stigmatizing group settings to facilitate optimal social reintegration and aid functional recovery.

Education

JCEP also aims to increase knowledge, public awareness, and enhance positive attitudes about psychosis among the general public in Hong Kong. Public education work (e.g. development of educational materials, training workshops and seminars, media reports, and events about early psychosis) was carried out extensively. Specific training was also provided to a network of professional gatekeepers, such as teachers, security guards, and the police, to provide them with the knowledge and skills necessary for early detection work in the community.

The effectiveness of public awareness campaigns was evaluated through two public attitude phone surveys conducted in 2009 and 2014 (Chan et al., 2016). The study revealed some reduction in common misconceptions about individuals with psychosis. However, general misconceptions and the discrimination associated with psychosis were still pervasive.

Outcome evaluation

A randomized controlled trial of 360 psychosis patients aged 26 to 55 years (clinicaltrials.gov identifier: NCT 00919620) was conducted to study the efficacy of JCEP early intervention, as well as to resolve issues concerning the optimal intervention period, sustainability of improved outcome, and the cost-effectiveness of early intervention. Patients were randomized into one of the three treatment groups: standard care, two years of case management, and four years of case management in addition to standard care. Results suggested that 4-year early intervention was associated with better social functioning outcomes compared with standard care only during the initial two years (Hui et al., 2022). Similarly, benefits in social functioning and clinical symptoms were only observed in the initial two years in the 4-year early intervention group compared with the 2-year early intervention group. The finding suggests that while service provision for at least the initial two years is crucial, subsequent treatment beyond two years confers few benefits for patients in this age range. Meanwhile, analyses also suggested that these functional benefits are more pronounced for patients aged ≤40 years with a long DUP.

Review of selected research programmes

Since EASY was launched, not only has it demonstrated its efficiency, but also shown its effectiveness in bettering multifaceted outcomes for patients with psychosis. A cohort study examined the three-year outcome of 700 patients who received early intervention from EASY and 700 who received standard care (Chen et al., 2011). A comparison of the two cohorts revealed that patients who received early intervention reported fewer positive and negative symptoms, enhanced functional and occupational outcomes, had fewer days of hospitalization, and a reduced suicide rate (Chen et al., 2011). While early intervention promoted better outcomes, the DUP and rate of relapse between the two groups did not differ. Rather than being an indication of ineffectiveness, this could be evidence that EASY engaged a number of patients who previously had difficulties accessing relevant services. Though no specific reduction of DUP was found in the younger population, a significant reduction of DUP in the adult population (age ≥ 25) over the longer term was found (Chan et al., 2018a). The comparable rates of relapse between the early intervention and standard care groups may be attributable to the two-year duration of intervention—before the end of which relapse rates are generally not high (Robinson et al., 1999).

Following the examination of EASY's 3-year outcome, another study was set up to explore the sustainability of the programme's effectiveness. Chan et al. (2015) investigated the 10-year outcomes of the same two cohorts, by retrieving medical records of 148 matched pairs of patients at three-month intervals, and conducting semi-structured interviews at the 10-year time point. Compared with patients who received standard care, EASY's service users had fewer and shorter durations of hospital admissions and longer periods of employment. With a 12-year follow up of 1,234 patients with half of them receiving the EASY service, a significantly lower rate of suicide mortality was found in patients who received the EASY service compared with the standard care patient group, though the main effect was during the initial three years (Chan et al., 2018b). It should, however, be noted that the two groups did not show significant differences in rates of symptomatic remission and functional recovery at the 10-year time point. Furthermore, a specific group of patients had a drop in employment rate after transition from the EASY service to the standard care service (Chan et al., 2020). While some of the impact of the EASY programme appears to be maintained at 10 years, the dilution of its short-term effects called for the re-evaluation of its operation duration.

As mentioned previously (refer to 'EASY: First Local Early Intervention Programme for Psychoses'), the EASY programme has undergone service extension to accommodate more patients. Chang et al. (2015) then conducted an RCT to compare the outcomes of patients who received two years versus three years of early intervention care. Results of the trial showed that a three-year long intervention programme is more effective than a two-year programme in reducing treatment default rates, negative symptoms, depression symptoms, and in improving functional outcomes (Chang et al., 2015; 2016). However, later follow-up of this cohort suggests that the therapeutic gains accomplished by the three-year intervention could not be sustained two years after patients return to standard psychiatric care (Chang et al., 2017b). Additionally, a territory-wide evaluation study was conducted to examine the effectiveness of the three-year EASY programme, which has been implemented since 2011, and demonstrated superior efficacy of extended EASY over standard care among adult FEP patients in terms of shortening of DUP, reduced symptom severity, and better quality of life (Chang et al., 2018).

A research agenda to address knowledge gaps

Currently, early intervention for psychosis patients of all ages is in place throughout the territory of Hong Kong. While well-regulated programmes are available in the city, they are still in their infancy. Being one of the first cities in Asia to establish early intervention services for psychosis, researchers and policymakers in Hong Kong could refer to the operations of other programmes, including: the Support for Wellness Achievement Programme (SWAP) in Singapore; Personal Assessment and Crisis Evaluation (PACE) in Melbourne, Australia, Cambridgeshire, and Peterborough; Assessing, Managing and Enhancing Outcomes (CAMEO) in Cambridge, UK; and Outreach and Support in South London, UK (OASIS). Knowledge exchange with experts operating these initiatives and incorporating certain aspects of these establishments could better inform the further development of local services. For instance, the naming of SWAP makes no reference to mental health issues, and its clinics are designed to resemble general polyclinics, minimizing the stigma associated with help-seeking. Another element worth highlighting is the Care Programme Approach adopted by CAMEO, which emphasizes the engagement of carers and service users themselves in any processes of decision-making (Department of Health, 1995).

Additionally, crucial to the delivery of effective services is the further enrichment of our knowledge base about psychoses. Local research efforts should be centred on clinically relevant topics, in order to develop data-driven intervention initiatives. To enhance service provision for people in need, the following research areas should be investigated among others: the identification of detectable and modifiable risk factors; methods of determining an individualized, optimal dose of antipsychotics; pinpointing biological or other measurable precursors to relapse; and developing a more cost-effective means of delivering psychosocial treatment.

The advancement of early intervention services in Hong Kong serves no purpose if societal barriers continue to stand in the way of help-seeking. Therefore, additional resources should be put into educating the public and raising awareness about psychosis. For more effective dissemination of knowledge, rather than relying on publicity events, campaigns could also utilize trending social media such as Instagram and Facebook to circulate non-stigmatizing information. More importantly, collaboration with the media to restrict the publication of stereotyping and inaccurate news is also crucial to reducing stigma.

References

Australian Bureau of Statistics (2011). First release media fact sheets—average household size. Retrieved from https://www.abs.gov.au/websitedbs/censushome.nsf/home/media factsheetsfirst

Chan, S. K. W., et al. (2017). Newspaper coverage of mental illness in Hong Kong between 2002 and 2012: impact of introduction of a new Chinese name of psychosis. *Early Interv Psychiatry*, *11*(4), 342–345.

Chan, S. K. W., et al. (2016). A population study of public stigma about psychosis and its contributing factors among Chinese population in Hong Kong. *Int J Soc Psychiatry*, *62*(3), 205–213.

Chan, S. K. W., et al. (2016). Web-based psychoeducation program for caregivers of first-episode of psychosis: an experience of Chinese population in Hong Kong. *Front Psychol*, 7. doi:10.3389/fpsyg.2016.02006

Chan, S. K. W., et al. (2018a). Long term effect of early intervention service on duration of untreated psychosis in youth and adult population in Hong Kong. *Early Interv Psychiatry*, *12*(3), 331–338.

Chan, S. K.W., et al. (2015), 10-year outcome study of an early intervention program for psychosis compared with standard care service. *Psychol Med*, *454*(6), 1181–1193.

Chan, S. K. W., et al. (2018b). Association of an early intervention service for psychosis with suicide rate among patients with first-episode schizophrenia-spectrum disorders. *JAMA Psychiatry*, *75*(5), 458–464.

Chan, S. K. W., et al. (2020). Ten-year employment patterns of patients with first-episode schizophrenia-spectrum disorders: comparison of early intervention and standard care services. *Br J Psychiatry*, *217*(3), 491–497.

Chang, W. C., et al. (2015). Optimal duration of an early intervention programme for first-episode psychosis: randomised controlled trial. *Br J Psychiatry*, *206*(6), 492–500.

Chang, W. C., et al. (2016). Prediction of functional remission in first-episode psychosis: 12-month follow-up of the randomized-controlled trial on extended early intervention in Hong Kong. *Schizophr Res*, *173*(1–2), 79–83.

Chang, W. C., et al. (2017a). Lifetime prevalence and correlates of schizophrenia-spectrum, affective, and other non-affective psychotic disorders in the Chinese adult population. *Schizophr Bull*, *43*(6), 1280–1290.

Chang, W. C., Kwong, V. W. Y., Lau, E. S. K., So, H. C., Wong, C. S. M., Chan, G. H. K., Jim, O. T. T., Hui, C. L. M., Chan, S. K. W., Lee, E. H. M., & Chen, E. Y. H. (2017b). Sustainability of treatment effect of a 3-year early intervention programme for first-episode psychosis. *Br J Psychiatry*, *211*, 37–44.

Chang, W. C., et al. (2018). Treatment delay and outcome comparison of extended early intervention service and standard psychiatric care for adults presenting with first-episode psychosis in Hong Kong. *Schizophr Bull*, *44*(suppl.1), S215.

Chen, E. (2004). *Developing an early intervention service in Hong Kong. Best care in early psychosis intervention*. London: Taylor & Francis, 125–130.

Chen, E. Y. H., Chan, G. H. K., Wong, G. H. Y., & Lee, H. (2013). *Early psychosis intervention: a culturally adaptive clinical guide (vol. 1)*. Hong Kong: Hong Kong University Press.

Chen, E. Y. H., et al. (2005a). A prospective 3-year longitudinal study of cognitive predictors of relapse in first-episode schizophrenic patients. *Schizophr Res*, *77*(1), 99–104.

Chen, E. Y. H., et al. (2005b). The impact of family experience on the duration of untreated psychosis (DUP) in Hong Kong. *Soc Psychiatry Psychiatr Epidemiol*, *40*(5), 350–356.

Chen, E. Y., et al. (2010). Maintenance treatment with quetiapine versus discontinuation after one year of treatment in patients with remitted first episode psychosis: randomised controlled trial. *BMJ*, *341*, c4024.

Chen, E. Y., et al. (2011). Three-year outcome of phase-specific early intervention for first-episode psychosis: a cohort study in Hong Kong. *Early Interv Psychiatry*, *5*(4), 315–323.

Cheung, E. (2016, 13 February). Breaking point: Hong Kong's overburdened mental health care system in need of a fix. Retrieved fromhttps://www.scmp.com/news/hong-kong/health-environment/article/1912457/breaking-point-hong-kongs-overburdened-mental

Chiu, C. P. Y., et al. (2010). Naming psychosis: the Hong Kong experience. *Early Interv Psychiatry*, *4*(4), 270–274.

Chung, K. F. & Wong, M. C. (2004). Experience of stigma among Chinese mental health patients in Hong Kong. *Psychiatr Bull*, *28*(12), 451–454.

Department of Health (1995). *Building bridges: a guide to arrangements for interagency working for the care and protection of severely mentally ill people*. London: HMSO.

Harris, M. J. & Jeste, D. V. (1988). Late-onset schizophrenia: an overview. *Schizophr Bull*, *14*(1), 39–55.

Hospital Authority (2019, 30 September). Waiting time for new case booking at psychiatry specialist out-patient clinics. Retrieved from https://www.ha.org.hk/visitor/ha_visitor_index.asp?Content_ID=214197&Lang=ENG&Dimension=100&Parent_ID=10053

Hui, C. L., et al. (2022). Effectiveness and optimal duration of early intervention treatment in adult-onset psychosis: a randomized clinical trial. *Psychol Med*, *11*, 1–13. doi:10.1017/S0033291721004189

Hui, C. L., et al. (2014). Early intervention and evaluation for adult-onset psychosis: the JCEP study rationale and design. *Early Interv Psychiatry*, *8*(3), 261–268.

Hui, C. L., Wong, G. H., Lam, C. Y., Chow, P. P., & Chen, E. Y. (2008). Patient–clinician communication and needs identification for outpatients with Schizophrenia in Hong Kong: role of the 2-COM instrument. *Hong Kong J Psychiatry*, *18*(2), 69–75.

Knifton, L., et al. (2010). Community conversation: addressing mental health stigma with ethnic minority communities. *Soc Psychiatry Psychiatr Epidemiol*, *45*(4), 497–504.

Lam, L. C. W., et al. (2015). Prevalence, psychosocial correlates and service utilization of depressive and anxiety disorders in Hong Kong: the Hong Kong Mental Morbidity Survey (HKMMS). *Soc Psychiatry Psychiatr Epidemiol*, *50*(9), 1379–1388.

Lee, S., Chiu, M. Y., Tsang, A., Chui, H., & Kleinman, A. (2006). Stigmatizing experience and structural discrimination associated with the treatment of schizophrenia in Hong Kong. *Soc Sci Med*, *62*(7), 1685–1696.

Lee, S., Lee, M. T., Chiu, M. Y., & Kleinman, A. (2005). Experience of social stigma by people with schizophrenia in Hong Kong. *Br J Psychiatry*, *186*(2), 153–157.

Office for National Statistics (2013). Families and households in the UK: 2013. Retrieved from https://www.ons.gov.uk/peoplepopulationandcommunity/birthsdeathsandmarriages/families/bulletins/familiesandhouseholds/2013-10-31

Pearlson, G. D., et al. (1989). A chart review study of late-onset and early-onset schizophrenia. *Am J Psychiatry*, *146*(12), 1568–1574.

Population Census Office (2012). 2011 population census summary results. Retrieved from http://www.censtatd.gov.hk/hkstat/sub/sp170.jsp?productCode=B1120055

Robinson, D., et al. (1999). Predictors of relapse following response from a first episode of schizophrenia or schizoaffective disorder. *Arch Gen Psychiatry*, 56(3), 241–247.

So, S. H. W., Chen, E. Y. H., Lee, H., Wong, G. H. K., & Wong, G. H. Y. (2013). Implementing psychological intervention programme in early psychosis (PIPE). In Chen, E. Y., Lee, H., Chan, G. H., & Wong, G. H. (eds) *Early psychosis intervention: a culturally adaptive clinical guide*. Hong Kong: Hong Kong University Press, 137–157.

Tang, J. Y., et al. (2010). Early intervention for psychosis in Hong Kong—the EASY programme. *Early Interv Psychiatry*, 4(3), 214–219.

United States Census Bureau (2015). Families and living arrangements: table HH-4. Households by size: 1960 to present. Retrieved from https://www.census.gov/data/tables/time-series/demo/families/households.html

Wong, G. H., et al. (2012). Early intervention for psychotic disorders: real-life implementation in Hong Kong. *Asian J Psychiatry*, 5(1), 68–72.

Wong, K. K., et al. (2011). Cost-effectiveness of an early assessment service for young people with early psychosis in Hong Kong. *Aust N Z J Psychiatry*, 45(8), 673–680.

Yung, A. R., Yuen, H. P., Phillips, L. J., Francey, S., & McGorry, P. D. (2003). Mapping the onset of psychosis: the comprehensive assessment of at-risk mental states (CAARMS). *Schizophr Res*, 1(60), 30–31.

18

Psychoses and mental health services in mainland China

Shuiyuan Xiao and Lu Niu

Introduction

This chapter provides a brief overview of the epidemiology of psychotic disorders and the provision of mental healthcare, with a focus on the general profile of individuals with psychotic disorders, in mainland China. This includes how individuals with psychotic disorders live in the sociocultural context and how they are cared for.

Prevalence and burden of psychotic disorders

The China Health Statistics Yearbook (2019) is the only available official resource reporting national prevalence of psychosis in mainland China (National Health Commission of China, 2019). Data are from the National Health Service Surveys conducted in 2003, 2008, and 2013, using a multistage cluster-area sampling in 31 provinces across mainland China. A total of 210,000 respondents in 2003, 180,000 in 2008, and 273,7000 in 2013 completed the surveys. As shown in Table 18.1, from 2003 to 2013, the reported prevalence of psychosis increased from 0.8% to 1.7% (two-week prevalence) and 1.9% to 3.0% (six-month prevalence). This trend of increasing prevalence may be best explained by more psychotic patients being diagnosed in this period, as patients with psychosis were defined as those who self-reported having a clinical diagnosis of any psychotic disorder in the past two weeks or six months before the survey. However, it is of course unclear from this what specific diagnoses individuals who responded positively to this question have received.

There are also some published epidemiological data on psychotic disorders by researchers. Phillips et al. (2009) conducted an epidemiological survey in four provinces of China (Shangdong, Gansu, Zhejiang, Qinghai) and found that the one-month prevalence of DSM-IV psychotic disorders (including schizophrenia, schizoaffective disorder, schizophreniform disorder, delusional

Table 18.1 Prevalence of psychosis in Mainland China, 2003, 2008, and 2013 (%)

	2003	2008	2013
Two-week prevalence			
Urban	0.9	1.7	1.7
Rural	0.8	1.2	1.4
Total	0.8	1.3	1.5
Six-month prevalence			
Urban	2.4	2.3	3.1
Rural	1.8	2.0	3.0
Total	1.9	2.1	3.0

disorder, brief psychotic disorder, and psychotic disorder Not Otherwise Specified) was 0.9% (95% CI: 0.7–1.1%) (Phillips et al., 2009). Recently, the China Mental Health Survey (CMHS), the first psychiatric epidemiological study sampled from all provinces of mainland China, reported a lifetime prevalence of schizophrenia and other psychotic disorders of 0.7% (95% CI: 03–1.2%) (Huang et al., 2019). The diagnostic assessments were conducted by psychiatrists with the Structured Clinical Interview for DSM-IV.

While epidemiological surveys rarely report psychosis or psychotic disorders as a single category of mental disorders, the prevalence of schizophrenia has been widely reported. In a systematic review (Chan et al., 2015), the prevalence of schizophrenia in China more than doubled between 1990 and 2010: the number of people affected by schizophrenia in their lifetime increased by 132% from 1990 to 2010, while the total population in China only increased by 18%. The contribution of cases from urban areas to the overall burden increased from 27% in 1990 to 62% in 2010. These changes might be partially attributed to the remarkable improvement of mental health services and increasing mental health use in China. However, further explorations are needed to explain this phenomenon.

Based on the Global Burden of Disease Study 2010, the all-age disability-adjusted life years (DALY) lost as a result of schizophrenia in China increased by 35.6% from 1990 to 2010 (Table 18.2). After adjusting for age, the DALY rate showed a decreasing pattern which was largely due to the decreased death rate. In 2010, schizophrenia accounted for 1.1% of total DALYs, 1.4% of DALYs due to non-communicable diseases, and 11.6% of DALYs due to mental and behavioural disorders (Yang et al., 2013). The age-standardized death rate for schizophrenia decreased by 57.7% during this period.

Table 18.2 Burden of schizophrenia and bipolar affective disorders, 1990 and 2010

	All-age DALYs, thousands (95% confidence intervals)			Age-standardized DALY rate, per 100,000 (95% confidence intervals)		
	1990	2010	Median %Δ	1990	2010	Median %Δ
All causes	365,390.8 (342,403.1–390,433.0)	316,616.1 (292,429.2–341,996.6)	–13.4	34,627.6 (32,546.7–36,963.9)	22,805.6 (21,125.1–24,630.4)	–34.2
Non-communicable diseases	217,135.5 (202,900.7–234,686.3)	243,787.7 (224,298.4–264,558.7)	12.3	22,358.9 (20,943.7–24,144.9)	17,021.8 (15,673.6–18,458.5)	–23.8
Mental and behavioural disorders	24,450.5 (20,025.4–29,182.9)	29,954.1 (24,451.7–35,839.5)	22.7	2173.9 (1,779.6–2,591.3)	2091.6 (1708.3–2502.6)	–3.8
Schizophrenia	2,554.2 (1,756.7–3,396.2)	3,472.3 (2,307.5–4,719.6)	35.6	250.8 (172.5–333.4)	225.5 (150.1–305.9)	–10.4
Bipolar affective disorder	2192.2 (1,352.7–3,238.7)	2758.5 (1,700.3–4,021.4)	26.0	193.7 (119.6–286.3)	185.8 (114.9–270.9)	–3.9

Note %Δ= percentage change

Psychotic disorders impose a huge economic burden on both families and society in China. By using the health records of two psychiatric hospitals and a prevalence-based bottom-up approach, it is estimated that the average total annual costs of mental disorders in China increased from USD $1,094.8 per patient in 2005 to USD $3,665.4 in 2013, and from $21.0 billion to $88.8 billion for the whole society. The total costs of mental disorders in 2013 accounted for more than 15% of the total health expenditure in China, and 1.1% of China's gross domestic product (Xu et al., 2016). In terms of schizophrenia, researchers used the Economic Burden Questionnaire (EBQ) to collect the economic cost data of patients with schizophrenia, and they estimated that the per case per annum direct costs and indirect costs of schizophrenia amounted to USD $862.81 and USD $1,723.40, respectively (Zhai et al., 2013). Additionally, researchers assessed the household economic burden of patients with schizophrenia after being unlocked and treated in rural China. They found that mean direct and indirect household economic burdens were USD $31.7 and USD $1,670 per year, respectively, while family total income was on average USD $1,913 per year (Xu et al., 2019).

Mental healthcare in China

Traditional Chinese medicine was historically widely used as a treatment for psychosis in China. However, there were no asylums or similar institutions until the first psychiatric hospital of China was founded in Guangzhou in 1898 by John Kerr, a Presbyterian medical missionary from the United States. After that, fewer than 30 psychiatric hospitals were opened in the large urban centres of the mainland in the first half of the twentieth century. Since 1950, China has gradually developed its mental healthcare system. However, the rapid development of mental healthcare has only happened in the past two decades.

The National Mental Health Law

The first National Mental Health Law of China was issued in 2012 and put into effect in May 2013 (Chen et al., 2012). The law covers almost all issues related to mental health, including mental health promotion, prevention, treatment and rehabilitation of mental disorders, protection of the rights of patients with mental disorders (privacy, informed consent, voluntary admission, etc.), prohibition of social stigma, and discrimination towards patients with mental disorders. The substantial influences of the law so far could be summarized into three aspects. First, national and local governments have paid greater attention to mental health; second, investment in mental health facilities and programmes has increased significantly; third, 'Construction of a Psychosocial

Service System', which mainly deals with mental health promotion and prevention of mental disorders outside of the traditional healthcare system and is targeted at vulnerable populations, such as children, adolescents, and older people, has been initiated nationwide. A major problem in the implementation of the law is the protection of patients' rights in general and the right to voluntary admission in particular.

Hospital care

The Chinese mental health system mainly consists of psychiatric hospitals and mental health centres at provincial, municipal, and county levels. Currently, there are more than 1,000 mental health institutes all over the country, mainly invested in and owned by the government, as private mental health institutes have emerged only recently. All psychiatric hospitals in China provide both outpatient and inpatient services. Some large general hospitals provide clinical mental health services, and a few also provide inpatient services. As shown in Table 18.3, the number of beds per 100,000 was 24.29 in 2016, very close to the number of the United States and Australia, about 10% of the capacity of Japan and four times that of India (World Health Organization, 2018). While pharmaceutical therapy remains the major treatment in most psychiatric hospitals, psychotherapies, physical therapies, rehabilitation, etc. are also available in many large psychiatric hospitals. The average time spent hospitalized by patients has gradually decreased from months to weeks in the last two decades, but there are still a small number of patients, usually with psychotic disorders, who are hospitalized for years. Some large hospitals, generally located in large urban centres, have thousands of beds and most wards are locked; many small hospitals, generally at county-level, have less than 100 beds and sometimes one bed is shared by two patients, reflecting the gap between demand for inpatient care and available resources.

Community care

Although there were a few programmes that provided community care for patients with psychosis in the 1960s and 1970s, these programmes only covered a small proportion of communities in selected provinces and cities and were interrupted in the 1980s and 1990s because of market economy reforms. A new wave of community care was started in 2004, when the national government of China announced the 'Management and treatment project of severe mental diseases' programme. Initially, 6,860,000 RMB (approximately 980,000 USD) were invested in this programme in 2004, so it is known as the '686 programme' in China. This programme, which aimed to decrease the social and economic

Table 18.3 Psychiatric beds per 100,000 in mainland China, compared with selected countries

Countries	Psychiatric beds per 100,000			
	Psychiatric hospitals	General hospitals	Community facilities	Total
China (mainland)	24.29	NA	NA	24.29
The United States	18.66	11.14	NA	29.80
Australia	7.21	21.76	10.38	28.97
Japan	196.63	66.15	NA	262.78
India	1.43	0.56	5.18	7.17

Source: data from WHO ATLAS 2017.

burden of psychotic disorders and prevent aggressive and criminal behaviour by patients with psychosis, was the first national mental health programme and was subsidized by the central government. The 686 programme has evolved to become one of the nine essential public health services in 2009, named as 'management of patients with severe mental diseases', covering schizophrenia, paranoid disorder, schizoaffective disorder, bipolar disorder, epilepsy with psychotic symptoms, and severe mental retardation. Community centres (urban areas) and Xiang/township health stations (rural areas) take the major responsibility for this task, with supervision and technical help from county or city centres for disease prevention and control as well as technical help from professional mental health facilities. The main activities of these essential public health services include: (1) identifying residents with the abovementioned 'severe mental diseases'; (2) collecting and reporting basic demographic information of these patients; (3) following up with patients four times a year to evaluate them, including symptoms, social function, and possible risk behaviour (mainly suicide and aggressive behaviours); (4) basic physical examination; and (5) supervision of treatment adherence. In many communities of the country, free antipsychotic drugs are also provided. Up to 2019, more than 6 million patients with severe mental disorders are registered in a national database, most of whom are diagnosed with schizophrenia. Generally, experts in the mental health field and the public believe the '686' and other mental health programmes have greatly improved the care of people with psychotic disorders (Good & Good, 2012). However, there has been no rigorously designed study to evaluate the effectiveness, benefits, and utility of these programmes, possibly because of the poor quality of the database, and government officials are reluctant to support evaluation studies (Patel et al., 2016).

Mental health resources

According to official statistics, there are about 22,000 clinical psychiatrists in mainland China. However, most of these psychiatrists have received only three years of junior college medical education or five years of general medicine education at university level, and only a small proportion of them have received specialty training in psychiatry. In order to meet demand, some Chinese medical schools provide five-year mental health education at bachelor level, and the government has encouraged general practitioners to apply for an additional licence in clinical psychiatry after one year of training in the past decades. There are no nurses trained specifically for psychiatry; clinical psychologists, psychological counsellors, and social workers in psychiatry have only recently begun to be employed by psychiatric hospitals. Table 18.4 shows China's mental health human resources, compared with selected countries (World Health Organization, 2018).

Medical insurance

In 1998 China started a new medical insurance scheme named the 'Basic Medical Insurance Scheme for urban employees' to replace the previous Government Medical Insurance Scheme (GHI) and Labour Medical Insurance Scheme (LHI), which were discontinued in the 1980s and 1990s. About ten years later, the government initiated the New Rural Cooperative Medical System (for rural residents) and basic medical insurance scheme for urban residents, now integrated into a single basic medical insurance for urban and rural residents, which is designed for people who are not formally employed (including children), with the ratio of individual to governmental contribution to be 1:4 in 2019. At the same time, employed or retired people are required to participate in the 'basic medical insurance scheme for urban employees'. It is reported that over

Table 18.4 Mental health human resources per 100,000 in mainland China, compared with selected countries

Countries	Psychiatrists*	Nurses*	Social workers*	Psychologists*
China (mainland)	2.20	5.42	NA	NA
The United States	10.54	4.28	60.34	29.87
Australia	13.53	90.58	NA	103.04
Japan	11.87	83.81	8.33	3.04
India	0.29	0.80	0.07	0.07

* per 100,000

Source: data from WHO ATLAS 2017.

95% of Chinese people have been covered with basic medical insurance since 2011, including people with psychotic disorders. According to the general regulation of basic medical insurance for urban and rural residents, 50% to 75% of expenditure for inpatient care could be reimbursed. In many areas, this scheme also provides specific arrangements for patients with psychotic disorders; for example, reimbursement for outpatient costs and a higher proportion of expenditures for inpatient services. Outside of medical insurance, there are four kinds of national and local plans to help patients with psychoses, including: (1) Subsidies for inpatient services for patients from low-income families; (2) Free treatment for homeless patients with psychotic disorders; (3) Priority to obtain a basic living allowance; and (4) Subsidies for family members who provide care for psychotic patients.

Perceptions of and attitudes toward patients with psychotic disorders

In traditional Chinese medicine, the term 'diankuang (癲狂)' is approximately equivalent to psychosis or psychotic disorders in modern psychiatry, with 'dian' indicating disorganization of the mind and 'kuang' meaning behavioural disturbance. 'Diankuang' is attributed to the influence of 'qi qing (七情)', which literately means seven human emotions, including joy, anger, worry, pensiveness (thinking too much or obsessing about a topic), sadness, fear, and shock (Larre et al., 1996). The main mechanism of 'diankuang' is pathological problems of 'the liver' (not the liver in anatomy), which is believed to be the organ that deals with emotions. In folk Chinese culture, however, 'diankuang' is more related to being possessed or bewitched by supernatural forces.

The lay explanatory models of psychosis in modern Chinese society tend to be multifaceted, including major life events (mainly interpersonal conflicts), strong emotions, being possessed or bewitched by supernatural forces, heredity, imbalance of life or nutrients, and pathological changes of the brain (for example, meningitis). Judgement of the nature of psychological and behavioural abnormalities, help-seeking behaviours, and social reactions towards the person with the perceived abnormalities are further determined by the explanatory model employed by the patient, the family, and the community, explicitly or implicitly.

Further, psychotic symptoms, as well as emotional problems such as depression and anxiety, are frequently perceived by the patient, the family, and the community as normal reactions to stress, especially interpersonal conflicts or heavy burdens resulting from school studies or work, in the early stages of the disorder. This explanatory model could decrease the possible stigmatization of the patient, leading to efforts to resolve problems in people's day-to-day lives, but it also impedes patients from seeking professional treatment.

In the past two or three decades, psychotic disorders have increasingly been perceived as a treatable in Chinese societies. However, the spiritual model is still used to explain psychotic symptoms such as hallucinations and delusions, especially among the less educated and in remote areas. It is still common for family members of the patient to seek help from witches, Buddhist monks, Taoist priests or folk healers, and psychiatrists simultaneously. In some cases, the patient is believed to be possessed or bewitched because of his or her unethical, miscreant, or at least wrong behaviours. In these cases, more stigma may be imposed on the patient than other patients, they may be punished by the family or community, and they could be refused or delayed in seeking professional help.

Stigma

Stigma is commonly imposed on patients with psychotic disorders. The word 'psychosis' (Shengjingbing in Chinese) is frequently used to insult people in everyday life, meaning the insulted person is mentally 'abnormal'. Often, patients with a diagnostic label of psychosis may be deprived of education, job opportunities, social interaction, marriage, etc. Institutional stigma and discrimination are also imposed on patients with psychotic disorders; for example, they are officially prohibited from taking high-speed trains and flights and cannot apply for a driving licence. The stigma may further influence the family members of the patient. With this strong culture of stigma, patients with psychotic disorders often—understandably—internalize the belief that they are dangerous, unreliable, shameful, a burden on their family and society, unable to make decisions, and even believe themselves to be morally wrong or have done something unethical previously in their life. Under this sociocultural pressure and the internalized stigma, patients with psychotic disorders are often reluctant to seek professional help from mental health facilities and refuse to adhere to treatment.

Family care

A large proportion of psychotic patients are dependent on the care of other people. In China, patients with psychosis are traditionally taken care of by their family members, while community and hospital care only play a complementary role. However, the situation has been changing very rapidly in the past few decades. The traditional extended family structure has been largely replaced by the nuclear family structure, resulting in no spare person in the family to take care of the patient with a psychotic disorder; at the same time, more and more young people are embracing values of individualism and liberalism and are no longer willing to take care of other family members who are unwell.

Conclusion

According to official estimates, China had about 16 million people with a psychotic disorder in 2012, which is more than the population size of many countries in the world. How to provide appropriate mental health services and improve the living conditions of this huge population is a major challenge to the Chinese government and to mental health professionals. The National Mental Health Law, the '686', and other programmes and efforts have significantly improved mental healthcare for people with a psychotic disorder. However, there is still a great gap between the demand for mental health services and the available resources, and ongoing challenges include quality of care and equity of care, public awareness of mental health, and stigma, which remains a major obstacle preventing patients from receiving adequate services. Additionally, the cost-effectiveness, and cost-benefits of mental health policies and programmes need to be evaluated systematically and scientifically to further promote the development of mental healthcare in China, and to provide experiences or lessons for other countries, especially middle- or low-income countries.

References

Chan, K.Y., et al. (2015). Prevalence of schizophrenia in China between 1990 and 2010. *J Glob Health*, *5*, 010410.

Chen, H., et al. (2012). Mental health law of the People's Republic of China (English translation with annotations). *Shanghai Arch Pyschiatry*, *24*, 305–321.

Good, B. J. & Good, M. J. (2012). Significance of the 686 Program for China and for global mental health. *Shanghai Arch Psychiatry*, *24*, 175–177.

Huang, Y., et al. (2019). Prevalence of mental disorders in China: a cross-sectional epidemiological study. *Lancet Psychiatry*, *6*, 211–224.

Larre, C., Valle, E. R. D. L., & Root, C. (1996). *The seven emotions: psychology and health in Ancient China*. Taos, NM: Redwing Book Co.

National Health Commission of China (2019). *The China health statistics yearbook (2019.* Beijing, Peking: Univon Medical College Press.

Patel, V., et al. (2016). The magnitude of and health system responses to the mental health treatment gap in adults in India and China. *Lancet*, *388*, 3074–3084.

Phillips, M. R., et al. (2009). Prevalence, treatment, and associated disability of mental disorders in four provinces in China during 2001–05: an epidemiological survey. *Lancet*, *373*, 2041–2053.

World Health Organization (2018). *Mental health atlas 2017*. Geneva: World Health Organization.

Xu, J., Wang, J., Wimo, A., & Qiu, C. (2016). The economic burden of mental disorders in China, 2005–2013: implications for health policy. *BMC Psychiatry, 16*, 137.

Xu, L., et al. (2019). Household economic burden and outcomes of patients with schizophrenia after being unlocked and treated in rural China. *Epidemiol Psychiatr Sci, 29*, e81.

Yang, G., et al. (2013). Rapid health transition in China, 1990–2010: findings from the Global Burden of Disease Study 2010. *Lancet, 381*, 1987–2015.

Zhai, J., Guo, X., Chen, M., Zhao, J., & Su, Z. (2013). An investigation of economic costs of schizophrenia in two areas of China. *Int J Ment Health Syst, 7*, 26.

19

Future directions

Tessa Roberts, Alex Cohen, and
Craig Morgan

There is a simple but critically important thread that runs through this volume: our knowledge and understanding of psychotic disorders are derived, overwhelmingly, from research conducted in populations in Europe, North America, and Australia. This is apparent in the volume's thematic chapters (Part 1), which draw almost exclusively on evidence from this relatively small, somewhat homogenous set of contexts. This severely limits our ability to generalize the findings to heterogenous populations living in Africa, Asia, and South America—and indeed to other parts of Europe (e.g. Central and Eastern Europe). The country-specific chapters begin to address this imbalance but, at the same time, demonstrate the patchiness of research and how sparse research on psychosis is—particularly population-based research with representative samples—in most countries of the world. There are notable gaps in the countries covered, and the absence of evidence from whole regions such as the Middle East severely limits our understanding. This lack of evidence from most of the world not only creates important limitations for the development of evidence-based services and policy, but it also means our assumptions about incidence, prevalence, risks, and short- and long-term course and outcome, must be tested in more diverse settings. This is essential if locally relevant systems of care and interventions are to be developed and implemented. Several challenges to achieving this goal remain.

First, a major barrier to comparing findings across settings is methodological heterogeneity. Even when considering, for example, the incidence of schizophrenia (Morgan et al., 2016), it is difficult to draw conclusions from the available research in diverse settings due to heterogeneity in inclusion criteria (e.g. in diagnostic group, age, and duration of untreated psychosis criteria) and strategies used to identify samples of individuals meeting these criteria. Thus, we need a global conversation to reach consensus about the methods that will generate comparable data from global research on psychoses, especially research conducted in those settings that have historically been neglected. One step to achieving this consensus is to establish a global consortium for psychosis research, with the aims to: (1) develop and agree on a core set of methods that will serve as a platform for global research on psychosis, much like the World Mental Health Survey Initiative for common mental disorders (Kessler et al., 2006); and (2) promote and coordinate efforts to conduct research that produces comparable evidence about psychosis in diverse settings.

Second, there is a fundamental tension between generating data that is comparable across settings and generating data that maximizes local validity. Isaac et al. (2007) call attention to the many challenges associated with trying to assess levels of disability and 'functioning' and the reliance on hospitalization as a measure of illness course and severity in different cultural settings. Research in India (Srinivasan & Thara, 1997; Srinivasan & Thara, 1999) and Ethiopia (Habtamu et al., 2015) illustrates the difficulty of assessing disability and 'functioning' status in specific local contexts, and a 35-year follow-up study (Rangaswamy & Cohen, 2020) suggests that hospitalization, at least in Chennai, India, is not a useful indicator of illness relapse. Addressing this tension will require resources that promote communication and collaboration of researchers across the world with the goal of producing directly comparable epidemiological and clinical research about psychosis.

Third, people with lived experience of psychosis, and their families, must be central to these endeavours—to defining relevant research questions (Asher et al., 2015), designing research programmes, shaping measures that capture outcomes that matter most (Balaji et al., 2012), interpreting and disseminating findings, developing and implementing interventions, and evaluating services in terms of their capacity to promote not just clinical remission but the ability to lead fulfilling lives (Chatterjee et al., 2012). In the Global North, people with lived experience have become increasingly involved in research, although there are ongoing debates about the nature and extent of such collaborations, while avoiding tokenism. In the Global South, the GMH Mental Health Peer Network (https://www.givengain.com/c/lived_experience_engagement_fund/about) and the creation of self-help groups for caregivers (e.g. in Ghana; see Cohen et al., 2012) are important steps in that direction, but more needs to be done. Resources are needed to support peer and family-led organizations in Asia, Africa, Latin America, Eastern Europe, and the Middle East, which often struggle for funding to sustain activities. There is much work to be done to enable meaningful dialogue between researchers and people with lived experience of psychosis, and their families and carers, especially in settings where there are cultural expectations to defer to those with medical training or with higher levels of training and qualifications.

Fourth, an understanding of the lived experiences of individuals with psychosis, and their families and carers, requires longitudinal, ethnographic research that documents the day-to-day realities of lives in a wide range of local settings (Cohen, 1992). Understanding of those realities can guide the development of interventions that effectively meet the needs of specific populations.

Fifth, there is now extensive literature about genetic (Legge et al., 2021) and environmental (Kirkbride et al., 2008; Morgan et al., 2014; Tarricone et al., 2021) risk factors for the development of psychosis. However, as already noted, what we know is based mostly on evidence from North America and Western Europe (and indeed, the genetic evidence arises mostly from white populations within these regions). Research about risk for psychosis is slowly emerging from other areas of the globe—e.g. urbanicity and psychosis in low- and middle-income countries (Del-Ben et al., 2019; DeVylder et al., 2018), but evidence is needed from research in a wide diversity of populations living in a range of cultural, socioeconomic, and physical settings. Only such evidence will allow us to critically test our assumptions.

The field of global mental health, to a great extent, has not focused on psychotic disorders. We hope this textbook and other contributions (Kleinman, 2009), will prove to be a corrective. By presenting the available evidence, and the gaps therein, we hope to stimulate efforts that will provide a greater understanding of psychosis and how it affects the lives of those who experience it, as well as those who are tasked with providing care and support and with intervening. By doing so, we hope to contribute—however indirectly—to improving the lives of those who experience psychosis through the production of evidence that will shape more effective social and biomedical interventions, both locally and globally.

References

Asher, L., et al. (2015). Development of a community-based rehabilitation intervention for people with schizophrenia in Ethiopia. *PLoS One*, *10*(11), e0143572.

Balaji, M., Chatterjee, S., Brennan, B., Rangaswamy, T., Thornicroft, G., & Patel, V. (2012). Outcomes that matter: a qualitative study with persons with schizophrenia and their primary caregivers in India. *Asian J Psychiatr*, *5*(3), 258–265.

Chatterjee, S., Pillai, A., Jain, S., Cohen, A., & Patel, V. (2009). Outcomes of people with psychotic disorders in a community-based rehabilitation programme in rural India. *Br J Psychiatry*, *195*(5), 433–439.

Cohen, A., et al. (2012). Sitting with others: mental health self-help groups in northern Ghana. *Int J Ment Health Syst*, *6*(1), 1.

Cohen, A. (1992). Prognosis for schizophrenia in the third world: a reevaluation of cross-cultural research. *Cult Med Psychiatry*, *16*(1), 53–75; commentaries & response 7–106.

Del-Ben, C. M., et al. (2019). Urbanicity and risk of first-episode psychosis: incidence study in Brazil. *Br J Psychiatry*, *215*(6), 726–729.

DeVylder, J. E., Kelleher, I., Lalane, M., Oh, H., Link, B. G., & Koyanagi, A. (2018). Association of urbanicity with psychosis in low- and middle-income countries. *JAMA Psychiatry*, *75*(7), 678–686.

Habtamu, K., Alem, A., & Hanlon, C. (2015). Conceptualizing and contextualizing functioning in people with severe mental disorders in rural Ethiopia: a qualitative study. *BMC Psychiatry*, *15*, 34.

Isaac, M., Chand, P., & Murthy, P. (2007). Schizophrenia outcome measures in the wider international community. *Br J Psychiatry Suppl*, *50*(suppl. 50), s71–s77.

Kessler, R. C., Haro, J. M., Heeringa, S. G., Pennell, B. E., & Ustun, T. B. (2006). The World Health Organization world mental health survey initiative. *Epidemiol Psychiatr Soc*, *15*(3), 161–166.

Kirkbride, J. B., et al. (2008). Testing the association between the incidence of schizophrenia and social capital in an urban area. *Psychol Med*, *38*(8), 1083–1094.

Kleinman, A. (2009). Global mental health: a failure of humanity. *Lancet*, *374*(9690), 603–604.

Legge, S. E., Santoro, M. L., Periyasamy, S., Okewole, A., Arsalan, A., & Kowalec, K. (2021). Genetic architecture of schizophrenia: a review of major advancements. *Psychol Med*, *51*(13), 2168–2177.

Morgan, C., et al. (2014). Adversity, cannabis use and psychotic experiences: evidence of cumulative and synergistic effects. *Br J Psychiatry*, *204*(5), 346–353.

Morgan, C., et al. (2016). The incidence of psychoses in diverse settings, INTREPID (2): a feasibility study in India, Nigeria, and Trinidad. *Psychol Med*, *46*(9), 1923–1933.

Rangaswamy, T. & Cohen, A. (2020). Invited commentary from a LAMIC country: thirty-five years of schizophrenia—the Madras Longitudinal study. *Schizophr Res*, *220*, 27–28.

Srinivasan, T. N. & Thara, R. (1997). How do men with schizophrenia fare at work? A follow-up study from India. *Schizophr Res*, *25*(2), 149–154.

Srinivasan, T. N. & Thara, R. (1999). The long-term home-making functioning of women with schizophrenia. *Schizophr Res*, *35*(1), 97–98.

Tarricone, I., et al. (2021). Migration history and risk of psychosis: results from the multinational EU-GEI study. *Psychol Med*, 1–13. doi: 10.1017/S003329172000495X. Online ahead of print.

Index

For the benefit of digital users, indexed terms that span two pages (e.g., 52–53) may, on occasion, appear on only one of those pages.

Tables are indicated by t following the page number